W0018812

Optical Coherence Tomography in Dentistry

Optical Coherence Tomography (OCT), a method to "see inside of things" without destroying them, has been applied to subjects ranging from materials science to medicine. This book focuses on the biomedical application of OCT in dentistry, covering topics from dental materials to clinical practice.

Since the introduction of the OCT method in ophthalmology in 1991, and then dentistry in 1998, developments in OCT methods, particularly in bio-medical areas, have led to its dissemination worldwide. The chapters of this book cover the basics and recent global advances of OCT in dentistry, including an overview of the method and its use in cariology, restorative dentistry, dental materials, endodontics, pediatric dentistry, orthodontics, prosthodontics, soft oral tissues and nanodentistry.

This book will be of interest to both newcomers in the field as well as those already working in OCT, either in research and/or the clinic. It will be of great use in courses on optical imaging applied to biomedical areas, particu-larly where it can provide real-life examples of the application of OCT.

For more information about this series, please visit:
www.crcpress.com/Series-in-Optics-and-Optoelectronics/book-series/
TFOPTICSOPT

Optical Coherence Tomography in Dentistry

Scientific Developments to Clinical Applications

Edited by
Anderson S. L. Gomes
Denise M. Zezell
Cláudia C. B. O. Mota
John M. Girkin

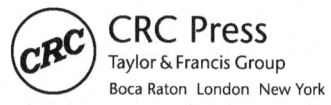

CRC Press
Taylor & Francis Group
Boca Raton London New York

CRC Press is an imprint of the
Taylor & Francis Group, an **informa** business

Designed cover image: courtesy of Anderson S. L. Gomes and Denise Valente

First edition published 2024
by CRC Press
6000 Broken Sound Parkway NW, Suite 300, Boca Raton, FL 33487-2742

and by CRC Press
4 Park Square, Milton Park, Abingdon, Oxon, OX14 4RN

CRC Press is an imprint of Taylor & Francis Group, LLC

© 2024 Taylor & Francis Group, LLC

Reasonable efforts have been made to publish reliable data and information, but the author and publisher cannot assume responsibility for the validity of all materials or the consequences of their use. The authors and publishers have attempted to trace the copyright holders of all material reproduced in this publication and apologize to copyright holders if permission to publish in this form has not been obtained. If any copyright material has not been acknowledged please write and let us know so we may rectify in any future reprint.

Except as permitted under U.S. Copyright Law, no part of this book may be reprinted, reproduced, transmitted, or utilized in any form by any electronic, mechanical, or other means, now known or hereafter invented, including photocopying, microfilming, and recording, or in any information storage or retrieval system, without written permission from the publishers.

For permission to photocopy or use material electronically from this work, access www. copyright.com or contact the Copyright Clearance Center, Inc. (CCC), 222 Rosewood Drive, Danvers, MA 01923, 978-750-8400. For works that are not available on CCC please contact mpkbookspermissions@tandf.co.uk

Trademark notice: Product or corporate names may be trademarks or registered trademarks and are used only for identification and explanation without intent to infringe.

ISBN: 9781138477537 (hbk)
ISBN: 9781032487175 (pbk)
ISBN: 9781351104562 (ebk)

DOI: 10.1201/9781351104562

Typeset in Palatino
by Newgen Publishing UK

Contents

Preface

Optical coherence tomography was born to see inside the eye, and it is has evolved to be "the eye seeing" throughout most parts of the human body. OCT, as it is commonly known, is one of the most fast growing optical imaging techniques, which provides real-time images capable of submicron resolution with penetration depths up to few millimeters. It can be used not only in hard and soft tissues, but has also been widely exploited on materials evaluation, including biomaterials.

The motivation to this book arose from the fast growing OCT applications in dentistry, which is opening new opportunities for early, noninvasive diagnostics or treatment follow-up for oral diseases. This will hopefully complement the state-of-the-art literature on OCT applications in life sciences, which is presently available.

The book is designed for professionals working in clinical practice, undergraduate, graduate students and post-docs performing research in this field, as well as industry professionals who are on the frontiers of optical based instrumentation for health diagnostics. It has been written to be used at all levels, with background chapters as well as updated bibliography on all areas of dental OCT. It can also be used in courses such as optical imaging techniques, lasers in dentistry, photobiomodulation, among others. Professional societies, such as SPIE and OPTICA, who provides annual short courses on biophotonics, will certainly benefit from this book. The core physical background will be present in one chapter but this will not be required for comprehension of the other more applied and practical chapters.

The chapters are organized in three main parts: two chapters are devoted to the principles of optical imaging, and the basics of OCT, both from a nontechnical and technical perspective and its early applications to dental science.

Ten chapters are devoted to OCT applications in specific areas of dentistry, from cariology and dental materials to the recent research field of nanodentistry.

Then, it ends with a chapter on what can be expected for developments in dental OCT. Each chapter will highlight the basic anatomy or features of the studied subject, then the conventional methods of diagnosis or analysis – in the case of materials – and then the literature results on the subject, with insights by the authors own research. Where applicable, clinical developments will be highlighted. The sequence follows the way that, in general, undergraduate syllabus courses are given.

We hope you have an enjoyable read!

Anderson S. L. Gomes
Denise M. Zezell
Cláudia C. B. O. Mota
John M. Girkin

Editor Biographies

Anderson S. L. Gomes is Professor of Physics at Universidade Federal of Pernambuco, Brazil, PhD in Physics from Imperial College of Science, Technology and Medicine (1986), post-doc from Brown University (1992). His research interests are in nonlinear optics, nanophotonics and biophotonics. He co-authored more than 300 scientific publications, is a Fellow of OPTICA, and Member of the Brazilian Academy of Sciences, Member of The World Academy of Science (TWAS) and the Brazilian Order of Scientific Merit.

Denise M. Zezell is Fellow of OPTICA and Senior Researcher at Nuclear and Energy Research Institute IPEN-CNEN, Sao Paulo, Brazil. She has a PhD in Physics from State University of Campinas in Lasers in Medicine (1991) and a post-doc from ICTP-Triste, Italy (1992). Her research interests are in biophotonics, tumor diagnosis via FTIR and lasers in dentistry, an area that she has pioneered in Brazil.

Cláudia C. B. O. Mota is a professor of Dentistry at Universidade de Pernambuco and Centro Universitário Tabosa de Almeida, DSc in Dentistry from Universidade Federal de Pernambuco (2014). Her research interests are focused on dental materials, imaging diagnostic and biophotonics.

John M. Girkin is Professor of Biophysics at Durham University, UK. He is internationally recognized for his expertise in the development of optical instrumentation for the life sciences and the clinic. He has previously developed commercially successful instruments for ophthalmology and researches on the development of optical methods for use in dentistry including OCT.

Contributors

Carlos Menezes Aguiar
Universidade Federal de
  Pernambuco
Brazil

Ana Marly Araújo Maia Amorim
Universidade Estadual da Paraíba
Brazil

Patricia Aparecida Ana
Federal University of ABC
Brazil

Alistair Bounds
Durham University
United Kingdom

**Vanda Sanderana Macêdo
Carneiro**
Universidade de Pernambuco
Brazil

Luiz Alcino Gueiros
Universidade Federal de
  Pernambuco
Brazil

**Cecília Maria de Sá Barreto Cruz
Falcão**
Universidade Federal de
  Pernambuco
Brazil

Marcelo Giannini
State University of Campinas
Brazil

John M. Girkin
Durham University
United Kingdom

Anderson S. L. Gomes
Universidade Federal de
  Pernambuco
Brazil

Jair Carneiro Leão
Universidade Federal de
  Pernambuco
Brazil

Mônica Schäffer Lopes
Universidade Federal de
  Pernambuco
Brazil

Patrícia Makishi
State University of Campinas
Brazil

Gabriela Monteiro
Universidade de Pernambuco
Brazil

Paulo Ney Lyra de Moraes
Nuclear and Energy Research
  Institute
Brazil

Marcia Cristina Dias de Moraes
Instituto de Pesquisas Energéticas
  e Nucleares
Brazil

Cláudia C. B. O. Mota
Centro Universitário Tabosa de
  Almeida and Universidade de
  Pernambuco
Brazil

Alireza Sadr
University of Washington
USA

Yasushi Shimada
Okayama University
Japan

Junji Tagami
Tokyo Medical and Dental
  University
Japan

Mariana Torres
International Iberian
  Nanotechnology Laboratory
Portugal

Denise Valente
Universidade Federal de
  Pernambuco
Brazil

Denise M. Zezell
Instituto de Pesquisas Energéticas e
  Nucleares
Brazil

1

Overview of Optical Imaging Methods Used in Dentistry

John M. Girkin and Alistair Bounds

Department of Physics, Durham University, Durham, UK

CONTENTS

1.1 Introduction

The first action of any dentist is to ask the patient to open their mouth so that they can undertake a visual inspection of the exposed surfaces of the tooth. Optical imaging, using the clinician's eyes as the detector, is still, therefore, the most important diagnostic tool employed. As well as looking at the tooth

DOI: 10.1201/9781351104562-1

surface, the skilled practitioner will also move their head around using the way that the light is returned from the tooth to make clinical judgments on the status of the teeth being observed. They are unlikely to consider deeply the way that the electromagnetic radiation, light, is interreacting with the molecular and crystal structure of the tooth, but it is this interaction that they are observing, and crucially how this interaction changes when there are local changes in the tooth. The aim of the instrument developer is therefore to provide the clinician with information that they cannot see directly with their eyes to enhance their decision making. This extra information may be to provide details on the internal structure of the tissue through to microscopic changes that are taking place dynamically on the surface of the tooth. In order to deliver these extra clinical insights different wavelengths (colors) of light may be used or methods that help to separate out the surface reflections from light scattered back from greater depths. Crucially though this information needs to be taken with minimal perturbation to the tooth, rapidly and a frequently over looked complication, with a live patient present in the dentist's chair.

Before considering the physical details of such interactions and instrumentation it is important to consider what the dentist actually wants. In relation to hard tissue, ideally, they would like to be able to detect, and quantify, early caries lesions assessing the level, and rate, of mineral loss from the tooth. These measurements should be rapid and provide information on not just the surface interactions but also what is taking place at deeper levels within the tooth. The method should clearly be non-invasive and "patient friendly" but present no risk to the subject such as that in the case of ionizing radiation (X-rays). Implicit in these comments is the requirement to detect problems early when the treatment will be as minimally invasive as possible, ideally using re-mineralization of the tooth to heal early lesions. A further practical consideration is that the method should be cost effective, and relatively fast providing real-time information to the clinician and patient. There is little point in taking several minutes to image each tooth with very high resolution as this would increase patient "chair time" making the method impractical in a real clinical setting. If the method is ever going to reach the clinic it will also need to be commercialized meaning it must be easy to operate, reliable and fit within the cost structure of the dental practice.

As well as the detection of early caries, a focus throughout this book, instruments are also required to assess the status of the gum and softer tissue – a growing area of concern as fluoride toothpastes improve the general status of dentition around the world. Here the requirement may be less of obtaining images but providing indications of levels of infection and blood flow through the tissue as a guide towards the vitality of the tissue. There are also requirements for methods that might be used during more invasive treatments to ensure that the correct level of diseased tissue has been removed and thus minimizing the risk of re-infection and further, even more invasive, treatment.

Before considering more details of practical physics and optics behind the various methods to be discussed, it is worth taking a moment to think about the difference between detecting, diagnosing and treating a condition. Although the terms are often, incorrectly, used interchangeably some thought should be given here for any long-term practical devices that may be dreamt up. In basic terms, detection is the identification of a problem, diagnosis is then the quantification of the problem and the initial consideration of a treatment plan, and then one moves onto the treatment phase, which is then the implementation of the diagnosis clinical pathway. In the case of the dental surgery, it is possible that these tasks may be undertaken by different people from dental nurses, dental hygienists through to dental surgeons. Each will have subtly different requirements and thus, in the long term, a suite of imaging methods may be required to deliver the best possible solution to each specialty. In all research work it is always worthwhile to keep these considerations in mind as it can help to increase the longer-term impact of any practical research.

The chapter will now go on to provide the basics on the physics of light and the way that it interacts with tissue. This understanding will then be used to show such interactions can help provide information that cannot just be seen with the dentist's eyes alone, explaining how several of the most recent optical methods, applied to dentistry, operate (Hall et al. 2004). All of this will, as far as possible, be set in the context of how such instrumentation can help the clinician improve patient care, which in the long term must be the aim of all such instrumentation.

1.2 Basic Properties of Light

At the heart of all the methods described in this book is light as a source of energy. It is then subtle changes in the properties, or quantity, of the light that is then seen by the detector that is then related back to the status of the sample. As a source of energy, light is part of the electromagnetic spectrum, but crucially in the region in which our eyes operate as a detector. This visible portion of the spectrum extends from around 400 to 700 nm (violet to deep red). At shorter wavelengths one enters into the region of UV excitation and longer than 700 nm is in the near infrared region. The wavelength of the light plays a very important role in the way that it interacts with the tissue. The exact nature of light has also been a subject of controversy since the 16th century, is light a wave (classical physics) or a particle (quantum mechanics or Newton's "Corpuscles")? Numerous experiments have been undertaken over the intervening 400 years and the conclusion is the light can exist in both "forms". Throughout this chapter, and indeed the entire book, explanations of the interaction of light with tissue will be given using both waves and particles. Generally, the one that provides the clearest explanation of a particular phenomenon will be used.

As a wave light obeys the equation $c = v\lambda$, where v is the frequency of the light, λ is the wavelength and c the speed of light in a vacuum (defined in 1983 as being 299, 792, 458 ms^{-1}). The other fundamental equation related to light is the energy present for an individual photon (particle of light). In Planck's equation $E = hv$ where E is the energy of an individual photon, h is Planck's constant (6.63 × 10^{-34} Js) and v again the frequency of the light. As a wave light has (a) wavelength: the distance from one peak (or trough) on the wave to the next one, and (b) frequency: the number of waves passing a point in a second. The height of the wave is known as the amplitude. These are illustrated in Figure 1.1.

As mentioned above the speed of light, in a vacuum, is now defined and according to Einstein nothing can travel faster than this velocity. However, when light passes through a material it is slowed down and the ratio of the velocity of light in a vacuum to its velocity in a material is known as the material's refractive index "n". For water this value is around 1.33, for glass 1.5 (or a velocity of around 2 × 10^8 ms^{-1}) but for dental enamel it is as high as 1.62. The exact value of the refractive index depends on the wavelength and thus different wavelengths of light will be slowed to greater or lesser extent. Generally, the longer the wavelength of light, the less the light is slowed. The high refractive index of dental enamel leads to the light being guided through the tooth as explained later.

The final property of light we need to consider is that of polarization. Polarization is the property of the direction of the wave's oscillation. For a

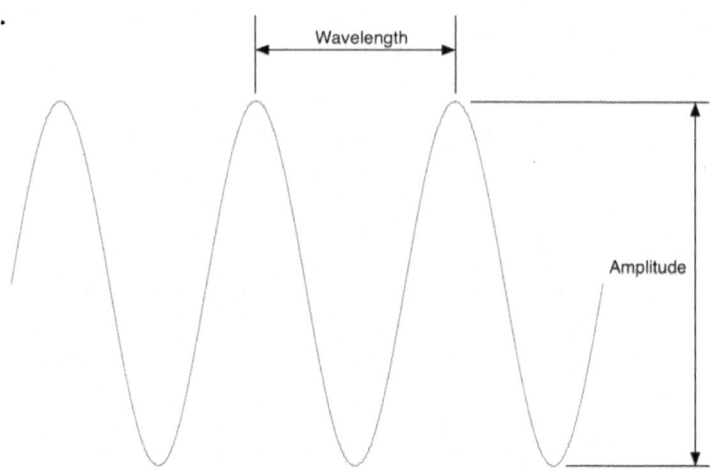

FIGURE 1.1
Diagrammatic representation of a light wave.

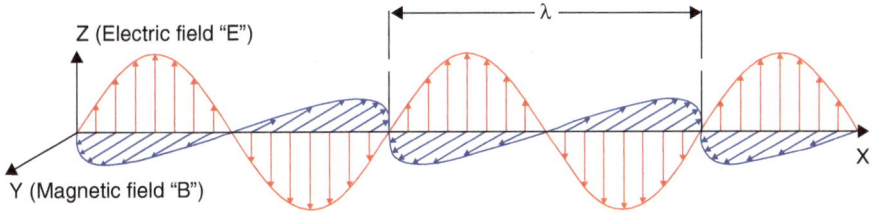

FIGURE 1.2
Representation of a wave illustrating the property of polarization.

wave traveling in the x direction, the waves can either oscillate in the y or z directions, or a mixture of the two. In the case of light, which is a combination of oscillating electric and magnetic fields, it is the direction of the electric fields' oscillations, which defines the direction of polarization. In Figure 1.2 the light is vertically polarized. A beam is *linearly polarized* if all of the waves are oscillating in the same direction, and *un-polarized*, or *randomly polarized*, light is a combination of waves oscillating in all directions. Light that is un-polarized can be separated into two polarization states (vertical and horizontal) using several components including specially coated optics, certain crystals and a specific polarization selected using special plastics (such as that used in sunglasses).

1.3 Interaction of Light, Matter and Tissue

Having described the basic properties of light we now need to consider how these properties are affected by interactions with materials, including both soft and hard tissue. In any optical detection system it is changes in the properties of light that produce the contrast in the data, or images, that can then be related back to clinical problems. All of the interactions of light are illustrated in Figure 1.3.

1.3.1 Reflection

Reflection occurs when light hits a surface and is then directly "thrown back" off the surface at a well-defined angle. Indeed the angle of the incoming light, relative to a line drawn normally to the surface, is equal to the outgoing angle, the other side of the normal as illustrated in Figure 1.3(a). Apart from the change in direction of the light there is no other alteration to its properties. In particular, the wavelength and polarization are not affected. The fact that the polarization is not affected can be used to remove surface reflections if a polarized light beam is incident on a reflective surface. Using a polarizing

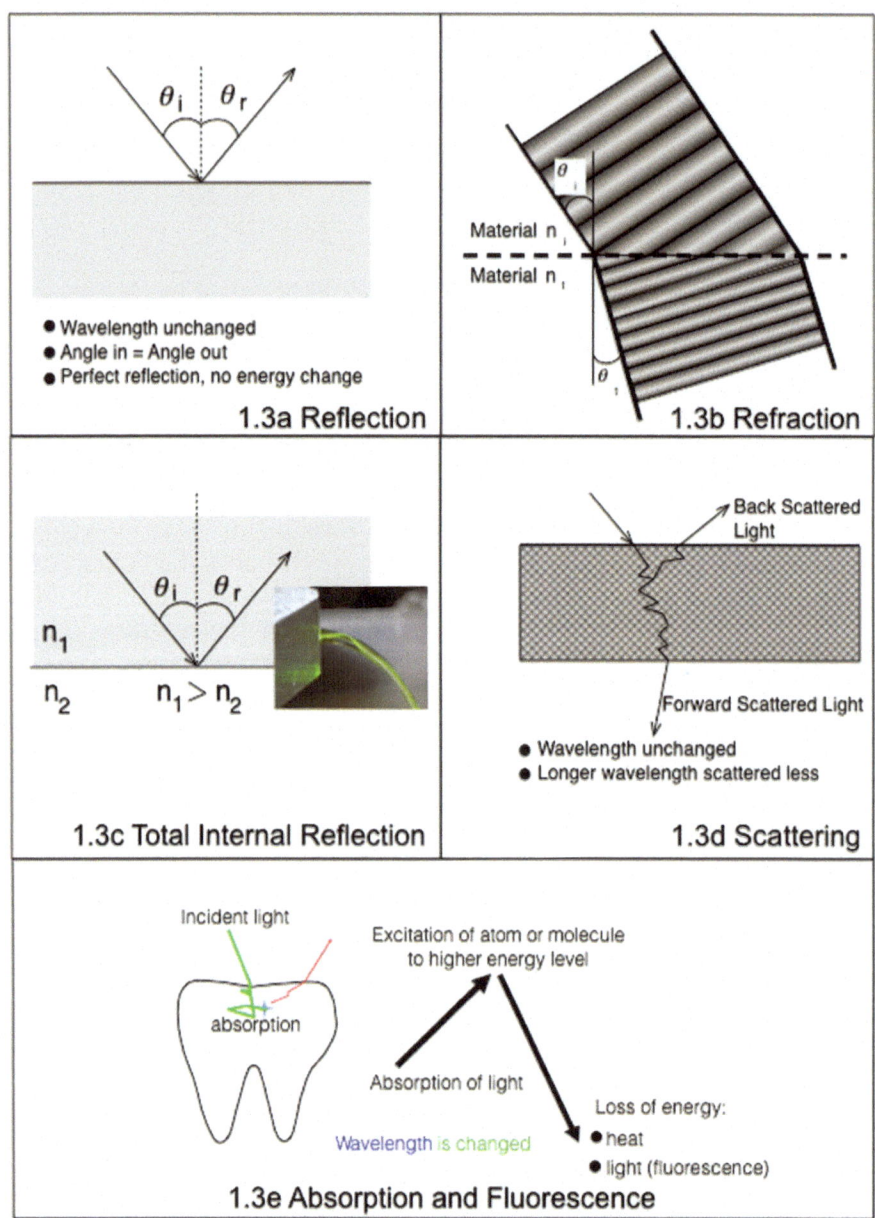

FIGURE 1.3
Interactions of light with matter. (a) Reflection. (b) Refraction. (c) Total internal reflection (inset shows TIR in a water flow). (d) Scattering. (e) Absorption and fluorescence.

filter, which is at ninety degrees (crossed) with the incoming polarization of light the reflected light will be rejected. This is a method frequently
used in optical coherence tomography (OCT) systems to remove the surface
reflections.

The most common reflective materials are metals and thin coatings of
aluminum and silver are frequently used to coat glass surfaces to produce
mirrors. Gold is also highly reflective but due to its atomic structure certain wavelengths are transmitted and hence the reflected light has a gold
rather than white color. However, all surfaces that are not highly absorbing
do reflect a certain quantity of incoming light unless they are specially
coated. This reflection is due to their refractive index and is known as
Fresnel reflection. If light hits glass at normal incidence then 4% of the
light will be reflected from the surface, with this percentage increasing
as the angle of incidence increases. This effect can be seen in the type of
mirror used in the home when one sometimes sees a double image, with
a strong reflection off the back silver-coated surface and weaker almost
"ghost" image from the reflection from the front of the glass. Although
Fresnel reflection does not change the polarization of the incoming light
one polarization is preferentially reflected and again this effect can be used
in certain optical instruments. This preferential reflection is the reason
that polarized sunglasses enable you to see more clearly through water
on a sunny day. The light reflected off the surface is partially polarized
and by using sunglasses, which reject this polarization, one removes the
reflected light.

1.3.2 Refraction

Refraction of light is due to a material's refractive index, which causes a
light beam to "bend" as it moves from one material to another. Figure 1.3(b)
illustrates the reason for this. If one considers a plane wave of light reaching
a transparent material where the refractive index is higher, the first part of
the light will enter the material but will be slowed down. This means that
light that has not yet entered the material and will start to "catch up" with
the part of the wave already inside. This means that the wave will appear
to pivot, or bend, towards the normal of the surface. On exiting the block,
the light will travel in the opposite manner such that when the wave fully
emerges it will be parallel with the input beam. The level of bending depends
on the relative refractive indices between the two materials and is given by
Snell's law:

$$\frac{\sin \theta_i}{\sin \theta_t} = \frac{n_1}{n_2} \qquad (1.1)$$

As mentioned earlier the refractive index of a material varies with the wavelength of the light so although the actual wavelength and properties of the light are unchanged, white light can be spread spectrally into its component colors due to the refractive index of a material. This is how a prism produces a "rainbow" from white light. Thus refraction only changes the direction of the light, and also the time that light may take to traverse a particular distance (as the light may be traveling more slowly).

1.3.3 Total Internal Reflection

The refractive index of a material also leads to two particular effects within dental tissue. The first is known as total internal reflection and plays an important role in the way that light is guided through a tooth. The effect can be predicted from Snell's law. For a fixed pair of refractive indices, there will be a point where the sine of the angle of the transmitted beam will become greater than 1, which is not possible (Figure 1.3(c)). The point at which this value becomes 1 is known as the critical angle and is given by

$$\theta_c = \arcsin\left(\frac{n_2}{n_1}\right) \tag{1.2}$$

For glass with a refractive index of 1 and where air ($n_2 = 1.00$) is the second medium the critical angle is 41.8°. If light hits the interface at an angle greater than this then it will be reflected rather than transmitted. This effect is illustrated in the inset in Figure 1.3(c) where a laser is being guided down a water flow (in air) due to total internal reflection. This is also the way in which optical fibers work and in teeth the enamel rods, or prisms, guide light in exactly the same way. In fact, the dimensions of an enamel rod are very similar to those of a single mode optical fiber, though the refractive index is higher in the case of enamel. This has the effect of helping to guide the light through the tooth towards the dentine where the light is scattered. There is in fact some guiding within the dentinal tubules but this is due to multiple scattering (Kienle et al. 2006). As will be described later, these two effects are the cause of early lesions appearing to the eye as a "white spot".

1.3.4 Scattering Including Raman Scattering

Scattering occurs due to differences in the local refractive index of the sample and is illustrated in Figure 1.3(d). The level of scattering depends on (a) the local difference in refractive index; (b) the size of the particle or feature; (c) the wavelength of the light. In a scattering process there is no change of wavelength with the exception of Raman scattering, which is discussed later. Light at longer wavelengths is scattered less than shorter wavelengths, which is one of the reasons near-infrared light is used for imaging in OCT as it penetrates as a well-structured beam further into the tissue.

The exact way (level of scattering and angular range of scattering) that light scatters depends on the relative size of the particle to the wavelength of light, and different scattering regimes use different approximations to solve the complex mathematical equations, which describe the process. At a larger scale scattering can be considered as being probabilistic and a value assigned to the chance of a photon being scattered over a particular angular range.

It should also be noted that the level of scattering is affected by the polarization of the light entering the sample relative to the orientation of the feature causing the scattering, and scattered light does have its polarization changed. Thus, through an examination of the polarization angle of the light, further contrast enhancements are possible to separate out highly scattered from less strongly scattered light and even reflections.

In general, the scattering processes do not change the wavelength of the light being scattered; the exception to this is in certain materials, which are described as being Raman active. The first observation of inelastic light scattering (change of wavelength) was made in 1928 by C.V. Raman and K.S. Krishnan and led to the award of the Nobel Prize in physics in 1930. Sir Chandrasekhara Venkata Raman, an Indian, was the first Asian and non-white person to receive a scientific Nobel Prize and the effect was rapidly named after him. As only around one photon in 10 million is Raman scattered (Raman scattering probability ~ 1×10^{-7}) the technology at the time was not sensitive enough for widespread practical application of the method. Instead near-infrared spectroscopy became the standard analytical tool used to help determine molecular composition. The laser and more recently charge-coupled device detectors have radically transformed this position.

The Raman effect can be explained both using a photon or electromagnetic wave approach. In the latter, the electric field of the light wave deforms the electric field of the molecule, causing the latter to oscillate at the same frequency as the light wave. The molecular oscillating field then acts as a dipole oscillator emitting light at the same frequency as the light field (conventional scattering) when there are no Raman active vibrational modes. An alternative, is that when the molecule is Raman active, part of the electromagnetic wave is used to excite a vibrational mode in the molecule and the resulting molecular dipole oscillates at a lower frequency, emitting light at a slightly longer wavelength than the incoming light. This emitted Raman light is known as the Stokes wavelength as it emerges at a longer wavelength. If the molecule is already in a more energetic state that when the light is re-emitted it may have gained energy leading to a shorter emission wavelength and anti-Stokes scattering, which has an even lower probability of occurring.

The Raman effect can also be considered, and perhaps more easily appreciated, using a quantum mechanical approach. The incoming photon excites the sample into a virtual energy state from which a photon is subsequently emitted with the molecule returning to its ground state that explains Rayleigh scattering. In the Stokes situation, the molecule does not return to its ground state but to a vibrational state that is at a slightly higher energy, leading to the emitted photon having a slightly lower energy, or longer wavelength. The final alternative is for the incoming photon to be taken to a virtual energy state but the molecule here is already in a vibrationally excited state and hence the emitted photon has greater energy than the incoming photon and therefore appears at a shorter wavelength.

The end result of Raman scattering is a spectrum for a molecule with a series of discrete wavelengths and this is known as the molecular fingerprint. Using computer-based methods it is now possible to use these spectral fingerprints to identify the molecules present within a sample and hence analyze complex spectra. This has been applied to dental tissue with the first recorded example probably being in 2000 (Hill et al. 2000).

1.3.5 Absorption and Fluorescence

The other major effect that can take place with light and tissue is the absorption of the light (Figure 1.3(e)). Here light of the correct wavelength is absorbed by a molecule either causing an electron to be excited up to a higher energy level, or a change in the molecular vibrational levels in the case of infrared light. The molecule will then lose this energy by one of two routes. In the first, all of the energy will be lost in the surrounding molecules and tissue causing a local heating effect. In the second, there will be a slight loss of energy, and then a photon will be re-emitted containing the remaining energy. This emerging light will be at a longer wavelength than the incoming light and is the well known fluorescent phenomena.

1.3.6 Thermal Emission

Although not really a practical method for any form of dental imaging, thermal emission is included here for completeness. Any material that is above absolute zero will emit some level of electromagnetic radiation, with the wavelength being determined by the temperature. Clearly for light in the visible one is looking for the sample to be several hundred degrees Celsius (red hot coals in a fire) but at lower temperatures the emission is in the mid to far infrared. These temperatures can be seen on a thermal imaging camera and these have been used to investigate clinical challenges in the oral cavity (Kaneko et al. 1999). The problem, however, is that the body is at 37°C and breath from the subject tends to confound the thermal image when applied in a clinical setting. In the oral cavity, hard tissue is slightly fluorescent when excited in the ultra-violet and violet portion of the optical spectrum.

1.4 Applications to Dental and Oral Disease

Having described in outline how light interreacts with matter we now need to consider how these interactions can be used to help improve methods of dental and oral disease detection. The optical properties of dental tissue can be found in a paper published in 1975 (Spitzer et al. 1975). Although the main focus of the book is on OCT, the applications and methods are well described in the individual contributions. This section will look, in outline, at other methods that are being explored for clinical applications in dentistry. This is not intended as a fully comprehensive review of the current work but much more as an outline to some of the work that has been undertaken and may, in the long term, be combined with OCT-based methods to provide a comprehensive diagnostic toolkit.

Before discussing how these optical methods can be used for dental diagnosis, we need to consider, in basic terms, the effect that dental caries have on the structure of the tooth. The process is illustrated in Figure 1.4. Initially a bacterial biofilm builds up on the enamel surface. The typical caries forming bacteria in the mouth (such as *Streptococcus mutans*) consume sugars and then eject an acidic liquid. If the biofilm is in place for long enough this acid will slowly start to dissolve the enamel surface. Initially due to the structure of the biofilm it makes the outer surface of the enamel porous. If the acid attack

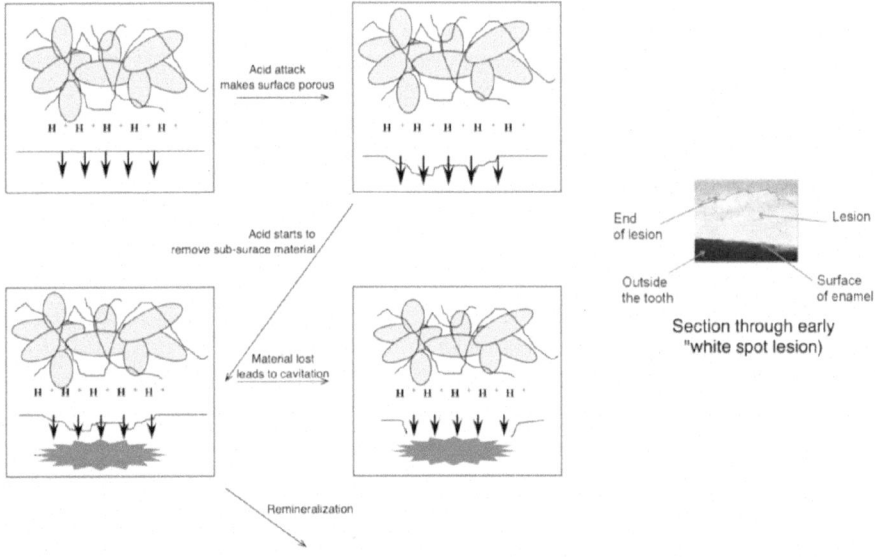

FIGURE 1.4
Basic cycle in the development of dental caries.

continues then material is now dissolved from beneath the surface of the tooth breaking down the enamel rods.

At this stage in the caries development process, the process can be reversed with the biofilm being removed and calcium ions (and frequently fluoride ions) moving through the porous surface to enable the enamel crystals to reform through a process known as protein-guided crystal growth. This is an important aspect of dental disease progression as it provides the reason for having methods to detect early caries at the point in which they can still be re-mineralized. It also indicates why a dentist would like to be able to take repeated measurements to assess if a lesion is growing, or re-mineralizing.

However, if the early lesion develops further, eventually the supporting enamel rods give way causing the top of the lesion to collapse and a cavity to form. This now provides a space for the bacteria to form a more complex biofilm that is harder to clean. If left unchecked this lesion will now continue to grow eventually leading down to the dentine and requiring more complex dental treatment, including "drill and fill". At this stage the lesion can start to become brown and black as the bacteria grow in number and trap other materials.

1.4.1 White Light Observations

As was stated at the outset of the chapter, dentist's first diagnostic tool is their eyes. Early caries lesions are described as "white spot lesions" and said to have a "chalky white appearance" (Ekstrand et al. 1998). Using the above descriptions of the interaction of light with materials, this effect can now be explained. In healthy dental tissue the white illumination light is partially reflected from the tooth's surface and then transmitted through the enamel towards the dentine both by direct illumination and also by total internal reflection as described above. The white light is then highly scattered by the dentine with much of it being backscattered towards the observer, back through the enamel. This gives the tooth its generally uniform white appearance.

We now need to consider what happens to light as caries develop in the manner described above. The outer surface becoming slightly porous means that it has a slightly rough surface, meaning that it does not act as well as a reflector giving a duller appearance to the reflected light. In addition to this, the light that passes through the surface is no longer guided through the enamel rods but is backscattered close to the surface. This scattering leads to a higher level of white light, compared to the slightly longer wavelength, redder, light that comes from photons that have traveled through to the dentine before being back scattered. Thus these two effects, the change in surface, and the lack of light guiding lead to the "chalk white" appearance.

The appearance of the early lesion can also be increased by air drying the tooth. An early lesion is normally filled with saliva (water), which has a refractive index of around 1.34, compared to the enamel at 1.62 and air at 1.0. Thus, if the water is "blown out" the difference between the refractive index of enamel in the tooth and the surrounding material (now air) will be much higher leading to higher scattering. This is why during a visual inspection, a dentist may use the air to speed up the drying process and potentially help reveal early lesions. Thus, using the basic rules of light propagation, it is possible to explain what a dentist sees without any additional visual aids.

The other method that is used clinically utilizing white light is that of fiber optics transillumination or FOTI. This method was first demonstrated in 1973 (Barenie et al. 1973). Here a conventional multimode fiber (typically around 400–600 μm in diameter) is placed against the tooth at normal incidence from the other lingual or buccal direction. The dentist then looks down on the tooth seeing light that is scattered towards the observer. This method is particularly useful in helping to identify approximal caries. The method has also been improved with the use of a camera to image the tooth in a process known as DIFOTI, or digital-FOTI (Schneiderman et al. 1997). A commercial system was developed but has never entered widespread clinical practice.

1.4.2 Quantitative Light Fluorescence

The technique of quantitative light fluorescence (QLF) uses the natural fluorescence from dental tissue when excited around 405 nm. The first report detailing the use of fluorescence on dental tissue was in 1985 when a range of teeth were imaged spectroscopically (Sundström et al. 1985). It was noticed there was a reduction in fluorescence from areas with white spot lesions and in fact this had previously been seen with dentists using composite curing lights. This observation was then built into a clinically useful instrument (de Josselin de Jong et al. 1995) in a method originally known as qualitative laser fluorescence but which became quantitative light fluorescence or QLF.

In this technique the tooth is illuminated with light at 405 nm (which may be from a laser, high-intensity arc lamp or LED) and fluorescence longer at around 450 nm imaged onto a camera. Generally the illumination and camera system surrounds a single tooth in a device resembling a dental handpiece. The recorded image is then processed in a novel manner in order to quantify the mineral loss. The area surrounding a suspected lesion is used as the base line for the fluorescent signal and then a calculation is made for each pixel on the area of the lesion. This calculation determines the level that the pixel intensity would need to rise in order to provide a uniform fluorescent emission over the entire region of the lesion and surrounding tooth. A sum of all the individual "missing" pixel intensities is then made to determine the loss of fluorescence due to the lesion. Work has also shown that the majority of the fluorescence detected comes from the dentine/enamel junction, probably due to the change in local refractive index causing increased back scattering of the fluorescence generated within the tooth (Rousseau et al. 2002).

This technique has now been applied in a number of clinical trials and it has been demonstrated that re-mineralization can be followed as lesions "heal themselves". In addition, the method has been applied to measure the rate of water loss through a lesion as a form of quantifying the porosity of an early lesion (van der Veen et al. 1999). Using both natural and artificial lesions the loss of fluorescence has been linked to an exact loss of mineral when measured using transverse micro-radiography on extracted teeth. The main problem with QLF is that the process is slow if every tooth is imaged in this way, the cost of the instrumentation was high and the teeth need to be clean to ensure that staining or other factors do not alter the readings.

1.4.3 Infrared Imaging

As discussed earlier, near infrared light (around 850 nm or longer) can pass through a tooth with significantly lower scattering than visible light. Figure 1.5 illustrates a near-infrared transmission image of an extracted tooth. The areas in which the light only passes through the enamel appear almost transparent due to the light guiding effect described earlier. In the image, an early white spot lesion can be clearly seen appearing as a slightly darker spot as the light is more highly scattered and hence does not reach the detector on the far side of the tooth. Work has also been undertaken at longer wavelengths up to 1300 nm (Jones et al. 2003). Here the tooth is more transparent due to lower scattering, however, the detectors are significantly

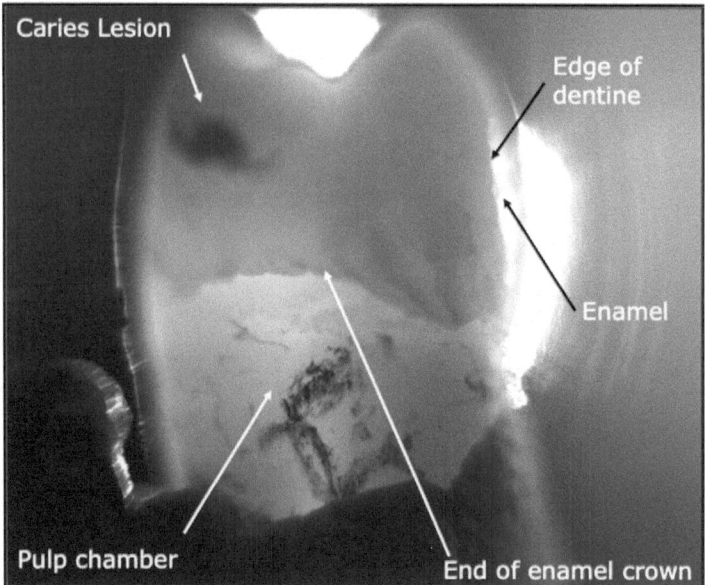

FIGURE 1.5
Infrared transmission image using light at 850 nm.

more expensive and generally larger as one needs to use materials that are more exotic than silicon, which works up to a wavelength of around 1000 nm. Work is on-going in this method of imaging and the images are easy for a clinician to appreciate as they appear to be very similar to an X-ray. Again it is unclear why this method has not had wider acceptance within the clinical community.

In a variation of a reflection confocal microscope, a depth profile has also been recorded using an infrared system and fiber optic light delivery and collection (Rousseau et al. 2007). Here a single mode optical fiber was used to deliver light to the tooth with a lens that focused the light down into the tooth. The light backscattered from the tooth was then collected by the same fiber and returned to the detector. In this configuration, the optical fiber acts as a confocal pinhole only letting light from the focus of the lens back through the system. Thus, by scanning the lens one can record a depth profile through the tooth. In this way, the team were able to distinguish between sound enamel, caries and re-mineralized enamel.

The use of near-infrared light has also been used to assess pulp vitality (Fein et al. 1997). It is known that blood has a different absorption coefficient depending on its level of oxygenation. Around 800 nm, the absorption of oxy-hemoglobin and deoxy-hemoglobin change significantly. Thus by sending light into a tooth at around 780 nm and 850 nm and measuring the relative attenuation, one can determine the level of blood and its status within the pulp cavity of a tooth. This is similar to the finger clamp that is used to measure blood oxygenation in the body as a whole. In the dental case, a special fiber optic system was used to deliver light precisely to points within the tooth and crucially to ensure correct collection of all wavelengths of transmitted light.

1.4.4 Fluorescence and Fluorescence Lifetime

The QLF method described earlier clearly uses fluorescence as the contrast mechanism for caries detection but there are several other methods that have been applied to dental tissue. The first method to be considered is that of a commercial system known as DIAGNOdent (Kavo Instruments Inc.). This system uses a red laser diode (around 650 nm) to excite bacterial fluorescence that are present in a carious lesion. Thus compared to QLF, which uses direct tissue fluorescence, this is more of an indirect measurement. The method was first applied in a clinical trial in 1999 (Reich et al. 1999) and for a few years was a huge commercial success. However, there are some limitations. The method was more suitable for later stage caries that had reached the dentine (Lussi et al. 2004) as this was when bacteria, and their porphyrin bi-products, could build up in large concentrations leading to a significant level of fluorescence. The system was also not just sensitive to bacterial-related fluorescence and other naturally occurring materials in the mouth (such as staining from tea) could provide false readings. However, when used with careful clinical judgement it did provide a method that gave the clinician extra information during both examinations and also during caries removal using a dental burr (Lussi et al. 2000) prior to restoration.

Work has also taken place using fluorescence in which the excitation, as with QLF, was in the violet portion of the spectrum. In this work, the aim was not just to detect the carious regions of the tooth but to also attempt to quantify the activity. The fluorescent light returned from the tooth was examined spectroscopically and certain spectral bands then used to assign the detect wavelength spectrum to the status of the lesion (Ribeiro et al. 2005). The team were able to distinguish between active and re-mineralizing and re-mineralized lesions though as a practical device there was again the complication of other fluorophores being present within the oral cavity confounding the results. Fluorescence spectroscopy has also been applied as a method to improve invasive treatments. The main focus here has been in determining if all the diseased tissue has been removed before a restoration is put in place and also for the detection and quantification of root caries (Buchalla et al. 2004). Although work has continued in the laboratory and in a few clinics, this has not been a method explored by commercial organizations to bring an instrument into wider clinical practice.

The other fluorescent-based method that has been used on dental tissue is that of fluorescent lifetime measurements. Here freshly extracted human teeth were hemisected and the fluorescent lifetime measured through the lesion (McConnell et al. 2007). The team demonstrated that the lifetime varied through a lesions and it is strongly suspected that this links to the local pH within the lesion. This could have important ramifications for monitoring activity with a lesion but the practical challenge is to return sufficient signal from deep within the tooth.

1.4.5 THz and Non-Linear Techniques

THz radiation is light present in the long infrared wavelength range typically around 100 μm. This portion of the optical spectrum is not significantly scattered by human tissue and will indeed pass through clothing and packaging material. It is however, absorbed by water, which does impose some limitations for clinical use. A group have used light at this wavelength to look at early dental lesions, in particular looking to measure the local refractive index and to match this to the presence of active caries (Crawley et al. 2003). The team demonstrated that the method does work and can provide highly sensitive measurements but again the challenge is to make this a practical method for caries detection and monitoring within the oral cavity, which is inherently wet! In addition at the time that this work was originally undertaken, THz sources were not compact using large femtosecond laser systems and complex detection systems. With applications being developed for THz in a range of security areas, these equipment challenges have now been met and the application to dentistry may be re-considered.

The other method that has used femtosecond lasers on teeth (beyond using their wide spectral bandwidth for OCT imaging) in generating two photon fluorescence (Girkin et al. 1999). In this technique, originally developed for optical microscopy, light at twice the wavelength (typically around 800 nm) of that required to generate fluorescence is directed onto the sample. Under normal circumstances, such light will not generate fluorescence, but when ultra-short pulses (around 100×10^{-15} s) are used the peak power is very high. This means that at the focus of the beam there is a significant probability of two photons being absorbed simultaneously leading to the local generation of fluorescence. As the probability of such an event taking place depends on the square of the laser intensity, this only takes place at the focus. If this focal point is then scanned around the sample one then has the ability to take an optical section through the tooth to build up a three-dimensional image. Areas of caries activity have been shown to generate different levels of detected fluorescence compared to healthy tissue and thus the multiphoton method can be used to detect caries.

1.5 Summary

In this chapter we have described the interactions that light has with any material and then related this to the effects that can then be seen in dental tissue. We have then explored how these interactions can be used to detect and diagnose early dental caries. As has been discussed, several of these methods have now made their way into advanced dental practice. This provides some advanced background into the OCT methods described else-where in the book.

References

Barenie, J., Leske, G., Ripa, L. W. 1973. The use of fiber optic transillumination for the detection of proximal caries. *Oral Surgery* 36: 891–897

Buchalla, W., Lennon, A. M., Attin, T. 2004. Comparative fluorescence spectroscopy of root caries lesions. *European Journal of Oral Sciences* 112: 490–496.

Crawley, D. A., Longbottom, C., Wallace, V. P., Cole, B. E., Arnone, D. D., Pepper, M. 2003. Three-dimensional terahertz pulse imaging of dental tissue. *Commercial and Biomedical Applications of Ultrafast and Free-Electron Lasers* 4633: 84.

de Josselin de Jong, E., Sundström, F., Westerling, H., Tranaeus, S., ten Bosch, J. J., Angmar-Mansson, B. 1995. A new method of in vivo quantification of changes in initial enamel caries with laser fluorescence. *Caries Research* 29: 2–7.

Ekstrand, K. R., Ricketts, D. N., Kidd, E. A., Qvist, V., Schou, S. 1998. Detection, diagnosing, monitoring and logical treatment of occlusal caries in relation to lesion activity and severity: an in vivo examination with histological validation. *Caries Research* 32:247–254.

Fein, M. E., Gluskin, A. H., Goon, W. W., Chew, B. B., Crone, W. A., Jones, H. W. 1997. Evaluation of optical methods of detecting dental pulp vitality. *Journal of Biomedical Optics* 2: 58–73.

Girkin, J. M., Hall, A. F., Creanor, S. L. 1999. Multi-photon imaging of intact dental tissue. *Early Detection of Dental Caries II. Proceedings of the 4th Annual Indiana Conference*, 155–168. Stookey GK, editor. Indianapolis: Indiana University School of Dentistry.

Hall, A., Girkin, J. M. 2004. A review of potential new diagnostic modalities for caries lesions. *Journal of Dental Research* 83: 89–94.

Hill, W., Petrou, V. 2000. Caries detection by diode laser Raman spectroscopy. *Applied Spectroscopy* 54: 795–799.

Jones, R., Gigi, H., Graham, J., Daniel, F. 2003. Near-infrared transillumination at 1310-nm for the imaging of early dental decay. *Optics Express* 11: 2259–2265.

Kaneko, K., Matsuyama, K., Nakashima, S. 1999. Quantification of early carious enamel lesions by using an infrared camera in vitro. *Early Detection of Dental Caries II. Proceedings of the 4th Annual Indiana Conference*, 83–100. Stookey GK, editor. Indianapolis: Indiana University School of Dentistry.

Kienle, A., Raimund H. 2006. Light guiding in biological tissue due to scattering. *Physical Review Letters* 97: 018104.

Lussi, A., Francescut, P., Achermann, F., Reich, E., Hotz, P., Megert, B. 2000. The use of the DIAGNOdent during cavity preparation. *Caries Research* 34: 327–328.

Lussi, A., Hibst, R., and Paulus, R. 2004. DIAGNOdent: an optical method for caries detection. *Journal of Dental Research* 83: C80–C83.

McConnell, G., Girkin, J. M., Ameer-Beg, S. M. et al. 2007. Time-correlated single-photon counting fluorescence lifetime confocal imaging of decayed and sound dental structures with a white-light supercontinuum source. *Journal of Microscopy* 225: 126–136.

Reich, E., Berakdar, M., Netuschil, L., Pitts, N., Lussi, A. 1999. Clinical caries diagnosis compared to DIAGNOdent® evaluations. *Caries Research* 33: 299.

Ribeiro, A., Rousseau, C., Girkin, J. M. et al. 2005. A preliminary investigation of a spectroscopic technique for the diagnosis of natural caries lesions. *Journal of Dentistry* 33: 73–78.

Rousseau, C., Poland, S., Girkin, J. M., Hall, A. F., Whitters, C. J. 2007. Development of fibre-optic confocal microscopy for detection and diagnosis of dental caries. *Caries Research* 41: 245–251.

Rousseau, C., Vaidya, S., Creanor, S. L. et al. 2002. The effect of dentine on fluorescence measurements of enamel lesions in vitro. *Caries Research* 36: 381–385.

Schneiderman, A., Elbaum, M., Schultz, T., Keem, S., Greenebaum, M., Driller, J. 1997. Assessment of dental caries with digital imaging fiber-optic transillumination (DIFOTI): in vitro study. *Caries Research* 31: 103–110.

Spitzer, D., Bosch, J. Ten. 1975. The absorption and scattering of light in bovine and human dental enamel. *Calcif Tissue Research* 17: 129–137.

Sundström, F., Fredriksson, K., Montan, S., Hafström-Björkman, U., Strom, J. 1985. Laser induced fluorescence from sound and carious tooth substance: spectroscopic studies. *Swedish Dental Journal* 9: 154–7.

van der Veen, M. H., de Josselin de Jong, E., Al-Khateeb, S. 1999. Caries activity detection by dehydration with quantitative light fluorescence. *Early Detection of Dental Caries II. Proceedings of the 4th Annual Indiana Conference*, 251–260. Stookey GK, editor. Indianapolis: Indiana University School of Dentistry.

2

Optical Coherence Tomography (OCT): From Basics to General Applications

Anderson S. L. Gomes* and Denise Valente

Department of Physics, Federal University of Pernambuco, Recife, Pernambuco, Brazil

* anderson.lgomes@ufpe.br

CONTENTS

2.1 Introduction

The birth of the OCT technique dates from 1991, when Huang and co-workers first described a tomographic image of the retina of the eye (Huang et al. 1991). Prior to that, related work on femtosecond optical ranging (Fujimoto et al. 1986), optical coherence domain reflectometry (Youngquist et al. 1987), and low-coherence reflectometry (Clivaz et al. 1992; Schmitt et al. 1993) had been published. Since then, there has been a fantastic development in the field, as reported on occasion of the 25th year of the first ophthalmic image (de Boer et al. 2017). Also important was the translation of OCT from basic research to commercially available systems, including clinical OCTs, with dissemination worldwide, as reviewed in (Swanson and Fujimoto 2017). With this level of maturity, there are several review articles (Baumann 2017; Kim et al. 2018; Yasin Alibhai et al. 2018; Israelsen et al. 2019; Leitgeb 2019; Song et al. 2021) and books (Drexler and Fujimoto 2015; Girach and Sergott 2016) on the subject, and the ones referenced here reflect the author's choice on prioritizing more recent publications. Earlier work can be found in the

DOI: 10.1201/9781351104562-2

cited references. Besides general books and reviews, there are also several more dealing with OCT in specific areas, which is beyond the scope of this book, and the reader is deferred to ref. (Kim et al. 2018) for further details.

This chapter follows, in a summarized way, ref. (Drexler and Fujimoto 2015), which is a very comprehensive book from basics to applications of optical coherence tomography.

2.2 Basic Setup and Theory

Optical coherence tomography is an interferometric technique that captures micrometer resolution from within optical scattering media by creating an interference pattern between light propagating in the sample and reference arms. One of the most common OCT setups resembles the Michelson interferometer, as shown in Figure 2.1(a). The light source is split into sample and reference arms and, in the sample arm, light is backscattered from internal structures at different depths while the second beam is reflected from a reference mirror. Both arms are recombined in the beamsplitter to form the interference fringes. For a coherent optical source, the interference pattern generated by an individual layer of the sample looks like the left figure in Figure 2.1(b), whereas for a low-coherence source, the pattern will look like that shown in the right of Figure 2.1(b).

Mathematically, the interference intensity can be written as

$$I_0 \propto |E_r|^2 + |E_s|^2 + 2 \cdot E_r \cdot E_s \cos(2k\Delta L) \tag{2.1}$$

where $E_r(t)$ and $E_s(t)$ are, respectively, the electric field of reference and sample beams, k is the wavevector and ΔL is the path difference between

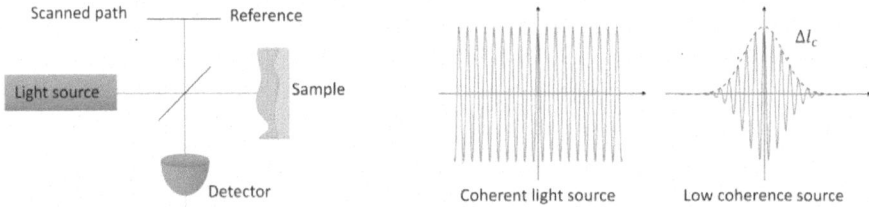

FIGURE 2.1

(Left) Schematic of a Michelson interferometer with scanned reference arm. (Right) Representation of interference fringes with a coherent and short-coherent light source. Interference only occurs when the path lengths are matched to within the coherence length.

reference and sample arms. The output electric field at the detector is the sum of the signal and reference fields, $E_r(t) + E_s(t)$. The interference fringes are then generated by either changing ΔL by scanning the reference arm (time domain OCT) or through k, by exploring the phase difference by different wavelengths (Fourier domain OCT).

Time domain OCT (TD-OCT) is the originally conceived operation principle (Huang et al. 1991) and is based on low-coherence interferometry by using a broadband light source. At this way, only light from a small depth range in the sample can contribute to an oscillatory signal due to the temporal coherence with the reference beam. Superluminescent diodes (SLDs) have been the most widely employed light source to TD-OCT (see chapters 17 and 18 in ref. (Drexler and Fujimoto 2015)), however, femtosecond optical sources have also been well exploited and preferred for some basic research and novel developments (Drexler and Fujimoto 2015; Taylor 2016).

Fourier domain OCT (FD-OCT) came around 10 years later than the time domain method (Fercher et al. 1995). The TD-OCT has as its main disadvantage the slow process to generate the data (up to several minutes), which hinders *in vivo* and real-time applications. In turn, FD-OCT systems rely on Fourier transformation between time and frequency or space, and are divided in two: the so-called spectral-domain OCT (SD-OCT), which is based on a measurement of the interference spectrum in space on a spectrometer, and the swept-source OCT (SS-OCT), also called optical frequency domain imaging (OFDI), which is a measurement of the interference spectrum in time during the wavelength sweep of a rapidly tunable narrow bandwidth light source. In either case, in FD-OCT a depth scan is achieved by calculating an inverse Fourier-transform on the interference spectrum, without the need to move the reference mirror. With this approach, the acquisition speed can be far higher. Another advantage of FD-OCT is its higher sensitivity than TD-OCT systems, by providing an improved signal-to-noise ratio. The sensitivity is enhanced by the ratio of the axial resolution to the axial imaging depth, which is ultimately limited by shot noise (Leitgeb et al. 2003).

However, FD-OCT technology has also its drawbacks. Standard FD-OCT cannot distinguish between positive versus negative time delays with respect to the zero delay. Therefore, features of the sample that cross the zero delay appears folded about this line producing a "mirror" artifact in the OCT image. Fourier domain detection is also more sensitive to reflections that are closer to the zero-delay position. This depth-dependent loss of SNR is called sensitivity roll-off and occurs due to the progressively higher frequency spectral oscillations with echoes that are further away from the zero-delay position, which eventually cannot be resolved by the finite spectral resolution of the system.

A more practical and typical laboratory layout of an OCT device is shown in Figure 2.2.

In this very illustrative figure, the process of image generation by OCT can be seen, as well as some practical features. The incident beam in each point

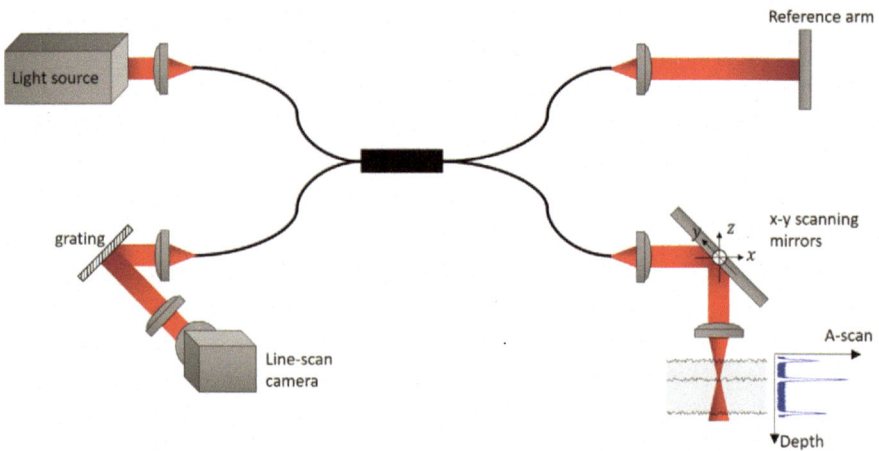

FIGURE 2.2

Schematic of a generic fiber optic SD-OCT system. Fiber paths are represented in black bold lines while free-space optical paths are represented in red.

of the sample gives rise to the depth profile of the sample reflectivity at the beam position, so-called A-scan (axial scan), whereas the lateral scanning of the tightly focused beam generates a 2D image, known as B-scan. A 3D image can then be generated by acquisition of sequential cross-sectional images by raster-scanning the beam on the sample. 3D-OCT data provides well defined volumetric structural information, which can be displayed like magnetic resonance or computed tomography images, being also referred to as the equivalent of an "optical ultrasound". Figure 2.3 shows examples of acquired A-scan (axial in the Z plan), 2D image B-scan (transverse X or Y scanning of A-scans) and 3D image after XY scanning. An *en face* OCT image can also be generated by summing the data in the axial direction.

One important aspect of any imaging systems is its spatial resolution. For OCTs, the axial and lateral resolutions are decoupled from each other. While the lateral resolution obeys the Rayleigh limit, depending on the wavelength and numerical aperture of the optical system, the axial resolution is based on the properties of the interferometric technique and therefore is independent of the optical system design itself, being given by the coherence length of the light source, determined by the optical source bandwidth. Table 2.1 shows the axial and transverse resolution expressions, at the diffraction limit, whose derivation can be found in ref. (Drexler and Fujimoto 2015).

It is noteworthy that, unlike microscopy, OCT can achieve fine axial resolution independent of the numerical aperture of the system. This feature is especially powerful for applications, such as ophthalmic imaging or catheter/endoscope imaging, where numerical apertures are limited.

Also, although traditional OCT images are derived from the absolute value of the electric field output at the detector, limited by the coherence length

A-Scan	B-Scan (512 A-Scans)	C-Scan (512 B-Scans)

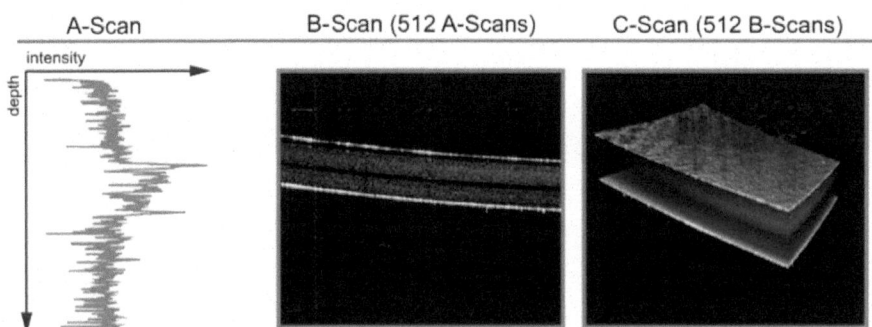

FIGURE 2.3

(Left) The OCT interference fringes gives rise to the axial profile (A-scans) of the sample of a given point. (Center) Scanning the OCT beam in a transverse direction and combining the A-scans generate cross-sectional images, called B-scans. (Right) From that, three-dimensional volumetric data sets can be acquired by raster scanning and attaching consecutive B-scans. The 3D-OCT contains comprehensive volumetric structural information and can be displayed similar to MR or CT images. Reprinted with permission from (Zechel. 2020) © tm-Technisches Messen.

and typically in the order of micrometers, recent works have shown that the phase sensitivity of OCT signals can be used to achieve nanometric axial resolution. One method consists in measuring the phase difference between two known layers in the sample as a function of time (Jonnal et al. 2012) with several applications including detection of neural activity (Akkin et al. 2004), measurement of vibrations in the auditory organs (Chen et al. 2011; Subhash et al. 2012), determining skin elasticity (Li et al. 2012), and *in vivo* measurements of optoretinography (ORG) (Jonnal et al. 2012, Dierck et al. 2016; Dubois et al. 2018; Zhang et al. 2019; Azimipour et al. 2020) where elongation of photoreceptors is observed in response to a stimulus of light. In another approach, the complex amplitudes of the Fourier components for different wavelengths and directions of illumination and scattering allows formation of a three-dimensional Fourier transform of the scattering potential, providing nanosensitivity to the spatial and temporal structural changes within the three-dimensional scattering objects (Alexandrov et al. 2014). As a 3D imaging system, penetration depth and depth of field (DOF) are also important parameters to be considered. The penetration depth is mainly determined by the sample absorption and scattering as well as the roll-off in FD-OCT. Meanwhile, the DOF is proportional to the square of the transverse resolution (Table 2.1). Consequently, a tradeoff occurs between the transverse resolution and the DOF in which a lower transverse resolution (higher δ_x) results in a larger DOF and vice versa.

A deeper theoretical insight with a proposed unified theory of OCT can be found in chapter 2 of ref. (Drexler and Fujimoto 2015), which discusses imaging performance in all three dimensions, besides treating both FD-OCT

TABLE 2.1

Optical Parameters for OCT

Mathematical expressions	Illustration	Comment
$$\delta z = \frac{2 ln 2}{\pi} \cdot \frac{\lambda^2}{\Delta\lambda}$$	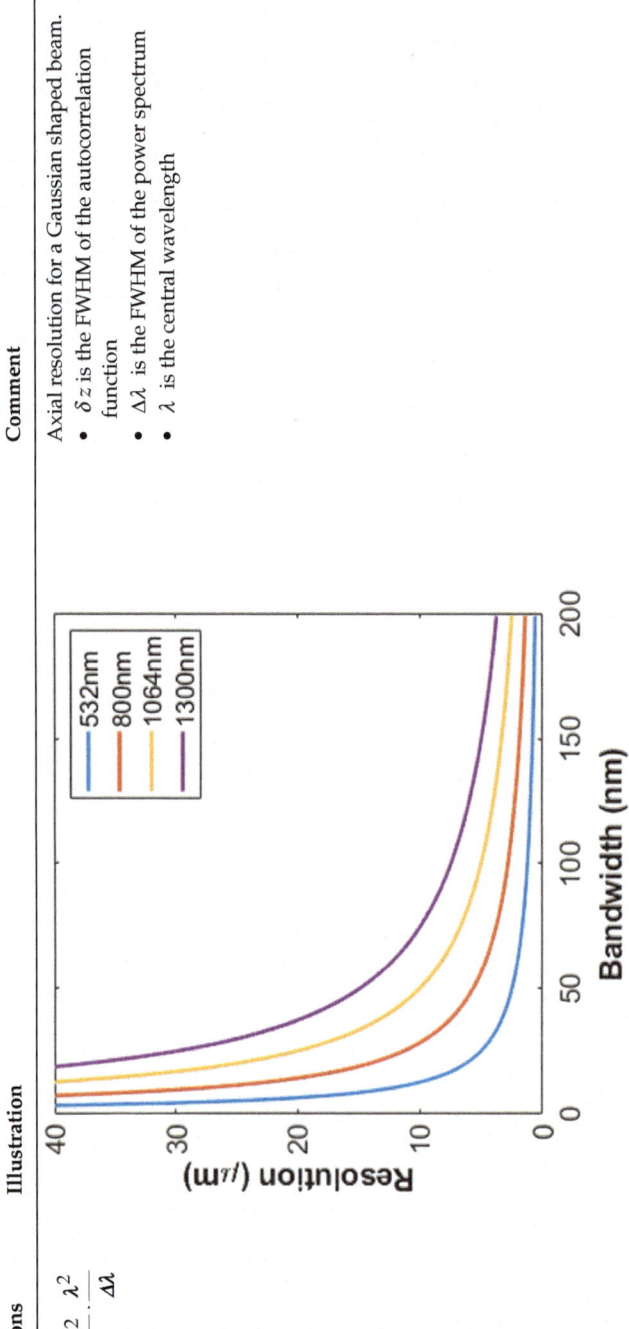	Axial resolution for a Gaussian shaped beam. • δz is the FWHM of the autocorrelation function • $\Delta\lambda$ is the FWHM of the power spectrum • λ is the central wavelength

Axial resolution as a function of light source bandwidths for center wavelengths of 532 nm, 800 nm, 1064 nm, and 1300 nm. This illustrates the need for a broadband light source for micrometer resolution and the impact of central wavelength on it.

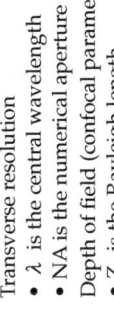

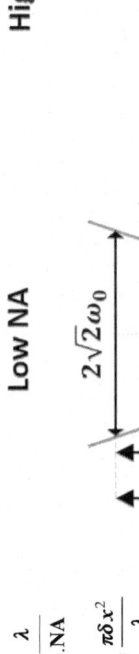

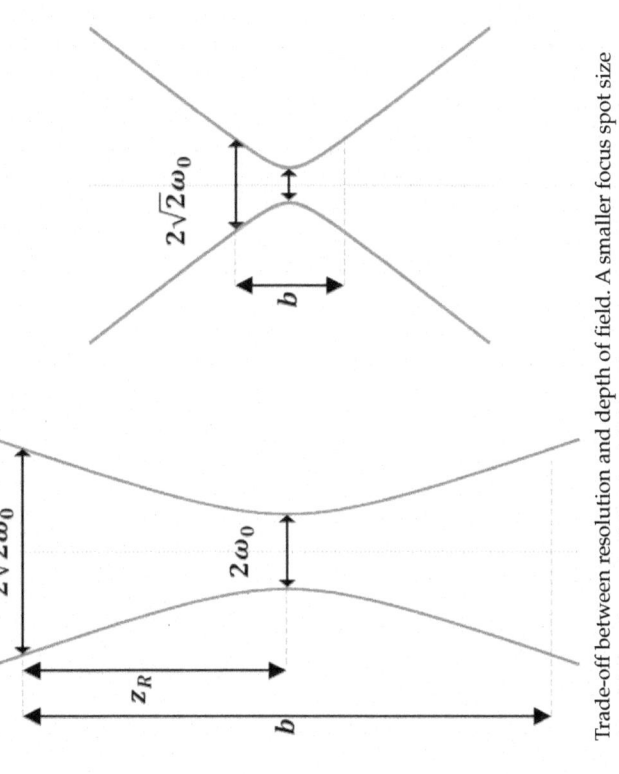

Transverse resolution
- λ is the central wavelength
- NA is the numerical aperture

Depth of field (confocal parameter)
- Z_R is the Rayleigh length

High NA

$2\sqrt{2}\omega_0$

b

Low NA

$2\sqrt{2}\omega_0$

$2\omega_0$

z_R

b

$$\delta x = 1.22 \frac{\lambda}{NA}$$

$$b = 2z_R = \frac{\pi \delta x^2}{\lambda}$$

Trade-off between resolution and depth of field. A smaller focus spot size implies reduction of depth of field and vice versa.

Source: Adapted from ref. Drexler and Fujimoto 2015.

and TD-OCT on the same theoretical grounds. There, it has been discussed that it is more appropriate to treat the sample arm of a conventional confocal OCT system as a "reflection-mode scanning confocal microscope". In this case, it can be realized that the single-mode optical fiber acts as a pinhole aperture both for light illumination and collection from the sample (see Figure 2.2). The intensity at the detector, considering an ideal reflection confocal microscope as a function of lateral position, can then be represented in terms of the Bessel functions as (Drexler and Fujimoto 2015):

$$I(v) = \left(\frac{2 \cdot J_1(v)}{v} \right)^4 \tag{2.2}$$

where $J_1(v)$ is a first-order Bessel function of the first kind, and v is the normalized lateral range parameter, which is related to x by $v = 2\pi \cdot x \cdot \sin(\alpha)/\lambda$ where x is the lateral distance from the optical axis, α is half the angular optical aperture subtended by the objective, and λ is the central wavelength of the optical source. Note that the numerical aperture of the objective is given by $NA = \sin(\alpha)$, for a properly filled objective. Lateral resolution is then given by the FWHM of equation 2.2 at the focal plane, given by $\delta x = 0.37 \cdot \lambda/NA$.

Figure 2.4 summarizes the results characterizing these quantities in lateral and axial directions in terms of numerical aperture (NA) and field of view (FOV). Only one lateral dimension is depicted since a cylindrically symmetric optical system is considered.

In practice, both clinically and in laboratory research, a relatively low NA objective is preferred in OCT, such that the lateral resolution δx is approximately matched to the axial resolution δz, defined by the low-coherence interferometer. However, for some applications, higher NA are desirable as they provide greater transverse resolution (Table 2.1), capable of resolving smaller and more compact structures in the sample.

Besides confocal OCT there are also the so-called full-field OCT (FF-OCT) and line-scan OCT (LS-OCT). In the first, the sample is illuminated in flood mode and the backscattered light is imaged at a CMOS camera, while the reference arm is collimated. In this configuration, each pixel of the camera is used as a point detector, acquiring A-scans simultaneously, whereby the complete *en face* slab of an OCT volume is obtained by the 2D camera array as the detector in a wide-field interferometer mode. This method was experimentally demonstrated in both time and Fourier domain (Beaurepaire et al. 1998; Dubois et al. 2002; Sarunic et al. 2006). Meanwhile, in line-scan OCT the sample is illuminated with a line-field and the backscattered light is either imaged in a line-scan camera (time domain LS-OCT) (Dubois et al. 2018) or goes through a diffraction grating, yielding a two-dimensional image at a 2D camera array, corresponding to the spatial and spectral components along the two axes (spectral domain LS-OCT) (Pandiyan et al. 2020).

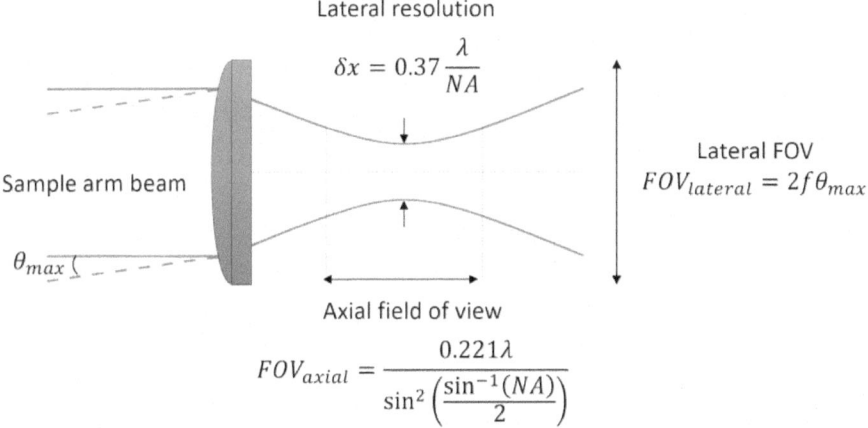

Lateral resolution

$$\delta x = 0.37 \frac{\lambda}{NA}$$

Sample arm beam

Lateral FOV

$$FOV_{lateral} = 2f\theta_{max}$$

θ_{max}

Axial field of view

$$FOV_{axial} = \frac{0.221\lambda}{\sin^2 \left(\frac{\sin^{-1}(NA)}{2} \right)}$$

FIGURE 2.4

Illustration of the main expressions and their meaning in a focused beam in lateral and axial directions in terms of numerical aperture (NA) and field of view (FOV). The axial field of view FOV_{axial} and lateral resolution δ_x expresssions assume that the system was diffraction limited (no significant optical aberration) and so, they are dominated by confocal geometric optics (Drexler and Fujimoto 2015). The lateral field of view $FOV_{lateral}$ assumes a simple *f*-theta scanning system.

Those new modalities arose by the advent of complementary metal-oxide-semiconductor (CMOS) cameras with high sensitivity and frame rates in the hundreds of kilohertz, allowing the parallelization of A-scans data acquisition that resulted in volume rates orders of magnitude higher than traditional raster scanning (flying spot) OCT systems.

Further considerations should be given to the designing of an OCT system, such as care with speckles, multiple scattering and crosstalk. The latter is generated when scattered light travels laterally and get mapped improperly at the detector, being more prominent in FF-OCT due to the lack of confocality (Karamata et al. 2004). These effects generate undesirable artifacts and limit the system resolution but they can be mitigated by exploiting optical sources with low spatial coherence (Drexler and Fujimoto 2015). For instance, SLDs are widely employed as an alternative optical source with desired coherence characteristics for OCT. In addition, another interesting approach – which has not been scaled up for OCT applications – is the use of random lasers (Gomes et al. 2021), which have already been shown to generate speckle-free laser imaging (Redding et al. 2012) in addition to crosstalk mitigation in FF-OCT (Redding et al. 2011). In ref. (Carvalho et al. 2016), the authors employed a RL as the optical source in an epi-illumination configuration and reported on its potential for biological imaging due to its image quality and spectral density. A random fiber laser has also been employed for transillumination imaging in dentistry (Guo et al. 2020), with the central wavelength at ~1550nm. Another alternative, to damp the crosstalk and scrambling of speckles uses a fast deformable membrane (Auksorius et al. 2019) or a multi-mode fiber (Auksorius et al. 2022) to create a spatial phase modulation to washes out fringes originating from multiply scattered light.

After data acquisition, signal processing must be performed and this includes different steps for TD-OCT and FD-OCT. The knowledge of proper signal processing is of paramount importance for obtaining high quality images and will be briefly discussed here. However, the details of this are beyond the scope of this introductory chapter and can be found elsewhere (Schmitt 1999; Fercher et al. 2003; Tomlins and Wang 2005; Drexler and Fujimoto 2015).

In SD-OCT the spectrometer generates an interference spectrum as a function of wavelength while in SS-OCT the source sweep speed is constant with respect to λ. Therefore, in both cases, the spectrum must be numerically resampled from wavelength to frequency or wavenumber $k = \dfrac{2\pi}{\lambda}$, using linear interpolation, before Fourier transforming.

Another issue that needs to be addressed is with respect to dispersion mismatch between sample and reference arm that causes a decreasing in the resolution and increases the depth misplacement. Dispersion artifacts can be compensated for by introducing glass such as BK7 or water in the reference arm. However, direct access to the spectrum in FD-OCT enables numerical dispersion compensation by adding k-dependent phase shifts, commonly defined as a third-order polynomial to the measured spectral fringe $I(x,y,k)$ (Wojtkowski et al. 2004).

Nonetheless, slow-sweeping SS-OCT systems might present higher-order chirp, possibly due to vibrations causing path length difference variations between reference and sample arms during single wavelength sweep. In that scenario, a method based on short-time Fourier transformation (STFT) can be employed to determine the appropriate k-dependent phase shifts to each OCT volume (Fercher et al. 2001; Valente et al. 2020).

In addition, in both time and Fourier domain scanning OCT systems the speed of the scanning mirrors may vary during volume acquisition. In resonant scanners for instance a sinusoidal scan speed is often used and desinusoiding is a key step to avoid distortions in the image. Desinusoiding transformation h_{des} can be determined by imaging a grid-pattern test target and the desinusoided reference image can be computed as $I_{des} = I_0 \cdot h_{des}$.

Several other issues are extremely important in setting up an OCT system, and these are reviewed in detail in ref. (Drexler et al. 2015). These include the axial ranging in low-coherence interferometry (LCI) systems and proper analysis of FD-LCI as well as TD-LCI systems. Among practical aspects of FD-OCT (most commonly used nowadays), care must be taken with sensitivity and sampling effects, besides the aforementioned artifact removal. Finally, regarding sensitivity and dynamic range, signal to noise analysis needs to be dealt with for both TD-OCT and FD-OCT.

2.3 Functional and Multimodal OCT

While traditional OCT creates depth-resolved reflectivity maps, functional information is not generally available. To overcome this, some changes can be made to the optical system or data processing to get further information. One example is the aforementioned phase-sensitive OCT, where during data processing not only the magnitude but also the phase of the interferometric signal is analyzed to provide nanometric axial or 3D resolution, capable of measuring vibrations or mechanical changes at the sample in response to a stimulus (Akkin et al. 2004; Chen et al. 2011; Jonnal et al. 2012; Li et al. 2012; Subhash et al. 2012; Alexandrov et al. 2014; Dierck et al. 2016; Dubois et al. 2018; Zhang et al. 2019; Azimipour et al. 2020; Vienola et al. 2022).

Phase changes of the OCT signal can also be used to determine the velocity of objects traversing the imaging beam, the phase-resolved Doppler OCT. There, multiple beams and sensors can be used in parallel to achieve 3D Doppler (Werkmeister et al. 2008; Haindl et al. 2016), but the complexity of those systems is increased by their parallelization, making them costly and prone to misalignment. An alternative approach would be the multiplexing of the OCT signal in a full-field setup either by hardware (Valente et al. 2021) or numerically (Spahr et al. 2018). Doppler frequency shift can also be measured with a time domain Doppler OCT by using a spectrogram method to create the image (Drexler and Fujimoto 2015).

In another approach, termed OCT angiography (OCTA), the retinal vasculature and blood flow can be examined by measuring the variance of the OCT signal collected in an area of the retina imaged multiple times in rapid succession to reveal the presence of moving scatterers, presumably blood cells moving in the vessels. This non-phase-sensitive method extracts quantitative velocity information by analyzing time varying speckle or intensity fluctuations of backscattered light with autocorrelation techniques. This technique is widely seen as a way to observe a functional aspect of the visual system: the perfusion of blood (Spaide et al. 2015; Gao et al. 2016; Chen and Wang 2017; Migacz et al. 2019).

Another technique that relies in data processing is the spectroscopic OCT (SOCT). There, a windowing method, such as the short-time Fourier transform (STFT) is used to separate the spectral fringes from wavelength-specific regions, creating a series of spectroscopically distinct tomograms to encode of spectral information into the tomographic images. The method has been shown valid to quantify burn severity (Zhao et al. 2015), retinal oximetry (Yi et al. 2013), microvascular hemoglobin mapping (Chong et al. 2015), examination of amyloid beta plaques in Alzheimer's disease brain samples (Lichtenegger et al. 2017) among others. However, the spectral windowing has a trade-off with depth resolution in the resulting image (Table 2.1).

Other properties of the scattered light like polarization and anisotropy can also be explored in OCT to improve contrast and allow differentiation between tissues. Polarization sensitive OCT (PS-OCT) was the first of these functional extensions, with reported measurements as early as 1992 (Hee et al. 1992) and have, since then, been applied in a varied of fields (de Boer et al. 1997; de Boer and Milner 2002; Pircher et al. 2004; Giattina et al. 2006; Gubarkova et al. 2020).

Meanwhile, directional OCT (dOCT) explores the anisotropy of the backscattered light. Light scattering is highly sensitive to alterations in scatterer properties, being a useful tool for the measurement of subcellular morphology. Angle-resolved light scattering has been used, for instance, to predict the presence of early carcinogenesis in goniometric measurements (Mourant et al. 1998). In ophthalmoscopy, dOCT is usually performed by varying the pupil entrance position of the OCT beam and has allowed measuring pointing direction of angular scatterers, such as the photoreceptors (Roorda and Williams 2002; Gao et al. 2008) as well as characterization of other directionally scattering retinal layers (Lujan et al. 2015; Meleppat et al. 2019; Marsh-Armstrong et al. 2022). Multi-channel OCTs have also been used for simultaneous probing of linearly independent orientations (Wartak et al. 2017). Scattering anisotropy can also be explored through path-length multiplexing element (PME) where a beam-dividing glass plate can be used, for instance, to encode different scattering angles (Ahn et al. 2007; Valente et al. 2021). An annular glass window (Wang et al. 2013; Gardner et al. 2020) or a multimode optical fiber has also allowed to separate the backscattered light from the sample into low and high angles, respectively the bright and dark-field OCT (Eugui et al. 2017).

Ultimately, OCT can also be combined with other techniques to provide a more comprehensive analysis of the sample. Multimodal imaging represents one of the current trends in the development of biophotonics imaging technologies and OCT has also been used in parallel with Raman (Wang et al. 2016), scanning laser ophthalmoscope (Azimipour et al. 2019), fluorescence laminar optical tomography (Chen et al. 2010), two-photon microscopy (Jeong et al. 2011), elastography (Larin and Sampson 2017), photoacoustic (Dadkhah et al. 2019) among others.

2.4 Applications: From Medical to Non-Medical

As already mentioned, OCT (or its close predecessors) started in non-medical applications, but it was in ophthalmology where the whole transformation started, leveraging further developments and popularizing the technique. Nowadays, OCT is wide spread with relevance in different fields. An overview of the diversity of applications for OCT can be found in ref. (Drexler and Fujimoto 2015), but also in the very reliable and trustable site OCT News

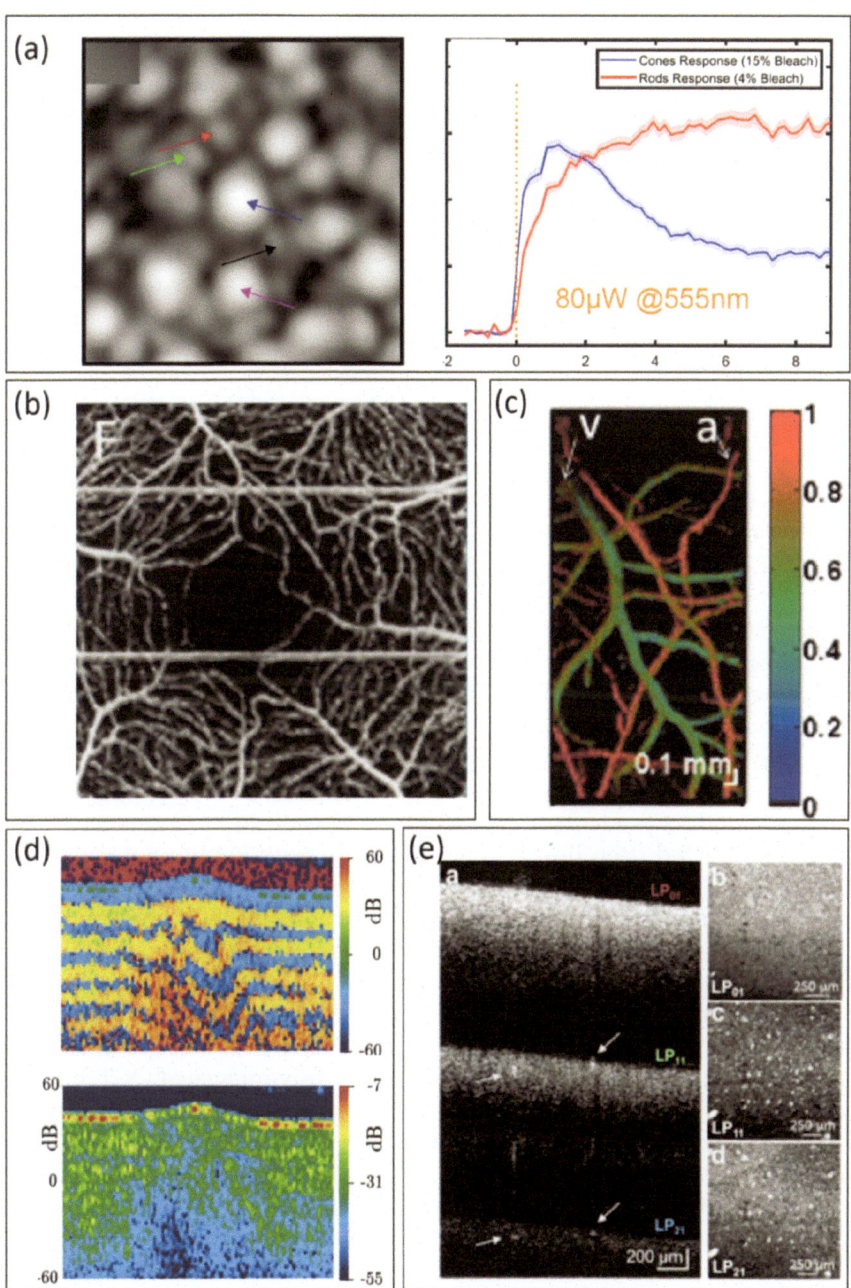

FIGURE 2.5
Functional OCT images. (a) Phase-sensitive OCT: despite the axial resolution of the system in
the order of micrometers, changes of photoreceptors length in human retina can be measured
in response to a stimulus of light with nanometric precision. (Reprinted with permission

from [Azimipour et al. 2020] © The Optical Society.) (b) OCT angiography projection of human retina showing detailed view of the vessels including the capillaries. (Reprinted with permission from [Migacz et al. 2019] © The Optical Society.) (c) Quantification of chromophores in the mouse brain in an *en face* view using a spectroscopic OCT to distinguish between arteries and veins. (Reprinted with permission from [Chong et al. 2015] © The Optical Society.) (d) OCT images of a fresh bovine tendon with (top) and without (bottom) polarization sensitivity. The birefringence of the tissue is clear in the colormap of the figure in the top. (Reprinted with permission from [de Boer et al. 1997] © The Optical Society.) (e) OCT image using a few-modes optical fiber to map scattering angles into different depths (right) of a cross-sectional OCT image of brain tissue. LP_{01} collects the scattered light at smaller angles, while LP_{11} and LP_{21} collects at intermediate and higher scattering angles. *En face* intensity projection images of the dark-field OCT components highlights the neuritic plaques of Alzheimer's disease. (Reprinted with permission from [Eugui et al. 2017] © The Optical Society.)

(Swanson 2022), organized and kept well updated by Eric Swanson. Their category list of OCT applications includes art, cardiology, dentistry, dermatology, developmental biology, gastroenterology, gynecology, microscopy, NDE/NDT (non-destructive testing and evaluation), neurology, oncology, ophthalmology, otolaryngology, pulmonology, urology and other non-medical applications. For completeness, in the site one can also find information on business (acquisition, clinical trials, funding, partnership, patents), technology and miscellaneous, which include jobs and studentships, student theses and textbooks.

Among non-medical applications, we would like to highlight the use of OCT to analyze the microstructures and other features in porous media, tested with oil source rock samples (Campello et al. 2014). Sedimentary rock samples extracted from Brazilian oil fields and with known porosity values (15% and 28%) were imaged, and the results compared with very good agreement with the traditional pycnometry method. The characterization included pore size distribution for the samples in three-dimensional plane. Figures 2.6 and 2.7 show the obtained results.

It is therefore clear that the results obtained indicate that the OCT is a reliable technique to obtain the pore size distribution in porous materials, limited to the OCT axial and lateral resolution. All the advantages of OCT, like non-invasiveness, non-destructiveness, relatively low cost and faster acquisition time than most of other techniques, confirms the expanding applications in the field.

Another interesting state-of-the-art OCT application comes from non-destructive inspection for semiconductor optical devices (Ozaki et al. 2020). There, OCT operating with a visible broadband light source allowed sub-micrometer axial resolution (Figure 2.8), used for high-resolution inspection of waveguides and stacked semiconductor thin layers. Comparative results obtained with OCT and with a scanning electron microscope system is shown in Figure 2.9.

OCT has also been employed for surface and internal fingerprint evaluation (Ding et al. 2020) as well as other applications in the forensic field (Nioi et al. 2019). Also, in the trending area of agriculture, OCT has been used for plant root growth in soil (Larimer et al. 2020), germination (Wijesinghe et al. 2017) and seed infection (Lee et al. 2012), among others.

Another very important advance comes from using an optical source in the mid-infrared (MIR), around 4 μm central wavelength (Israelsen et al. 2019). The main advantage of using longer wavelength is the strong reduction in scattering and deeper penetration in the sample when compared to shorter wavelengths, generally employed in OCT systems, as it scales with $1/\lambda^4$. There, the MIR-OCT is achieved using a broadband, high-brightness mid-IR supercontinuum (SC) source for illumination and a broadband frequency upconversion system for detection. Even though the MIR imposes somewhat complicated experimental setups and is demanding on optical parts (Figures 2.10 and 2.11), this represents a fantastic tool for research labs,

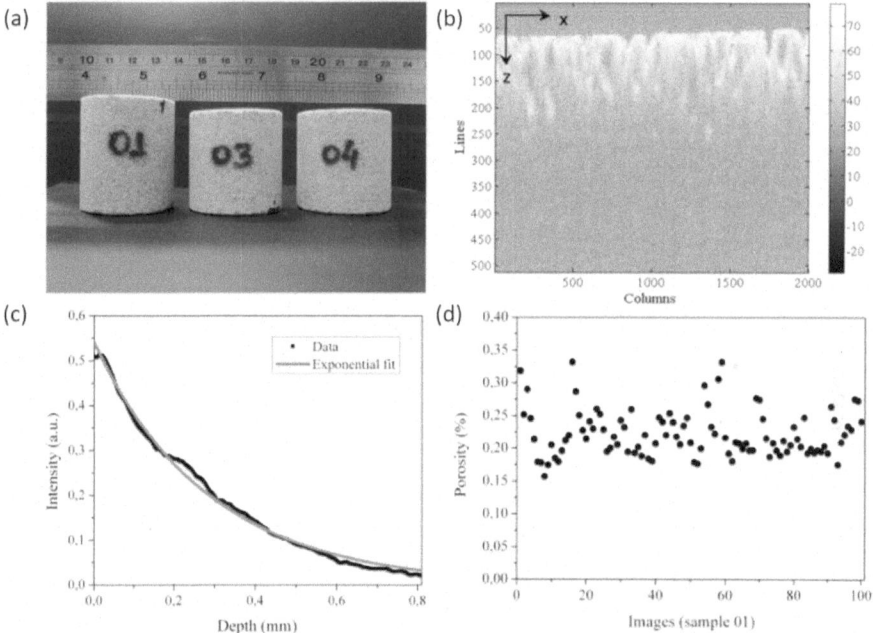

FIGURE 2.6

Analysis of porosity in sedimentary rocks using OCT. (a) Photographs of the specimens used in the study. The samples were provided by PETROBRAS (Petroleum Brazilian State Company). (b) Typical OCT image obtained. (c) Average signal decay: $I_s \propto \exp(-\mu L_{depth})$, where μ include contribution from scattering and absorption, and L_{depth} is the penetration depth. (d) Porosity for a given slice of the obtained OCT image. (Reprinted with permission from [Campello et al. 2014] © Elsevier.)

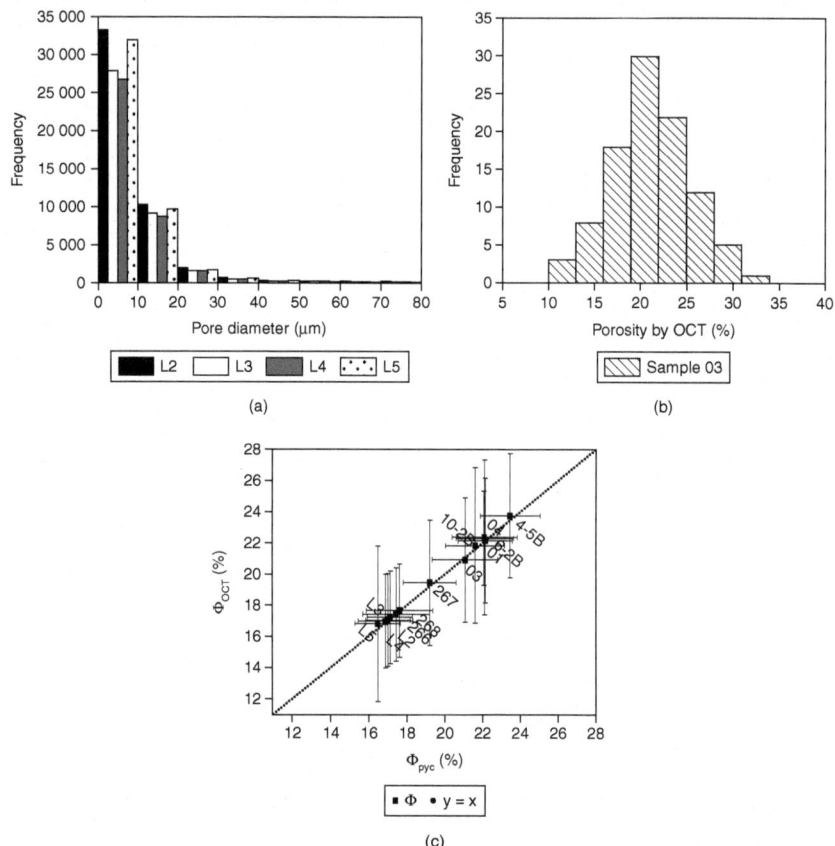

FIGURE 2.7

Histogram of the pore size distribution and porosity distribution are given in (a) and (b), respectively, whereas (c) shows the correlation between pore sizes measured by OCT and picnometry, in order to visualize the performance of the OCT method. The slope ≈ 1 shows good agreement between the two methods. (Reprinted with permission from [Campello et al. 2014] © Elsevier.)

from which further technological development and footprint reduction can come through.

Regarding the medical applications of OCT, ophthalmology is still the flagship in the field, but a variety of other studies ranging from developmental biology to oncology, as aforementioned, represents countless literature material. Therefore, trying to cover or even exemplify them in a didactical way is out-of-the-scope of this book, and the reader should refer to ref. (Drexler and Fujimoto 2015), as well as follow the OCT News website (Swanson 2022).

To complete this chapter, we depicted in Figure 2.12 the covered subject related to OCT in dentistry, the main subject of this book. Each topic will be described in the following chapters.

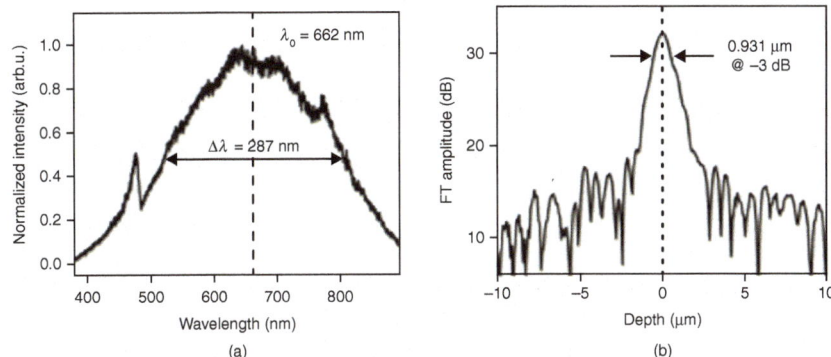

FIGURE 2.8

(a) Spectrum of the light source in the Vis-OCT. (b) The axial resolution (Δz) was estimated experimentally by measuring the full-width at half-maximum (FWHM) of the point spread function (PSF) with a mirror in the sample arm. (Reprinted with permission from [Ishida et al. 2018] © IOP Publishing.)

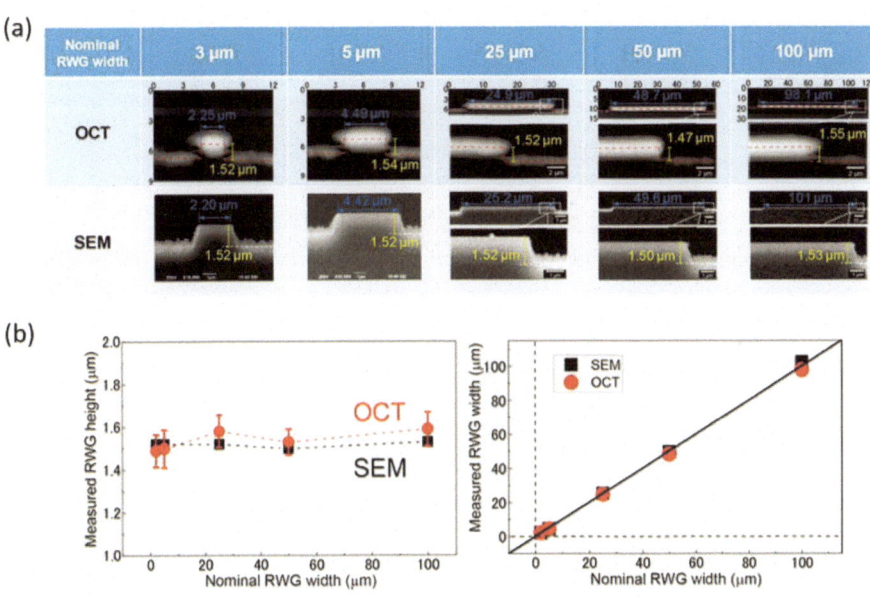

FIGURE 2.9

(a) Comparison of profile images using Vis-OCT and scanning electron microscopy (SEM) for ridge-type optical waveguides with various widths (Ozaki et al. 2020). (b) Measurements of height and width of the waveguides with various nominal widths using Vis-OCT and SEM. (Reprinted with permission from [Ishida. 2018] © IOP Publishing.)

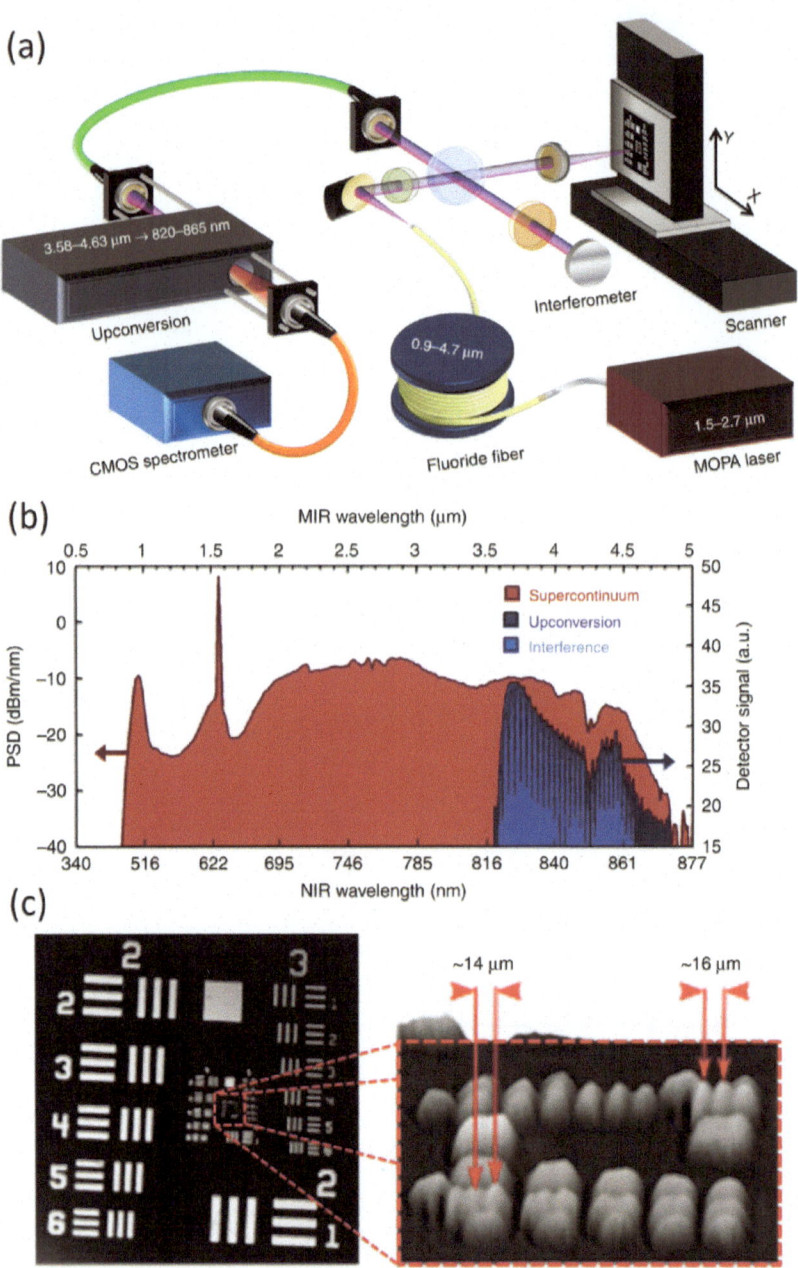

FIGURE 2.10
(a) Schematic of the experimental setup for the MIR-OCT. A frequency upconversion module is used to allow signal detector using a silicon CMOS-based spectrometer. (b) Superposition of the SC spectra before (red) and after (dark blue) upconversion together with an example of the interference spectrum (light blue). (c) An USAF 1951 target was used to determine the system's lateral spatial of ~15 μm (Israelsen et al. 2019).

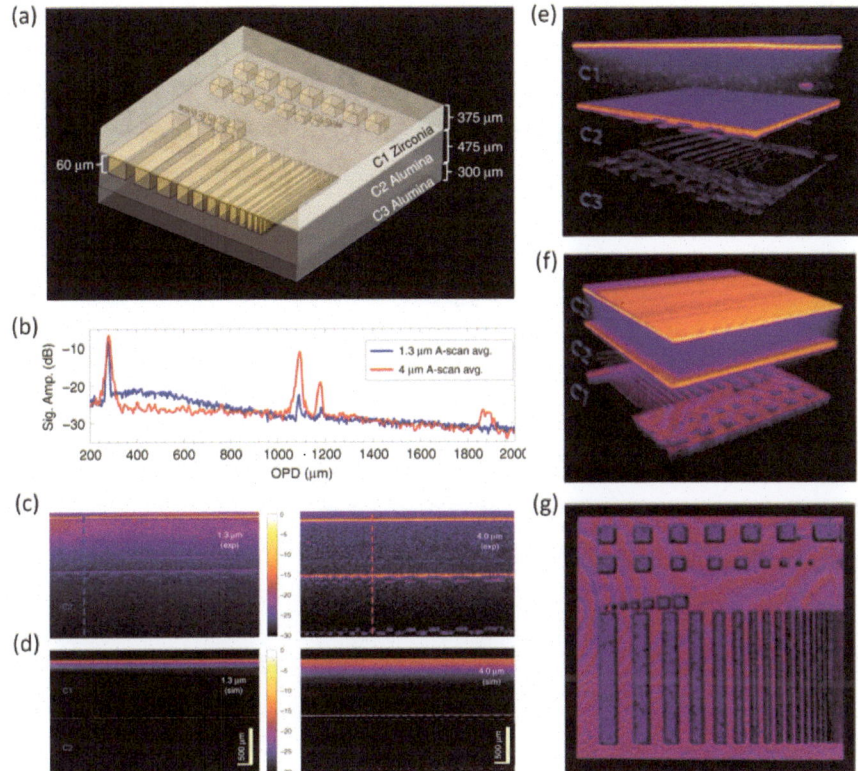

FIGURE 2.11

Proof-of concept for the MIR-OCT. (a) Schematic of the sample structure. (b) Average of ten representative A-scans for a NIR OCT and the MIR-OCT. (c) Comparison between B-scans using the 1.3-μm OCT (left) and 4-μm OCT systems (right). Dashed lines illustrate the position of the A-scans shown in (b). (d) Monte Carlo simulations for the depth penetration of the experiments in (c). (e) and (f) 3D 4-μm OCT volume visualizations of the sample illuminating from the top (C1 → C2 → C3) and the bottom (C3 → C2 → C1), respectively. (g) *En face* view of the microstructures imaged.

Source: Israelsen et al. 2019.

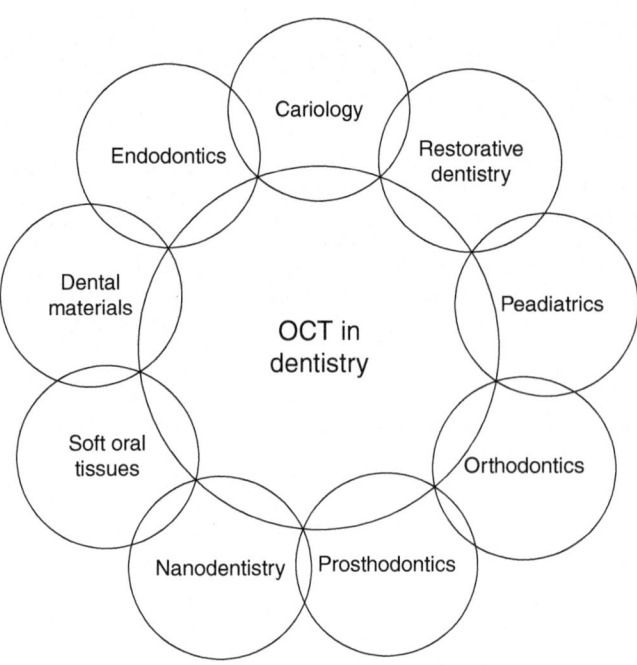

FIGURE 2.12
Topics of OCT in dentistry that will be discussed in this book.

References

Ahn, Y.-C., Jung, W. and Chen, Z. 2007 Quantification of a three-dimensional velocity vector using spectral-domain Doppler optical coherence tomography. *Optics Letters*. 32: 1587–1589.

Akkin, T., Davé, D.P., Milner, T.E. and Rylander III, H.G. 2004 Detection of neural activity using phase-sensitive optical low-coherence reflectometry. *Optics Express*. 12: 2377–2386.

Alexandrov, S., Subhash, H. and Leahy, M. 2014 Nanosensitive optical coherence tomography for the study of changes in static and dynamic structures. *Quantum Electronics*. 44: 657.

Auksorius, E., Borycki, D. and Wojtkowski, M. 2019 Crosstalk-free volumetric in vivo imaging of a human retina with Fourier-domain full-field optical coherence tomography. *Biomedical Optics Express*. 10: 6390–6407.

Auksorius, E., Borycki, D., Wegrzyn, P., *et al.* 2022 Multimode fiber as a tool to reduce cross talk in Fourier-domain full-field optical coherence tomography. *Optics Letters*. 47: 838–841.

Azimipour, M., Jonnal, R.S., Werner, J.S. and Zawadzki, R.J. 2019 Coextensive synchronized SLO-OCT with adaptive optics for human retinal imaging. *Optics Letters*. 44: 4219–4222.

Azimipour, M., Valente, D., Vienola, K. V, *et al.* 2020 Optoretinogram: optical measurement of human cone and rod photoreceptor responses to light. *Optics letters.* 45: 4658–4661.

Baumann, B. 2017 Polarization sensitive optical coherence tomography: a review of technology and applications. *Applied Sciences.* 7: 474.

Beaurepaire, E., Boccara, A.C., Lebec, M., Blanchot, L. and Saint-Jalmes, H. 1998 Full-field optical coherence microscopy. *Optics Letters.* 23: 244–246.

Campello, S.L., Dos Santos, W.P., Machado, V.F., *et al.* 2014 Micro-structural information of porous materials by optical coherence tomography. *Microporous and Mesoporous Materials.* 198: 50–54.

Carvalho, M.T., Lotay, A.S., Kenny, F.M., Girkin, J.M. and Gomes, A.S.L. 2016 Random laser illumination: an ideal source for biomedical polarization imaging?.in *Multimodal Biomedical Imaging XI.* SPIE.: 79–84.

Chen, C.-L. and Wang, R.K. 2017 Optical coherence tomography based angiography [Invited]. *Biomedical Optics Express.* 8: 1056–1082.

Chen, F., Zha, D., Fridberger, A., *et al.* 2011 A differentially amplified motion in the ear for near-threshold sound detection. *Nature Neuroscience.* 14: 770–774.

Chen, Y., Yuan, S., Wierwille, J., *et al.* 2010 Integrated optical coherence tomography (OCT) and fluorescence laminar optical tomography (FLOT). *IEEE Journal of Selected Topics in Quantum Electronics.* 16: 755–766.

Chong, S.P., Merkle, C.W., Leahy, C., Radhakrishnan, H. and Srinivasan, V.J. 2015 Quantitative microvascular hemoglobin mapping using visible light spectroscopic optical coherence tomography. *Biomedical Optics Express.* 6: 1429–1450.

Clivaz, X., Marquis-Weible, F. and Salathe, R.P. 1992 Optical low coherence reflectometry with 1.9 mu m spatial resolution. *Electronics Letters.* 28: 1553–1555.

Dadkhah, A., Zhou, J., Yeasmin, N. and Jiao, S. 2019 Integrated multimodal photoacoustic microscopy with OCT-guided dynamic focusing. *Biomedical Optics Express.* 10: 137–150.

de Boer, J.F. and Milner, T.E. 2002 Review of polarization sensitive optical coherence tomography and Stokes vector determination. *Journal of Biomedical Optics.* 7: 359–371.

de Boer, J.F., Leitgeb, R. and Wojtkowski, M. 2017 Twenty-five years of optical coherence tomography: the paradigm shift in sensitivity and speed provided by Fourier domain OCT. *Biomedical Optics Express.* 8: 3248–3280.

de Boer, J.F., Milner, T.E., van Gemert, M.J.C. and Nelson, J.S. 1997 Two-dimensional birefringence imaging in biological tissue by polarization-sensitive optical coherence tomography. *Optics Letters.* 22: 934–936.

Dierck, H., Hendrik, S., Clara, P., *et al.* 2016 In vivo optical imaging of physiological responses to photostimulation in human photoreceptors. *Proceedings of the National Academy of Sciences.* 113: 13138–13143.

Ding, B., Wang, H., Chen, P., *et al.* 2020 Surface and internal fingerprint reconstruction from optical coherence tomography through convolutional neural network. *IEEE Transactions on Information Forensics and Security.* 16: 685–700.

Drexler, W. and Fujimoto, J.G. 2015 *Optical coherence tomography: technology and applications.* Springer.

Dubois, A., Levecq, O., Azimani, H., *et al.* 2018 Line-field confocal time-domain optical coherence tomography with dynamic focusing. *Optics Express.* 26: 33534–33542.

Dubois, A., Vabre, L., Boccara, A.-C. and Beaurepaire, E. 2002 High-resolution full-field optical coherence tomography with a Linnik microscope. *Applied Optics*. 41: 805–812.

Eugui, P., Lichtenegger, A., Augustin, M., *et al.* 2017 Beyond backscattering: Optical neuroimaging by BRAD. *Biomedical Optics Express*. 9: 4007–4025.

Fercher, A.F., Drexler, W., Hitzenberger, C.K. and Lasser, T. 2003 Optical coherence tomography-principles and applications. *Reports on Progress in Physics*. 66: 239.

Fercher, A.F., Hitzenberger, C.K., Kamp, G. and El-Zaiat, S.Y. 1995 Measurement of intraocular distances by backscattering spectral interferometry. *Optics Communications*. 117: 43–48.

Fercher, A.F., Hitzenberger, C.K., Sticker, M., *et al.* 2001 Numerical dispersion compensation for partial coherence interferometry and optical coherence tomography. *Optics Express*. 9: 610–615.

Fujimoto, J.G., De Silvestri, S., Ippen, E.P., *et al.* 1986 Femtosecond optical ranging in biological systems. *Optics Letters*. 11: 150–152.

Gao, S.S., Jia, Y., Zhang, M., *et al.* 2016 Optical coherence tomography angiography. *Investigative Ophthalmology & Visual Science*. 57: OCT27–OCT36.

Gao, W., Cense, B., Zhang, Y., Jonnal, R.S. and Miller, D.T. 2008 Measuring retinal contributions to the optical Stiles-Crawford effect with optical coherence tomography. *Opt. Express*. 16: 6486–6501.

Gardner, M.R., Baruah, V., Vargas, G., *et al.* 2020 Scattering angle resolved optical coherence tomography detects early changes in 3xTg Alzheimer's disease mouse model. *Translational Vision Science & Technology*. 9: 18.

Giattina, S.D., Courtney, B.K., Herz, P.R., *et al.* 2006 Assessment of coronary plaque collagen with polarization sensitive optical coherence tomography (PS-OCT). *International Journal of Cardiology*. 107: 400–409.

Girach, A. and Sergott, R.C. 2016 *Optical coherence tomography*. Springer.

Gomes, A.S.L., Moura, A.L., de Araújo, C.B. and Raposo, E.P. 2021 Recent advances and applications of random lasers and random fiber lasers. *Progress in Quantum Electronics*. 78: 100343.

Gubarkova, E. V, Kiseleva, E.B., Sirotkina, M.A., *et al.* 2020 Diagnostic accuracy of cross-polarization OCT and OCT-elastography for differentiation of breast cancer subtypes: Comparative study. *Diagnostics*. 10: 994.

Guo, J.Y., Zhang, W.L., Rao, Y.J., *et al.* 2020 High contrast dental imaging using a random fiber laser in backscattering configuration. *OSA Continuum*. 3: 759–766.

Haindl, R., Trasischker, W., Wartak, A., *et al.* 2016 Total retinal blood flow measurement by three beam Doppler optical coherence tomography. *Biomedical Optics Express*. 7: 287–301.

Hee, M.R., Huang, D., Swanson, E.A. and Fujimoto, J.G. 1992 Polarization-sensitive low-coherence reflectometer for birefringence characterization and ranging. *Journal of the Optical Society of America B*. 9: 903–908.

Huang, D., Swanson, E.A., Lin, C.P., *et al.* 1991 Optical coherence tomography. *Science*. 254: 1178–1181.

Ishida, K., Ozaki, N., Ohsato, H., *et al.* 2018 Non-destructive and non-contact measurement of semiconductor optical waveguide using optical coherence tomography with a visible broadband light source. *Japanese Journal of Applied Physics*. 57: 08PE03.

Israelsen, N.M., Petersen, C.R., Barh, A., *et al.* 2019 Real-time high-resolution mid-infrared optical coherence tomography. *Light: Science & Applications.* 8: 1–13.

Jeong, B., Lee, B., Jang, M.S., *et al.* 2011 Combined two-photon microscopy and optical coherence tomography using individually optimized sources. *Optics Express.* 19: 13089–13096.

Jonnal, R.S., Kocaoglu, O.P., Wang, Q., Lee, S. and Miller, D.T. 2012 Phase-sensitive imaging of the outer retina using optical coherence tomography and adaptive optics. *Biomedical Optics Express.* 3: 104.

Karamata, B., Lambelet, P., Laubscher, M., Salathé, R.P. and Lasser, T. 2004 Spatially incoherent illumination as a mechanism for cross-talk suppression in wide-field optical coherence tomography. *Optics Letters.* 29: 736–738.

Kim, S., Crose, M., Eldridge, W.J., *et al.* 2018 Design and implementation of a low-cost, portable OCT system. *Biomedical Optics Express.* 9: 1232–1243.

Larimer, C.J., Denis, E.H., Suter, J.D. and Moran, J.J. 2020 Optical coherence tomography imaging of plant root growth in soil. *Applied Optics.* 59: 2474–2481.

Larin, K. V and Sampson, D.D. 2017 Optical coherence elastography–OCT at work in tissue biomechanics. *Biomedical Optics Express.* 8: 1172–1202.

Lee, S.-Y., Lee, C., Kim, J. and Jung, H.-Y. 2012 Application of optical coherence tomography to detect Cucumber green mottle mosaic virus (CGMMV) infected cucumber seed. *Horticulture, Environment, and Biotechnology.* 53: 428–433.

Leitgeb, R., Hitzenberger, C.K. and Fercher, A.F. 2003 Performance of Fourier domain vs. time domain optical coherence tomography. *Optics Express.* 11: 889–894.

Leitgeb, R.A. 2019 En face optical coherence tomography: a technology review. *Biomedical Optics Express.* 10: 2177–2201.

Li, C., Guan, G., Reif, R., Huang, Z. and Wang, R.K. 2012 Determining elastic properties of skin by measuring surface waves from an impulse mechanical stimulus using phase-sensitive optical coherence tomography. *Journal of the Royal Society Interface.* 9: 831–841.

Lichtenegger, A., Harper, D.J., Augustin, M., *et al.* 2017 Spectroscopic imaging with spectral domain visible light optical coherence microscopy in Alzheimer's disease brain samples. *Biomedical Optics Express.* 8: 4007–4025.

Lujan, B.J., Roorda, A., Croskrey, J.A., *et al.* 2015 Directional optical coherence tomography provides accurate outer nuclear layer and Henle fiber layer measurements. *Retina.* 35: 1511–1520.

Marsh-Armstrong, B., *et al.* 2022 Using directional OCT to analyze photoreceptor visibility over AMD-related drusen. *Scientific Reports.* 12.1: 9763.

Meleppat, R.K., Zhang, P., Ju, M.J., *et al.* 2019 Directional optical coherence tomography reveals melanin concentration-dependent scattering properties of retinal pigment epithelium. *Journal of Biomedical Optics.* 24: 1–10.

Migacz, J. V, Gorczynska, I., Azimipour, M., *et al.* 2019 Megahertz-rate optical coherence tomography angiography improves the contrast of the choriocapillaris and choroid in human retinal imaging. *Biomedical Optics Express.* 10: 50–65.

Mourant, J.R., Freyer, J.P., Hielscher, A.H., *et al.* 1998 Mechanisms of light scattering from biological cells relevant to noninvasive optical-tissue diagnostics. *Applied Optics.* 37: 3586–3593.

Nioi, M., Napoli, P.E., Mayerson, S.M., Fossarello, M. and d'Aloja, E. 2019 Optical coherence tomography in forensic sciences: A review of the literature. *Forensic Science, Medicine and Pathology.* 15: 445–452.

Ozaki, N., Ishida, K., Nishi, T., *et al*. 2020 OCT with a Visible Broadband Light Source Applied to High-Resolution Nondestructive Inspection for Semiconductor Optical Devices. In *Optical Coherence Tomography and its Non-medical Applications*. IntechOpen. 187–200.

Pandiyan, V.P., Jiang, X., Maloney-Bertelli, A., *et al*. 2020 High-speed adaptive optics line-scan OCT for cellular-resolution optoretinography. *Biomedical Optics Express*. 11: 5274–5296.

Pircher, M., Goetzinger, E., Leitgeb, R. and Hitzenberger, C.K. 2004 Three dimensional polarization sensitive OCT of human skin in vivo. *Optics Express*. 12: 3236–3244.

Redding, B., Cao, H. and Choma, M.A. 2012 Speckle-free laser imaging with random laser illumination. *Nature Photonics*. 6: 355–359.

Redding, B., Choma, M.A. and Cao, H. 2011 Spatially incoherent random lasers for full field optical coherence tomography. In *CLEO: Science and Innovations*. Optical Society of America: PDPC7.

Roorda, A. and Williams, D.R. 2002 Optical fiber properties of individual human cones. *Journal of Vision*. 2: 4.

Sarunic, M. V, Weinberg, S. and Izatt, J.A. 2006 Full-field swept-source phase microscopy. *Optics Letters*. 31: 1462–1464.

Schmitt, J.M. 1999 Optical coherence tomography (OCT): a review. *IEEE Journal of Selected Topics in Quantum Electronics*. 5: 1205–1215.

Schmitt, J.M., Knüttel, A. and Bonner, R.F. 1993 Measurement of optical properties of biological tissues by low-coherence reflectometry. *Applied Optics*. 32: 6032–6042.

Song, G., Jelly, E.T., Chu, K., Kendall, W.Y. and Wax, A. 2021 A review of low-cost and portable optical coherence tomography. *Progress in Biomedical Engineering*. 3: 032002.

Spahr, H., Pfäffle, C., Koch, P., *et al*. 2018 Interferometric detection of 3D motion using computational subapertures in optical coherence tomography. *Optics Express*. 26: 18803–18816.

Spaide, R.F., Fujimoto, J.G. and Waheed, N.K. 2015 Optical coherence tomography angiography. *Retina*. 35: 2161.

Subhash, H.M., Jacques, S.L., Nguyen-Huynh, A.T., *et al*. 2012 Feasibility of spectral-domain phase-sensitive optical coherence tomography for middle ear vibrometry. *Journal of Biomedical Optics*. 17: 60505.

Swanson, E. 2022 *OCT News*. www.octnews.org/.

Swanson, E.A. and Fujimoto, J.G. 2017 The ecosystem that powered the translation of OCT from fundamental research to clinical and commercial impact. *Biomedical Optics Express*. 8: 1638–1664.

Taylor, J.R. 2016 Tutorial on fiber-based sources for biophotonic applications. *Journal of Biomedical Optics*. 21: 61010.

Tomlins, P.H. and Wang, R.K. 2005 Theory, developments and applications of optical coherence tomography. *Journal of Physics D: Applied Physics*. 38: 2519.

Valente, D., Vienola, K. V, Zawadzki, R.J. and Jonnal, R.S. 2020 Kilohertz retinal FF-SS-OCT and flood imaging with hardware-based adaptive optics. *Biomedical Optics Express*. 11: 5995–6011.

Valente, D., Vienola, K. V, Zawadzki, R.J. and Jonnal, R.S. 2021 Simultaneous directional full-field OCT using path-length and carrier multiplexing. *Optics Express*. 29: 32179–32195.

Vienola, K. V., Valente, D., Zawadzki, R.J. and Jonnal, R.S. 2022 Velocity-based optoretinography for clinical applications. *Optica.* 9: 1100–1108.

Wang, B., Yin, B., Dwelle, J., *et al.* 2013 Path-length-multiplexed scattering-angle-diverse optical coherence tomography for retinal imaging. *Optics Letters.* 38: 4374–4377.

Wang, J., Zheng, W., Lin, K. and Huang, Z. 2016 Development of a hybrid Raman spectroscopy and optical coherence tomography technique for real-time in vivo tissue measurements. *Optics Letters.* 41: 3045–3048.

Wartak, A., Augustin, M., Haindl, R., *et al.* 2017 Multi-directional optical coherence tomography for retinal imaging. *Biomedical Optics Express.* 8: 5560–5578.

Werkmeister, R.M., Dragostinoff, N., Pircher, M., *et al.* 2008 Bidirectional Doppler Fourier-domain optical coherence tomography for measurement of absolute flow velocities in human retinal vessels. *Optics Letters.* 33: 2967–2969.

Wijesinghe, R.E.H., Lee, S.-Y., Kim, P., *et al.* 2017 Optical sensing method to analyze germination rate of Capsicum annum seeds treated with growth-promoting chemical compounds using optical coherence tomography. *Journal of Biomedical Optics.* 22: 1–7.

Wojtkowski, M., Srinivasan, V.J., Ko, T.H., *et al.* 2004 Ultrahigh-resolution, high-speed, Fourier domain optical coherence tomography and methods for dispersion compensation. *Optics Express.* 12: 2404–2422.

Yasin Alibhai, A., Or, C. and Witkin, A.J. 2018 Swept source optical coherence tomography: a review. *Current Ophthalmology Reports.* 6: 7–16.

Yi, J., Wei, Q., Liu, W., Backman, V. and Zhang, H.F. 2013 Visible-light optical coherence tomography for retinal oximetry. *Optics Letters.* 38: 1796–1798.

Youngquist, R.C., Carr, S. and Davies, D.E.N. 1987 Optical coherence-domain reflectometry: a new optical evaluation technique. *Optics Letters.* 12: 158–160.

Zechel, F., Kunze, R., König, N., Schmitt, R. H. 2020 Optical coherence tomography for non-destructive testing. *Technisches Messen.* 87: 404–413.

Zhang, F., Kurokawa, K., Lassoued, A., Crowell, J.A. and Miller, D.T. 2019 Cone photoreceptor classification in the living human eye from photostimulation-induced phase dynamics. *Proceedings of the National Academy of Sciences.* 116: 7951–7956.

Zhao, Y., Maher, J.R., Kim, J., *et al.* 2015 Evaluation of burn severity in vivo in a mouse model using spectroscopic optical coherence tomography. *Biomedical Optics Express.* 6: 3339–3345.

3

OCT *in Cariology:* In Vitro *and* In Vivo *Studies*

Denise M. Zezell[1] and Patricia Aparecida Ana[2]

[1]*Center for Lasers and Applications, Nuclear and Energy Research Institute IPEN-CNEN, Sao Paulo, Brazil.*

[2]*Center for Engineering, Modeling and Applied Social Sciences, Federal University of ABC, Sao Bernardo do Campo, Brazil.*

CONTENTS

3.1 Introduction

The advent of the paradigm of minimal intervention in dentistry has increased the need for early diagnosis real-time monitoring methods. Considering that the caries and erosion lesions can be reversed before the structural loss of the dental hard tissue occurs, optical techniques have emerged as excellent options over traditional clinical methods employed to date, such as tactile-visual inspection and imaging by radiography.

The most recognized method for clinical diagnosis of caries lesions is based on the ICDAS (International Caries Detection and Assessment) system. Although this method based on visual examination has demonstrated good accuracy and reproducibility (Ismail et al. 2007), it has some limitations regarding the diagnosis of lesions within outer enamel layers (Schneider et al. 2017), as well as it being time-consuming and not possible to assess the

DOI: 10.1201/9781351104562-3

extension of the lesion towards the pulp. Also, it does not have a clear relation between the clinical appearances with the activity of a lesion (Banting
1993). Better results have been obtained when it is supported with some other
auxiliary method, mainly optical ones (Iranzo-Cortés et al. 2017). Still, many
dentists have difficulty in differentiating between active and arrested incipient
lesions, which differ from one another because of the glossy appearance of
arrested lesions (Fejerskov et al. 2015).

In this way, the use of optical technologies based on electrical conductance, transillumination and fluorescence has become attractive, considering
that they have better spatial resolution than the conventional radiographic
imaging methods (Lussi et al. 2003) (dental radiography has resolution of
50 μm) (Wijesinghe et al. 2016), are easy to generate and detect, as well as
offering other advantages, such as the imaging of interproximal regions in
real time (considering the transillumination technique) and without the use
of ionizing radiation. Due to the use of ionizing radiation and its poor sensitivity (National Institute of Health 2001), the use of radiographic methods for
monitoring a short-term progression of caries lesions is not indicated.

The use of non-ionizing radiation is the main aspect to be considered for
monitoring the remineralization of hard tissue injuries, which allows the
imaging of structures in several sessions without risk to the health of the
patient, and it is an important advantage for pregnant patients and children. However, the optical methods are still not very popular among the
clinical professionals, since the obtained data sometimes are not easy for
interpretation; as well, the results given depend on the oral environment,
being influenced by the presence of saliva, stains or biofilm (Hall et al. 2004),
for example, or even by the positioning or protecting the probes during the
examination (Cabral et al. 2006).

The optical coherence tomography (OCT) is a novel technique that allows
the cross-sectional imaging of structures using a broadband near infrared
light. In this way, this technique becomes very attractive due to the real-time
imaging without ionizing radiation, providing caries diagnosis even for proximal lesions (Shimada et al. 2014), as well is less sensitive to the oral environment when compared to fluorescence-based methods. An advantage of OCT
in this aspect is that the enamel demineralization can be accurately measured
at wavelengths in the near infrared (above 1200 nm) because stains do not
interfere with the image obtained in this region (Almaz et al. 2016). Also, the
images can be further processed to facilitate interpretation (Maia et al. 2016)
and there is no overlap of structures in the image, as occurs in conventional
interproximal (Bite-wing) radiographs.

The equipment currently available employ different light wavelengths (780
up to 1500 nm), all in the near infrared region. This allows the imaging of
structures of greater depth (reaching up to 2.5 mm) with high lateral (below
15 μm) and axial (below 8 μm) (Boppart et al. 1999; Ding et al. 2002) resolution
because of weak scattering and absorption in this region, especially around

1310 nm. The transparency of enamel is highest in 1325 nm and the demineralization process alter the refractive indices of enamel and dentin (refractive index of dentin: 1.48–1.80; refractive index of enamel: 1.45–1.61) (Schneider et al. 2017), which allows the quantification of demineralization degree. In addition to that, increase in scattering and changes in light polarization are characteristics that allow the diagnosis of demineralization. Considering 830 nm, the optical penetration on enamel can reach up to 7 mm and, in this way, it is relatively easy to image dentin with high contrast (Jones et al. 2004).

Another advantage of the OCT technique is the possibility of obtaining a quantitative analysis and, thus, to ensure the effectiveness of preventive strategies or even monitoring treatments performed on dental hard tissues. For the diagnosis of caries lesions, the amount of mineral is frequently correlated with the optical attenuation coefficient (Popescu et al. 2008; Mandurah et al. 2013; Cara et al. 2014) or the integrated reflectivity index (Ngaotheppitak et al. 2005). For monitoring lesion progress or remineralization, also the measurement of the optical boundary depth is used (Natsume et al. 2011). For dental wear lesions, the determination of depth or areas of erosion lesions is very useful (Pereira et al. 2018). To maximize quantification, the use of the "en face" imaging systems allows the evaluation of the size and mineral distribution on the surface of the lesions, similar to that obtained by fluorescence imaging techniques (Maia et al. 2016).

OCT presents some limitations, mainly related to the signal approach, caused by the attenuation due to scattering and absorption. An *in vivo* study related that the progression of white spot lesions with boundary depths greater than 300 μm cannot be evaluated by SS-OCT (Sugiura et al. 2016). In the case of caries lesions, the imaging quality at deeper penetration depths can be altered due to multiple scattering. In this way, the use of optical clearing agents was studied in order to improve the optical penetration and contrast of OCT images, mainly in the subsurface caries lesions (Jones et al. 2005; Kang et al. 2014, 2016a, 2016b; Carneiro et al. 2018). It was showed that these agents should have higher refractive index than water and act as a scattering and reflection reducer, since they can fill pores and dentinal tubules (Yang et al. 2019). A small increase in enamel surface layer thickness decreases surface permeability significantly. Hence, measurements of sorptivity of water showed a linear correlation to the mineral distribution of the immediate enamel subsurfaces, verified by SS-OCT, which can guide clinical remineralization therapies for individual teeth (Gan et al. 2020).

The OCT technique has been tested in dentistry since 1998, when the first prototype of dental equipment was built by Colston & cols (Colston et al. 1998). The suggestion of the use of OCT in dentistry was based mainly on the possibility of real-time imaging, without ionizing radiation, with axial and lateral resolution comparable to the microscopy methods, which allows the diagnosis and monitoring of lesions about 100 times smaller than those detected by conventional radiographs. Still in 1998, Warren & cols (Warren et al. 1998) reported the first applications for diagnosing dental caries *in vitro*, while Feldchtein & cols (Feldchtein et al. 1998) demonstrated the first possibilities of using OCT for oral soft and hard tissue imaging, suggesting the diagnosis of caries and noncaries lesions, composite resin and compomers restorations, as well as treated tissues with drilling and acid etching. In 2000, the use of OCT for imaging oral soft tissue lesions as well as periodontal pockets and attachments was expanded (Otis et al. 2000). Since the publication of these first images, the increase in the number of publications that involve the use of OCT in dentistry is notable.

Nowadays, the applications of OCT in dentistry include the progression of periodontal disease, detection of oral cancer, caries and erosion lesions, calculus, the extent of fractures, thickness of cementum (Manesh et al. 2009) and other applications. Concerning dental hard tissues, OCT can differentiate enamel from dentin and cementum, as well as some anatomic details from these tissues, such as dento-enamel junction, cemento-enamel junction and mineralization defects (Walther et al. 2017).

In this chapter, we will review the main applications of OCT in cariology, mainly in the early diagnosis of carious and non-carious lesions, as well as in monitoring the progression or reversal of these lesions. Nevertheless, the development of technologies aimed at the applications of OCT in dental hard tissues will be approached.

3.2 OCT for Caries Diagnosis and Monitoring

Caries is a multifactorial disease whose clinical signs are manifested by the localized demineralization of dental hard tissues, which causes the so-called caries lesion. A caries lesion begins with a demineralization of the more superficial layers of the enamel and/or dentin, promoted by the acids produced by the biofilm bacteria. These acids cause the oral pH drop and the minerals (calcium and phosphate of the hydroxyapatite) are released from the tooth to the saliva. Saliva has an important buffer capacity when it is supersaturated in relation to the oral hard tissues; in this way the oral pH arises, the calcium and phosphate ions return to the tooth and thus remineralization occurs. The teeth are constantly submitted to cycles of demineralization and remineralization. However, when demineralization exceeds the buffer capacity of the saliva, incipient caries lesions, also termed "early" or "white spot" lesions, takes place (Fejerskov et al. 2015). Due to the backscattering of the incident white light in its porous regions, the incipient caries lesions appear whitish in the clinical examination.

The incipient lesions are not cavitated and can be remineralized, and this process occurs with the help of fluoridated agents and biofilm control. At this stage, the surface becomes hardened and the lesion is arrested, which represents fewer damages for the patient and the professional (Tenuta et al. 2010). However, the caries lesions often require restorative treatment when diagnosed late; so early diagnosis is indispensable in a non-invasive and efficient way, and also allows the monitoring of the remineralization process. The OCT is a very promising technique for that since the pores of the demineralized enamel increase 2 to 3 times the light scattering when considered the near infrared region (1300 nm) (Darling et al. 2006).

Early diagnosis techniques with high resolution are widely discussed in order to enable remineralization of very small lesions. OCT is a feasible technique to monitor the remineralization of lesions considering the changes in light scattering caused by fluoride treatment, which makes the remineralized tissue with hardness similar to that of sound one. In this way, the OCT is advantageous in relation to fluorescence-based methods (Ando et al. 2006) by allowing visualization of the tissues internally; also, it is possible to monitor the body of the caries lesions and to verify if there is still some activity or if they were in fact arrested. A comparison among OCT and other illumination devices such as near-infrared (NIR) and fiber optic technology (FOTI/ DIFOTI), showed the OCT has superior sensitivity to NIR and fiber-optic devices in detect initial caries (Macey et al. 2021). Compare to laser fluorescence (LF) and quantitative light-induced fluorescence (QLF), both were insensitive to less pronounced smooth-surface caries lesions while OCT allowed differentiation based on the penetration depth of the carious lesions (Park et al. 2021).

The image contrast obtained in PS-OCT systems allows a better spatial separation of the lesion body versus sound enamel (Fried et al. 2002). In addition, OCT is able to detect and measure the thickness of the remineralized layer after a remineralization treatment (Manesh et al. 2009). In Figure 3.1, a dentin caries lesion as viewed by OCT 930 nm is shown.

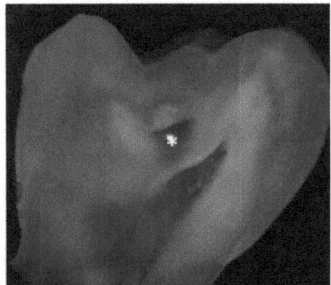 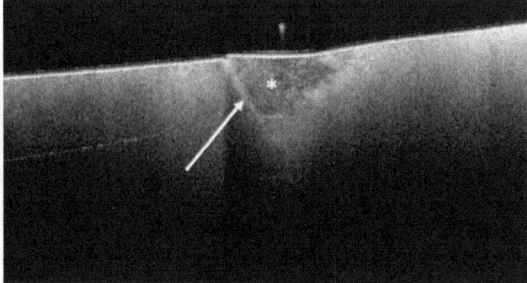

FIGURE 3.1

Dentin caries lesion (marked with an *) viewed by visual examination (left image) and by OCT 930 nm examination (right image). Note the differences in backscattered signal in caries lesion and the proximity to the pulp chamber (arrow).

It is possible to quantify the degree of demineralization in different ways, depending on the type of equipment used. The use of the integrated reflectivity is proposed for measurement of the activity of caries lesions using PS-OCT (polarization sensitive OCT system), taking into account that polarized light rapidly depolarizes when it returns from a demineralized tissue (Iijima et al. 1999). The integrated reflectivity in the perpendicular axis was positively related with the mineral loss measured by transverse microradiography (Jones et al. 2006). Also, the shrinkage of dentin lesions can be successfully measured and correlated to demineralization degree and lesion activity (Manesh et al. 2009).

The literature reports that PS-OCT has an advantage in relation to SS-OCT due to the fact that the incident light does not depolarize as a result of the reflection by the surface of the dental hard tissue, which has a high refraction index (Jones et al. 2006). The measurement of integrated reflectivity is summarily obtained after the separation of the backscattered polarized laser beam into parallel and perpendicular axes; then the obtained signals are modulated and series of integrations of line profiles are made, given in logarithmic reflectivity (dB), which evaluates the general gravity of the caries lesions. The calculation of the lesion depth and the integration of the perpendicular-axis image obtained determine the lesion severity (Ngaotheppitak et al. 2005) and can evaluate the remineralization of these lesions (Jones et al. 2006).

Using conventional OCT equipment, it is possible to detect incipient enamel caries lesions by analyzing the optical attenuation coefficient (OAC), whose method has sensitivity and specificity values close to 90% when using 850 nm wavelength (Popescu et al. 2008). For this, the decay of the *a-scan* signal obtained in the image of the lesion is evaluated. Considering that this decay is exponential, it can be easily fitted using an equation adapted from the Lambert-Beer law (Schmitt et al. 1994):

$$I_{(z)} - I_0 e^{-2\mu z} \qquad (3.1)$$

where $I_{(z)}$ is the OCT signal intensity at an optical distance z beneath the tooth surface, I_0 is the incident intensity of laser beam and μ is the attenuation coefficient (Popescu et al. 2008; Maia et al. 2016). Figure 3.2 shows a *b-scan* image and an *a-scan* signal printed in yellow, where it is possible to evidence the exponential decay as the tissue depth increases.

In the Cara & cols (Cara et al. 2014) study, when analyzing artificial caries lesions of greater severity with a 930 nm OCT system, a modification was proposed in Equation 1, adding a factor "C" that corresponds to the equipment signal (background):

$$I_{(z)} = I_0 e^{-2\mu z} + C \qquad (3.2)$$

where C is a constant (from signal background).

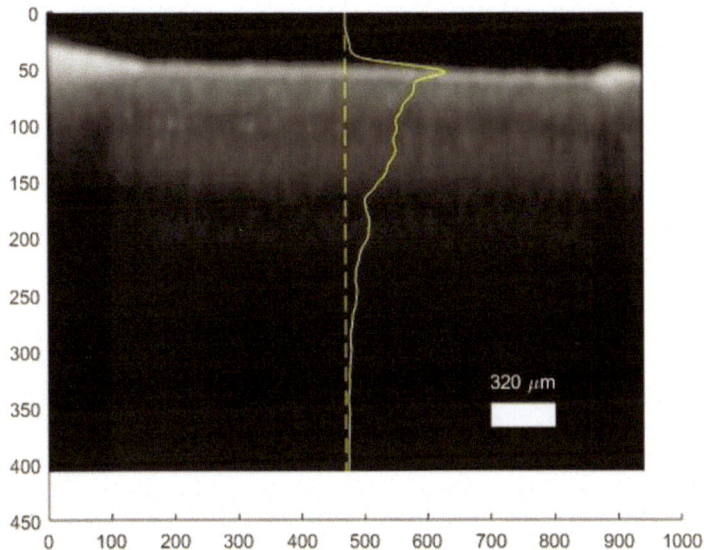

FIGURE 3.2

An OCT image (*b-scan*) of sound dentin with one representative *a-scan* (yellow line). It is observed the decay of laser signal across the tissue in an exponential way.

As with integrated reflectivity, OAC is positively correlated (99%) with loss of enamel microhardness due to caries lesion (Cara et al. 2014). Later work (Ana et al. 2017) has shown the feasibility of using OAC also to quantify the demineralization of root dentin.

Although the use of the OAC to quantify caries lesions is well established, the literature differs concerning the values obtained. Some authors report that attenuation of the OCT signal in healthy tissue is greater than attenuation as it propagates within a demineralization zone (Popescu et al. 2008; Sowa et al. 2011; Maia et al. 2016) because the propagation of light is hindered in the demineralized regions, which contain disorganized hydroxyapatite crystals and with a large volume of pore with many different sizes. At these interfaces with the pores, the light reflection occurs due to abrupt refractive index changes, as well as the effective reduction in scattering when light travels without being deviated through the space within the pores (Kienle et al. 2006). However, other studies report that the increase of the intercrystalline spaces and the disorganization of the prismatic structure of dental hard tissues promote a greater OAC (Jones et al. 2006; Cara et al. 2014).

Besides the mineral loss, the OAC is also a useful parameter to measure optical changes promoted by different treatments in the microstructure of hard dental tissues, such as the influence of high-power laser irradiation for caries prevention, for example (Figure 3.3).

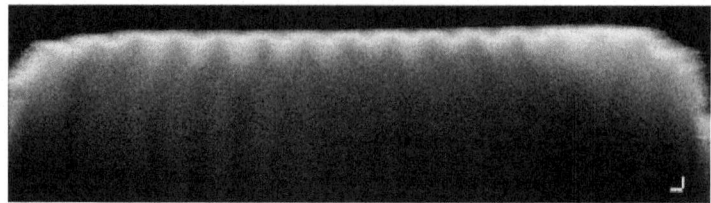

FIGURE 3.3

OCT image from root dentin after irradiation with pulsed Er,Cr:YSGG laser aimed at caries prevention. It is possible to evidence a higher backscattered signal in the dentin surface where the laser pulses interacted.

Another quantitative measurement proposed is the determination of an optical boundary (Natsume et al. 2011), which is especially useful in cavitated root caries lesions observed by SS-OCT. In this way, the boundary with higher reflectivity observed in OCT images corresponds to the lesion front, but it has modest correlation with the findings obtained by transverse microradiography mainly due to the subjective determination of the black-and-white border of the lesion, even when performed by a calibrated operator.

Using a customized SD-OCT system (1300 nm) with higher depth penetration, an *ex vivo* study performed by Wijesinghe & cols (Wijesinghe et al. 2016) proposed to monitor quantitatively the progression of early enamel caries using an algorithm that analyzes the total intensity fluctuation in depth, as well as to calculate the thickness and volume of remaining enamel in order to identify initial caries. However, the authors emphasize that the system has limitations concerning the quality of images and that it is a preliminary study that needs to be continued for future implementation.

In addition to the type of caries lesion, hard tissue and OCT equipment employed, it is important to note that some aspects should also be considered when using OCT for caries diagnosis: the presence of water or other high-refractive index fluids, which alter the penetration depth of OCT images (Jones et al. 2005), as well as angle of probe light (Park et al. 2017), surface roughness (Habib et al. 2018), porosity (De Oliveira Mota et al. 2013), color and the hydration of tissues, mainly concerning dentin caries lesions, which shrink when dried and change their optical properties (Zhou et al. 2018).

In order to improve the quality, contrast and sensitivity of OCT images, as consequences of deeper optical penetration (calculated as $1/e^2$), some authors propose the application of optical clearing agents on the surface of enamel and dentin. These agents have higher refractive index than the dental hard tissue and, in this way, reduce the scattering and reflection of the surfaces. The authors also say that the lower viscosity and biocompatibility are important for that in order to allow the material penetration into biological structures. The use of water, glycerol and propylene glycol were first suggested to improve the imaging of occlusal caries lesions (Jones et al. 2005) and, later, other agents such as BABB (33% benzyl alcohol + 67% benzyl benzoate), a Cargille Liquid (hydrogenated terphenyl 1-bromo-naphthalene, Cedar Grove, NJ) (Kang et al. 2014) and a vinyl polysiloxane impression material (Star VPS Clear Bite, Danville Materials, San Ramon, California) (Kang et al. 2016b) were successful tested to better detect occlusal hidden subsurface lesions. Recently, silver nanoparticles mixed in glycerol were applied together to SD-OCT 930 nm to better diagnosis enamel hidden lesions (Carneiro et al. 2018) and the glycerol and propylene glycol were combined with PS-OCT 1300 nm to allow the diagnosis of severity of root caries lesions as well as root fractures (Yang et al. 2019).

In dental literature, OCT was employed to diagnose natural and artificial caries lesions on smooth and occlusal surfaces of enamel and dentin using *in vitro* (Jones et al. 2006a, 2006b; Popescu et al. 2008; Manesh et al. 2009; Natsume et al. 2011; Sowa et al. 2011; Nakagawa et al. 2013; Mandurah et al. 2013; Cara et al. 2014; Maia et al. 2016; Wijesinghe et al. 2016; Ana et al. 2017; Park et al. 2017; Matsuura et al. 2018; Zhou et al. 2018), *ex vivo* (Feldchtein et al. 1998; Jones et al. 2005; Ngaotheppitak et al. 2005; Douglas et al. 2010; De Oliveira Mota et al. 2013; Yang et al. 2019) and *in vivo* (Lenton et al. 2012; Nakajima et al. 2012; Holtzman et al. 2015; Chan et al. 2016; Sugiura et al. 2016; Park et al. 2018) studies. A previous study shows that caries lesions located on smooth surfaces are relatively easier to diagnose using OCT, with significantly greater sensitivity than the visual inspection method alone depending on the extent of lesions (Nakagawa et al. 2013). Another study (Douglas et al. 2010) shows a greater correlation in the diagnosis of natural occlusal caries lesions using OCT after validation with polarized light microscopy (the correlation coefficient – Pearson – was $r = 0.63$) and transverse microradiography (the correlation coefficient was $r = 0.75$). OCT was also able to determine the severity of natural caries lesions on both smooth (Ngaotheppitak et al. 2005) and occlusal (Jones et al. 2006) surfaces. Radiation-related caries on enamel and dentin were detected by a SR-OCT (930 nm) system *ex vivo* (De Oliveira Mota et al. 2013), and an increase was evidenced in reflectivity on dentin caries, high light absorption in non-cavitated brown-discolored enamel, decreased view of the dentin-enamel junction, loss of cement and disorganization of cement-enamel junction. Also, a good agreement was observed with the images showed by polarized light microscopy.

Although the ability to detect non-cavitated fissure caries on occlusal surfaces by OCT has already been demonstrated, a recent *ex vivo* study (Zain et al. 2018) showed the possibility of diagnosis of these lesions in its slope and wall loci separately by PS-OCT, and the authors proposed an interpretation criteria based upon the location, thickness and pattern of the intensity range of –15 dB to –5 dB. Even though high values of sensitivity (0.98) and specificity (0.95) have been obtained, the authors caution that specular reflections may interfere with the diagnosis of slope lesions. Also, the authors found a high correlation between the results obtained by OCT and polarized light microscopy.

Thus, considering the ability of OCT to evaluate natural and artificial caries lesions, both on occlusal and smooth surfaces, with excellent correlation with gold standard techniques, such as sectional microhardness, transverse microradiography and polarized light microscopy, OCT also has been used as a tool to evaluate the effects of different treatments on caries lesions. Early studies (Fried et al. 2002; Chong et al. 2007; Abdelaziz et al. 2022) evidenced that OCT can detect the inhibition effects of fluoridated agents on enamel demineralization, as well as association with lasers such as CO_2 (Hsu et al. 2008), Er,Cr:YSGG (Ana et al. 2017) and Nd:YAG (Dias-Moraes et al. 2021). In the *in vitro* study of Nakata & cols (Nakata et al. 2018), OCT was used to confirm the increase of the enamel to demineralization after treatment with calcium-releasing anti-demineralization pastes or sodium fluoride solution. Also, OCT and microhardness test were used to demonstrate the potential of nanosilver fluoride to increase remineralization of deciduous enamel (Mota et al. 2018). By measurement of the maximum pixel value from CP-OCT images, it was possible to detect the capacity of the 45S5 bioglass on remineralization of non-cavitated lesions around orthodontic brackets *in vitro* (Bakhsh et al. 2018).

Most *in vivo* studies are performed on vestibular faces of anterior teeth due to the dimensions of the probes. The first clinical study (Louie et al. 2010) using PS-OCT was done to evaluate the formation and remineralization of incipient caries lesions around orthodontic brackets and other devices, on both smooth and occlusal surfaces. It was found a good correlation of PS-OCT results with those obtained from polarized light microscopy and transversal microradiography, which indicated that the OCT can be used clinically in a effectively way, since the other techniques require the exodontics of the tooth for preparation of the sample. In this study, the OCT presented better performance on occlusal surfaces because the specular reflection is higher on smooth surfaces and can generate artifacts that hamper accurate analysis. A study (Lenton et al. 2012) performed with a cross-polarized system (CP-OCT, 1310 nm) using an intraoral probe was efficient for isolating the perpendicular axis of light, which reduced the surface reflection signal and propitiated the use on infants. Also, it was possible to detect secondary caries lesions below composite restorations *in vivo*. In the study of Shimada & cols (Shimada et al. 2014), proximal caries of premolars and molars were evaluated using a SS-OCT (1300 nm) system also equipped with an intra-oral scanning probe. In this study, OCT presented higher sensitivity (0.92 for enamel demineralization, 0.84 for cavitated enamel lesions and 0.56 for dentin caries) than bitewing radiography (0.88, 0.65 and 0.35, respectively). The specificity values were also upper (the SS-OCT presented 0.58, 0.82 and 0.94 for enamel demineralization, cavitated enamel caries and dentin caries, whereas radiography presented 0.47, 0.73 and 0.91, respectively). Regarding the advantages of OCT (no overlap of images; the enamel is almost transparent at 1300 nm, which allows dentin to also be seen; the cavities appear with clear borders, which allows the differentiation of cavitated from non-cavitated lesions; it was possible to see lesions that extended to the dentin, because the demineralization always appears lighter than the healthy regions due to the increase in the number of pores, some limitations should be pointed out, mainly due to the thickness of dentin, which attenuates the OCT signal due to its microstructure. Therefore, the sensitivity in the diagnosis of dentin caries is low, besides the fact that it is not possible to visualize the pulp tissue and, consequently, the distance of the caries lesion of the pulp chamber.

A further clinical study (Lenton et al. 2012) that compared OCT findings with ICDAS classification, proved that a portable TD-OCT (1310 nm) system detects smooth and occlusal caries lesions with high sensitivity (95.1%) and specificity (85.8%). Another study (Chan et al. 2016) proved that the CP-OCT Santec (1300 nm) can be successfully applied to diagnose and monitor the remineralization of smooth lesions treated with fluoride and is able to detect the arrestment of lesions in patients with higher caries risk. Recently it was demonstrated that SS-OCT (1300 nm) can image and differentiate smooth lesions that have the same ICDAS classification (code 2, early caries), but that vary in extension and depth (Park et al. 2018).

Concerning the remineralization, it was demonstrated that OCT can monitor structural changes in lesions during the remineralization process on enamel (Jones et al. 2006) and dentin (Manesh et al. 2009) *in vitro*. A clinical trial demonstrated that OCT can been used for quantifying the effects of chewing gums containing phosphoryl oligosaccharides of calcium with or without fluoride on enamel, and detected that the treatments helped to arrest or reverse white spot lesions (Sugiura et al. 2016).

Another need for the use of OCT in cariology is to verify the quality of restorations, as well as the efficiency of the treatment over time, monitoring the onset of secondary caries lesions. An *in vitro* study showed the possibility of PS-OCT to detect demineralization under restorations and sealants (Jones et al. 2006), while the recent *in vitro* study performed by Matsuura & cols (Matsuura et al. 2018) evidenced that a hand probe 3D constructed for a SS-OCT system (1310 nm) can diagnose natural caries lesions below composite restorations up to 2 mm thick, and presented values of sensitivity and specificity significantly higher than those of digital radiography.

Although many papers show the viability and efficacy of OCT in the early diagnosis of caries lesions, clinical studies have not yet been found to prove that the method can be used alone (Sugiura et al. 2016). Therefore, the association of OCT with other traditional methods proves to be a much more efficient strategy.

3.3 OCT for Tooth Wear Diagnosis and Monitoring

Non-carious cervical lesions or tooth wear are lesions characterized by the loss of hard tissues, that have non-bacterial origin and affect the cervical regions of the teeth, with a higher prevalence on the vestibular surfaces. This classification includes erosion, abrasion, attrition and abfraction lesions. Dental erosion or erosive tooth wear is an irreversible loss of dental hard tissues, mainly caused by acids intrinsic to the oral environment (Ganss et al. 2014). The etiology of dental erosion is related to the ingestion of acidic beverages (soft drinks, isotonics) (Lussi et al. 2006) as well as to gastric reflux, eating disorders (regurgitation, alcoholism), psychic disorders (bulimia) and occupational causes (inhalation of acid vapors). This lesion is usually difficult to differentiate from abrasion or abfraction lesions, especially in its early stage (Lussi et al. 2006).

Dental abrasion is a wear that results by mechanical action involving tooth-foreign materials. In this way, dental brushing is the most important cause of abrasion, but this lesion can also be caused by some foods (Addy et al. 2006). Attrition is a lesion caused by the excessive contact between teeth and abfraction is characterized by cracks in cemento-dentinal junction caused by occlusal forces (bruxism or occlusal interferences) (Ganss 2006).

The increased prevalence of tooth wear lesions on the root surface may also be related to the presence of teeth in the oral cavity for a longer period of time, due to the increase in life expectancy and the improvement of the hygiene conditions of the individuals (Bartlett 2009). The clinical diagnosis and differentiation of wear lesions is based on visual examination (morphological aspects) and quantitative criteria, determined by Tooth Wear Index (TWI) (Smith et al. 1984) or based erosive wear examination (BEWE) (Ganss et al. 2014). The colorimetric method can also be used, in which the quantity of dissolved analyte is measured (Joshi et al. 2016). However, none of these techniques are accurate and can be performed alone because they do not provide all the information necessary (morphological + chemical) for a correct diagnosis.

In this way, there is a lack of objective clinical tools for diagnosing and monitoring tooth wear. Most methods that have high sensitivity and specificity are *in vitro* and destructive (such as scanning electron microscopy, optical perfilometry, polarized light microscopy, atomic force microscopy and others) (Joshi et al. 2016), which avoids long term monitoring. For this reason, the OCT presents the advantage due to the non-destructive visualization of morphological aspects of lesions, as well as can see and characterize very early demineralization (without loss of the surface) and remineralization. Thus, the early diagnosis of the lesions is essential for the implementation of strategies that minimize or prevent their progression.

The use of OCT for diagnosing tooth wear is based on the morphological changes (i.e., lesion aspect and depth, tissue thickness, texture and porosity) promoted by demineralization of enamel/dentin surfaces and immediate sub-surfaces (Huysmans et al. 2011), which alter the backscattered OCT signal. The signal of tooth wear differs from those obtained by caries lesions due to the greater demineralization of caries, promoting a deeper sub-surface lesion that changes the refractive index. OCT is able to differentiate between non-carious cervical lesions and root caries (Wada et al. 2015), as well as allows the visualization of morphological changes due to wear lesions, such as flattening, concavities and roughness.

The literature show that *en face* OCT can be used to characterize various degrees of attrition (Mărcăuteanu et al. 2009), as well as the presence of cracks under non-carious cervical lesions (Demjan et al. 2010). Also, it is possible to notice morphological signs of occlusal overload on teeth with normal morphology (Marcauteanu et al. 2011); OCT also allows a dynamic evaluation of pathological incisal wear (Marcauteanu et al. 2014) and can be used to calculate the volumes of non-carious cervical lesions (Stoica et al. 2014). OCT can evaluate and characterize the transparent dentin due to attrition, which presents a sclerotic layer that is more resistant to acid pretreatment (Mandurah et al. 2015). As well, OCT is able to differentiate erosion from attrition, abfraction and abrasion lesions, since they have some morphological particularities, that varies from shallow depressions appearing as saucer-shaped to broad wedge-shaped defects, as described by Mercut & cols (Mercuţ et al. 2017). This last study related, in *ex vivo* erosion lesions, that OCT showed cavities with a weak signal on lesion borders, due to the absence of dentin support on the enamel edges. Where demineralization was more intense, there was an increase in the backscattered signal, just as occurs in caries lesions. In the attrition lesions, the OCT revealed the presence of cracks in the dentin enamel junction, as well as an intense signal was observed on the external surface of the lesions. In the abfraction lesions the OCT indicated a great loss of tissue on the affected surfaces, as well as extensive cracks and an intense signal on the glossy surface. It was also possible to notice the proximity of the lesion with the pulp chamber. In the abrasion lesions, a homogeneous OCT signal was shown on the external surface of the lesions, with fewer cracks; in these lesions, the OCT signal was weaker on the cervical surface.

As in the diagnosis of caries lesions, the OCT also shows the optical changes that occur after the treatment of non-carious lesions (Figure 3.4), which allows

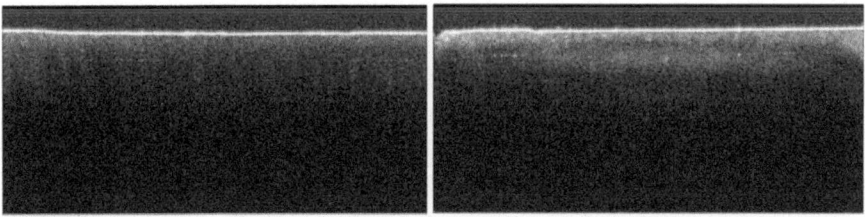

FIGURE 3.4
OCT image of eroded root dentin without treatment (left image) and after acidulated phosphate fluoride gel application (right image). It is possible to note a higher backscattered signal in the right image due to the remineralization of lesions.

determination of how effective the treatment was as well as monitoring of the progress of the lesions. The occlusal overload in bruxing patients can also be detected and monitored by OCT (Demjan et al. 2010).

The literature shows the possibility of measuring the progression of abfraction and attrition lesions by SS-OCT (1060 nm), suggesting that a color chart can be made to identify the distance between the incisal edge and the smooth surface affected by attrition, as well as it being possible to measure the areas and volume losses by 3D reconstruction of OCT images (Marcauteanu et al. 2014b). In the same way, the progression of non-cavitated erosion lesions can be successfully monitored by SS-OCT (1325 nm), in which the backscattered intensity at 40 μm depth provided useful information about the degree of demineralization in an orange juice erosive model, as well as it being possible to monitor the lesion depth in a positive relation with the porosity of enamel (Chew et al. 2014). The authors state that the backscattered signal measurements in shallower regions more than 40 μm are easily confused with specular surface reflectance; however, although the OCT allowed the analysis of the lesions in depth and did not confuse lesions with surface staining, the authors observed that the OCT presented a low correlation with the erosion intervals used in the study, thus suggesting that the quantitative light fluorescence (QLF) is still the most appropriate technique to monitor the progression of erosion.

For quantification of dental erosion lesions, OCT is a useful tool to determine the depth of the lesions, as well as the area and volume of them (de Moraes et al. 2017; Pereira et al. 2018) (Figure 3.5). The OAC can be also applied to determine the degree of demineralization of the lesions, as well as to verify the effectiveness of preventive strategies or treatments (Pereira et al. 2018).

Recently, it was noticed that the OAC can also be related with surface roughness (Habib et al. 2018), which is indispensable to distinguish the erosion lesions from sound or abraded surfaces (Hara et al. 2016). In this way, it is possible not only to quantify the demineralization in depth but also to determine the progression of lesions.

Another proposed way to quantify and monitor enamel erosion is to determine the enamel thickness. The study of Wilder-Smith & cols (Wilder-Smith

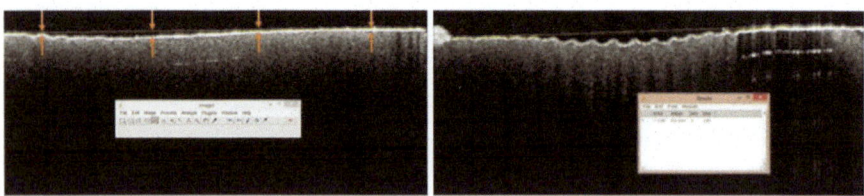

FIGURE 3.5
Analysis of root dentin erosion area (right image) and depth (left image) on OCT images.

et al. 2009) used the dentinal enamel junction (DEJ) as a reference in advanced stages of dental erosion, while Chan & cols (Chan et al. 2014) used a 9.3 µm CO_2 laser irradiated enamel surface as a reference for monitoring erosion in early stages, since laser irradiation can prevent dental erosion and demineralization. More recently, in a standardized *in vitro* study (Algarni et al. 2016), it was demonstrated that the PS-OCT is a powerful technique to be clinically used for measurement of enamel thickness, presenting good agreement with both microtomography (µ-CT) and histology methods, even with lower resolution than µ-CT.

The OCT can also be used to evaluate the effects of different treatments on dental on enamel and dentin erosion inhibition and progression, including high-intensity laser irradiation such as CO_2,[90] and Nd:YAG (de Moraes et al. 2017; Pereira et al. 2018) lasers. Later, Cassimiro-Silva & cols (Cassimiro-Silva et al. 2016) confirmed a good correlation of OCT (930 nm) with optical profilometry, and the possibility of OCT to detect the reduced mineral loss promoted by a SnF_2/NaF toothpaste on an erosive challenge.

The clinical studies that use OCT to diagnose tooth erosion are more recent than those assessing caries lesions. Wilder-Smith & cols (Wilder-Smith et al. 2009) proposed that OCT can effectively detect the effectiveness of a proton pump inhibitor on gastroesophageal reflux disease and consequent dental erosion in a 3-week follow up, by measuring enamel thickness and changes in optical reflectivity on depth on enamel, with standardization of measurement sites over time. They found significant differences on enamel thickness on treated patients, as well as increase in optical reflectivity due to the demineralization promoted by reflux. The increase in optical reflectivity is due to the increase on enamel pores, in the same way that it occurs in the diagnosis of caries lesions with OCT. Afterwards, the study of Wada & cols (Wada et al. 2015) showed that SS-OCT can measure the non-carious cervical lesions in buccal surfaces of teeth, as well as can detect the presence of cracks and demineralization, using a previous OAC determined previously *in vitro*, which was correlated with the mineral content measured by microradiography. The authors explain that the SS-OCT presents some advantages such as better detection of cracks and can provide information about demineralization depth, as well as can effectively detect dentin demineralization as a highlighted zone due to increased pores in the site, as occurs in caries lesions. Recently, the clinical study performed by Austin & cols (Austin et al. 2017) showed a SS-OCT (1305 nm) backscattered signal significantly higher ($p<0.0001$) in dental enamel of incisor teeth that were subjected to an early erosive challenge with orange juice. In this study, the authors proposed an algorithm to evaluate the signal without the interferences of optical artifacts and detected changes in the immediate sub-surface enamel. In the same year, a pilot study (Sugita et al. 2017) showed the possibility of SS-OCT (1310 nm) to determine and quantify the progression of non-carious cervical lesions *in vivo* during 4 or 5 years. For that, the depth and axial length of lesions were measured after the achievement of several buccolingual outlines of each lesion.

Thus, even with few randomized clinical trials, OCT is a promising technique to accurately differentiate different types of non-carious cervical lesions, as well as quantify the severity, monitor the progression of the lesions, and evaluate different treatment strategies. Nevertheless, it is noticed that different types of equipment can be used successfully. However, the clinician should be aware of the signal produced, as well as standardize the positioning of the probe during the course of treatment. This last aspect is not yet fully defined in the literature, but the suggestions made are quite efficient and easily applicable.

3.4 Technologies

After the first use of OCT for caries diagnosis was suggested, several systems were developed aimed to improve the clinical access to tiny sites with sensitivity and accuracy. The literature reports the use of several OCT systems for caries diagnosis, such as polarization-sensitive OCT (PS-OCT), cross-polarization OCT (CP-OCT), non-polarization sensitive spectral domain system (SD-OCT) and swept-source OCT (SS-OCT).

The conventional OCT equipment provides a high spatial resolution in the micrometer range. The PS-OCT is a preferable system for differentiating sound tissues from demineralized ones because it allows better contrast images with fewer artifacts[68]. However, the SS-OCT and SD-OCT systems are still employed for assessment of carious lesions (Nakagawa et al. 2013; Wijesinghe et al. 2016), and both PS-OCT and SS-OCT were also used for assessing and monitoring occlusal enamel and dentin caries (Shimada et al. 2013; Popescu et al. 2022; Serban et al. 2022), due to their superior sensitivity and higher resolution.

3.5 Conclusion

OCT is a valuable technique in cariology because it allows the diagnosis of carious and non-carious lesions, cavitated or not in enamel, dentin or cementum, in a quick and efficient way, as well as allowing them to be differentiated. Due to in-depth imaging with comparable resolution to microscopy techniques, OCT allows reliable quantification of lesion size in depth and extent, as well as quantifies structural losses. *In vitro* and clinical studies show the possibility of evaluating the presence of sub-surface lesions in different sites, as well as quantifying their severity in distinct ways. Also, OCT allows the monitoring of treatment strategies and evaluates remineralized or arrested lesions. Although quite advantageous, there is still much to be done for the actual clinical implementation of the technology, such as the development of probes that allow the imaging of posterior interproximal regions with acceptable resolution and cost, as well as devices that allow the positioning of the probes in a standardized way and that allow the analysis of images taken in the same place but on different days. Nevertheless, although OCT allows a wide range of information to be obtained, it is a technique that should not be used alone, but together with an accurate clinical examination to define the best treatment strategy.

References

Abdelaziz, M., Yang, V., Chang, N.Y.N. et al. 2022. Monitoring silver diamine fluoride application with optical coherence tomography and thermal imaging: An in vitro proof of concept study. *Lasers Surg. Med.* 54:790–803.

Addy, M., Shellis, R.P. 2006. Interaction between attrition, abrasion and erosion in tooth wear. *Monogr. Oral Sci.* 20: 17–31.

Algarni, A., Kang, H., Fried, D., Eckert, G.J., Hara, A.T. 2016. Enamel thickness determination by optical coherence tomography: In vitro validation. *Caries Res.* 50: 400–406.

Almaz, E.C., Simon, J.C., Fried, D., Darling, C.L. 2016. Influence of stains on lesion contrast in the pits and fissures of tooth occlusal surfaces from 800-1600-nm. *Lasers Dent. XXII 9692*: 96920X.

Ana, P.A., Benetti, C., Bachmann, L., Maria Zezell, D. 2017. Structural characterization of dentin irradiated with Er,Cr:YSGG laser and fluoride for caries prevention. 2017 *Conf. Lasers Electro-Optics, CLEO 2017* – Proc. 2017-Janua, 1–2.

Ando, M., Stookey, G.K., Zero, D.T. 2006. Ability of quantitative light-induced fluorescence (QLF) to assess the activity of white spot lesions during dehydration. *Am. J. Dent.* 19: 15–18.

Austin, R.S., Haji Taha, M., Festy, F. et al. 2017. Quantitative swept-source optical coherence tomography of early enamel erosion in vivo. *Caries Res.* 51: 410–418.

Bakhsh, T., Al-batati, M., Mukhtar, M., Al-Najjar, M., Bakhsh, S. 2018. Effect of bioglass on artificially induced enamel lesion around orthodontic brackets: OCT study 1047302: 1.

Banting, D.W. 1993. Diagnosis and prediction of root caries. *Adv. Dent. Res.* 7: 80–86.

Bartlett, D. 2009. Etiology and prevention of acid erosion. *Compendium* 30: 616–620.

Boppart, S.A., Herrmann, J., Pitris, C., Stamper, D.L., Brezinski, M.E., Fujimoto, J.G. 1999. High-resolution optical coherence tomography-guided laser ablation of surgical tissue. *J. Surg. Res.* 82: 275–284.

Cabral, R.M.R., Mendes, F.M., Nicolau, J., Zezell, D.M. 2006. The Influence of PVC seal wrap and probe tips autoclaving on the in vitro performance of laser fluorescence device in occlusal caries in primary teeth. *J. Pediatr. Dent*. 30: 306–309.

Cara, A.C.B., Zezell, D.M., Ana, P.A., Maldonado, E.P., Freitas, A.Z. 2014. Evaluation of two quantitative analysis methods of optical coherence tomography for detection of enamel demineralization and comparison with microhardness. *Lasers Surg. Med*. 46: 666–671.

Carneiro, V.S.M., Mota, C.C.B. d. O., Gomes, A.S.L., Et, A. 2018. Optical clearing agents associated with nanoparticles for scanning dental structures with optical coherence tomography. *Br Dent J* 10507: 305–12.

Cassimiro-Silva, P.F., Maia, A.M.A., Monteiro, G.Q. de M., Gomes, A.S.L. 2016. Mitigation of enamel erosion using commercial toothpastes evaluated with optical coherence tomography. *Sixth Int. Conf. Lasers Med*. 9670, 96700Y.

Chan, K.H., Tom, H., Darling, C.L., Fried, D. 2014. A method for monitoring enamel erosion using laser irradiated surfaces and optical coherence tomography. *Lasers Surg. Med*. 46: 672–678.

Chan, K.H., Tom, H., Lee, R.C. et al. 2016. Clinical monitoring of smooth surface enamel lesions using CP-OCT during nonsurgical intervention. *Lasers Surg. Med*. 48: 915–923.

Chew, H.P., Zakian, C.M., Pretty, I.A., Ellwood, R.P. 2014. Measuring initial enamel erosion with quantitative light-induced fluorescence and optical coherence tomography: An in vitro validation study. *Caries Res*. 48: 254–262.

Chong, S.L., Darling, C.L., Fried, D. 2007. Nondestructive measurement of the inhibition of demineralization on smooth surfaces using polarization-sensitive optical coherence tomography. *Lasers Surg. Med*. 39: 422–427.

Colston, B.W., Sathyam, U.S., DaSilva, L.B., Everett, M.J., Stroeve, P., Otis, L.L. 1998. Dental OCT. *Opt. Express* 3: 230.

Darling, C.L., Huynh, G.D., Fried, D. 2006. Light scattering properties of natural and artificially demineralized dental enamel at 1310 nm. *J. Biomed. Opt*. 11: 034023.

de Moraes, M.C.D., Freitas, A.Z., Aranha, A.C.C. 2017. Progression of erosive lesions after Nd:YAG laser and fluoride using optical coherence tomography. *Lasers Med. Sci*. 32: 1–8.

De Oliveira Mota, C.C.B., Gueiros, L.A., Maia, A.M.A. et al. 2013. Optical coherence tomography as an auxiliary tool for the screening of radiation-related caries. Photomed. *Laser Surg*. 31: 301–306.

Demjan, E., Mărcăuțeanu, C., Bratu, D. et al. 2010. Analysis of dental abfractions by optical coherence tomography. *Lasers Dent*. XVI 7549: 754903.

Dias-Moraes, M.C., Castro, P.A.A., Pereira, D.L., Ana, P.A., Freitas, A.Z., Zezell, D.M. 2021. Assessment of the preventive effects of Nd: YAG laser associated with fluoride on enamel caries using optical coherence tomography and FTIR spectroscopy. *PLoS One* 16: 1–14.

Ding, Z., Ren, H., Zhao, Y., Nelson, J.S., Chen, Z. 2002. High-resolution optical coherence tomography over a large depth range with an axicon lens. *Opt. Lett*. 27: 243.

Douglas, S.M., Fried, D., Darling, C.L. 2010. Imaging natural occlusal caries lesions with optical coherence tomography. *Lasers Dent*. XVI 7549: 75490N.

Fejerskov, O., Nyvad, B., Kidd, E. 2015. Dental Caries: The Disease and its Clinical Management. Wiley-Blackwell, 3rd Edition. ed. Wiley-Blackwell.

Feldchtein, F.I., Gelikonov, G. V., Gelikonov, V.M. et al. 1998. In vivo OCT imaging of hard and soft tissue of the oral cavity. *Opt. Express* 3: 239.

Fried, D., Xie, J., Shafi, S., Feathersone, J.D.B., Breunig, T.M., Le, C. 2002. Imaging caries lesions and lesion progression with polarization sensitive optical coherence tomography. *J. Biomed. Opt.* 7: 618–627.

Gan, S.C., Fok, A.S.L., Sedky, R.A., Sukumaran, P., Chew, H.P. 2020. Sorptivity of water in enamel for categorizing caries lesions. *Dent. Mater.* 36: 1379–1387.

Ganss, C. 2006. Definition of erosion and links to tooth wear. *Monogr. Oral Sci.* 20: 9–16.

Ganss, C., Lussi, A. 2014. Diagnosis of erosive tooth wear. *Monogr. Oral Sci.* 25: 22–31.

Habib, M., Lee, K.M., Liew, Y.M., Zakian, C., Ung, N.M., Chew, H.P. 2018. Assessing surface characteristics of eroded dentine with optical coherence tomography: a preliminary in vitro validation study. *Appl. Opt.* 57: 8673.

Hall, A., Girkin, J.M. 2004. A review of potential new diagnostic modalities for caries lesions. *J. Dent. Res.* 83: 89–94.

Hara, A.T., Livengood, S. V., Lippert, F., Eckert, G.J., Ungar, P.S. 2016. Dental Surface Texture Characterization Based on Erosive Tooth Wear Processes. *J. Dent. Res.* 95: 537–542.

Holtzman, J.S., Kohanchi, D., Biren-Fetz, J. et al. 2015. Detection and proportion of very early dental caries in independent living older adults. *Lasers Surg. Med.* 47: 683–688.

Hsu, D.J., Darling, C.L., Lachica, M.M., Fried, D. 2008. Nondestructive assessment of the inhibition of enamel demineralization by CO_2 laser treatment using polarization sensitive optical coherence tomography. *J. Biomed. Opt.* 13: 054027.

Huysmans, M.C.D.N.J., Chew, H.P., Ellwood, R.P. 2011. Clinical studies of dental erosion and erosive wear. *Caries Res.* 45: 60–68.

Iijima, Y., Takagi, O., Ruben, J., Arends, J. 1999. In vitro remineralization of in vivo and in vitro formed enamel lesions. *Caries Res.* 33: 206–213.

Iranzo-Cortés, J.E., Terzic, S., Montiel-Company, J.M., Almerich-Silla, J.M. 2017. Diagnostic validity of ICDAS and DIAGNOdent combined: an in vitro study in pre-cavitated lesions. *Lasers Med. Sci.* 32: 543–548.

Ismail, A.I., Sohn, W., Tellez, M. et al. 2007. The International Caries Detection and Assessment System (ICDAS): an integrated system for measuring dental caries. *Oral Heal. Care – Pediatr. Res. Epidemiol. Clin. Pract.* 35: 170–178.

Jones, G.C., Jones, R.S., Fried, D. 2004. Transillumination of interproximal caries lesions with 830-nm light. *Lasers Dent.* X 5313: 17.

Jones, J.R., Fried, D. 2006. Remineralization of enamel caries. *J. Dent. Res.* 85: 804–808.

Jones, R. S., Darling, C.L., Featherstone, J.D.B., Fried, D. 2006a. Remineralization of in vitro dental caries assessed with polarization-sensitive optical coherence tomography. *J. Biomed. Opt.* 11: 014016.

Jones, R. S., Darling, C.L., Featherstone, J.D.B., Fried, D. 2006b. Imaging artificial caries on the occlusal surfaces with polarization-sensitive optical coherence tomography. *Caries Res.* 40: 81–89.

Jones, R.S., Fried, D. 2005. The effect of high-index liquids on PS-OCT imaging of dental caries. *Lasers Dent.* XI 5687: 34.

Joshi, M., Joshi, N., Kathariya, R., Angadi, P., Raikar, S. 2016. Techniques to evaluate dental erosion: A systematic review of literature. *J. Clin. Diagnostic Res.* 10: ZE1–ZE7.

Kang, H., Darling, C.L., Fried, D. 2014. Enhancing the detection of hidden occlusal caries lesions with OCT using high index liquids. *Lasers Dent. XX 8929*: 892900.

Kang, H., Darling, C.L., Fried, D. 2016a. Use of an optical clearing agent to enhance the visibility of subsurface structures and lesions from tooth occlusal surfaces. *J. Biomed. Opt.* 21: 081206.

Kang, H., Darling, C.L., Fried, D. 2016b. Enhancement of OCT images with vinyl polysiloxane (VPS). *Lasers Dent. XXII 9692*: 96920T.

Kienle, A., Hibst, R. 2006. Light guiding in biological tissue due to scattering. *Phys. Rev. Lett.* 97: 2–5.

Lenton, P., Rudney, J., Chen, R., Fok, A., Aparicio, C., Jones, R.S. 2012. Imaging in vivo secondary caries and ex vivo dental biofilms using cross-polarization optical coherence tomography. *Dent. Mater.* 28: 792–800.

Lopes, M.S., Mota, C.C.B.O., Pereira, D.L., Amaral, M.M., Zezell, D.M., Gomes, A.S.L. 2019. Effect of Nd:YAG laser and aluminum oxide sandblasting preconditioning on lingual enamel: Brackets shear bond strength and morphological characterization. *Opt. InfoBase Conf. Pap. Part F142*: 19–22.

Louie, T., Lee, C., Hsu, D. et al. 2010. Clinical assessment of early tooth demineralization using polarization sensitive optical coherence tomography. *Lasers Surg. Med.* 42: 898–905.

Lussi, A., Francescut, P. 2003. Performance of conventional and new method for the detection of occlusal caries in deciduous teeth. *Caries Res.* 37: 36–45.

Lussi, A., Hellwig, E., Zero, D., Jaeggi, T. 2006. Erosive tooth wear: Diagnosis, risk factors and prevention. *Am. J. Dent.* 19: 319–325.

Macey, R., Walsh, T., Riley, P. et al. 2021. Transillumination and optical coherence tomography for the detection and diagnosis of enamel caries. *Cochrane Database Syst. Rev.* 1: 1–110.

Maia, A.M.A., de Freitas, A.Z., de L. Campello, S., Gomes, A.S.L., Karlsson, L. 2016. Evaluation of dental enamel caries assessment using quantitative light induced fluorescence and optical coherence tomography. *J. Biophotonics* 9: 596–602.

Mandurah, M.M., Sadr, A., Bakhsh, T.A., Shimada, Y., Sumi, Y., Tagami, J. 2015. Characterization of transparent dentin in attrited teeth using optical coherence tomography. *Lasers Med. Sci.* 30: 1189–1196.

Mandurah, M.M., Sadr, A., Shimada, Y. et al. 2013. Monitoring remineralization of enamel subsurface lesions by optical coherence tomography. *J. Biomed. Opt.* 18: 046006.

Manesh, S.K., Darling, C.L., Fried, D. 2009. Polarization-sensitive optical coherence tomography for the nondestructive assessment of the remineralization of dentin. *J. Biomed. Opt.* 14: 044002.

Marcauteanu, C., Bradu, A., Sinescu, C. et al. 2014a. The advantages of a swept source optical coherence tomography system in the evaluation of occlusal disorders. *Fifth Int. Conf. Lasers Med. Biotechnol. Integr. Dly. Med.* 8925: 89250W.

Marcauteanu, C., Bradu, A., Sinescu, C., Topala, F.I., Negrutiu, M.L., Podoleanu, A.G. 2014b. Quantitative evaluation of dental abfraction and attrition using a swept-source optical coherence tomography system. *J. Biomed. Opt.* 19: 0211081–0211086.

Marcauteanu, C., Negrutiu, M., Sinescu, C. et al. 2009. Early detection of tooth wear by en-face optical coherence tomography. *Lasers Dent. XV 7162*: 716205.

Marcauteanu, C., Negrutiu, M., Sinescu, C. et al. 2011. Early characterization of occlusal overloaded cervical dental hard tissues by en face optical coherence tomography. *Opt. InfoBase Conf. Pap.* 8091: 1–6.

Matsuura, C., Shimada, Y., Sadr, A., Sumi, Y., Tagami, J. 2018. Three-dimensional diagnosis of dentin caries beneath composite restorations using swept-source optical coherence tomography. *Dent. Mater. J.* 37: 642–649.

Mercuţ, V., Popescu, S.M., Scrieciu, M. et al. 2017. Optical coherence tomography applications in tooth wear diagnosis. *Rom. J. Morphol. Embryol.* 58: 99–106.

Mota, C.C.B.O., Silva, A.V.C., Lins, E.C.C.C., Teixeira, J.A., Gomes, A.S.L., Rosenblatt, A. 2018. Potential of nano-silver fluoride for tooth enamel caries prevention. *Proc. of SPIE* 10507: 105071A1–10.

Nakagawa, H., Sadr, A., Shimada, Y., Tagami, J., Sumi, Y. 2013. Validation of swept source optical coherence tomography (SS-OCT) for the diagnosis of smooth surface caries in vitro. *J. Dent.* 41: 80–89.

Nakajima, Y., Shimada, Y., Miyashin, M., Takagi, Y., Tagami, J., Sumi, Y. 2012. Noninvasive cross-sectional imaging of incomplete crown fractures (cracks) using swept-source optical coherence tomography. *Int. Endod. J.* 45: 933–941.

Nakata, T., Kitasako, Y., Sadr, A., Nakashima, S., Tagami, J. 2018. Effect of a calcium phosphate and fluoride paste on prevention of enamel demineralization. *Dent. Mater. J.* 37: 65–70.

National Institute of Health 2001. Diagnosis and management of dental caries throughout life; National Institutes of Health Consensus Development.

Natsume, Y., Nakashima, S., Sadr, A., Shimada, Y., Tagami, J., Sumi, Y. 2011. Estimation of lesion progress in artificial root caries by swept source optical coherence tomography in comparison to transverse microradiography. *J. Biomed. Opt.* 16: 071408.

Ngaotheppitak, P., Darling, C.L., Fried, D. 2005. Measurement of the severity of natural smooth surface (interproximal) caries lesions with polarization sensitive optical coherence tomography. *Lasers Surg. Med.* 37: 78–88.

Otis, L.L., Everett, M.J., Sathyam, U.S., Colston, B.W. 2000. Optical coherence tomography: A new imaging technology for dentistry. *J. Am. Dent. Assoc.* 131: 511–514.

Park, K.J., Haak, R., Ziebolz, D., Krause, F., Schneider, H. 2017. OCT assessment of non-cavitated occlusal carious lesions by variation of incidence angle of probe light and refractive index matching. *J. Dent.* 62: 31–35.

Park, K.J., Schneider, H., Ziebolz, D., Krause, F., Haak, R. 2018. Optical coherence tomography to evaluate variance in the extent of carious lesions in depth. *Lasers Med. Sci.* 33: 1573–1579.

Park, K.J., Voigt, A., Schneider, H., Ziebolz, D., Haak, R. 2021. Light-based diagnostic methods for the in vivo assessment of initial caries lesions: Laser fluorescence, QLF and OCT. *Photodiagnosis Photodyn. Ther.* 34: 102270.

Pereira, D.L., Freitas, A.Z., Bachmann, L., Benetti, C., Zezell, D.M., Ana, P.A. 2018. Variation on molecular structure, crystallinity, and optical properties of dentin due to Nd:YAG laser and fluoride aimed at tooth erosion prevention. *Int. J. Mol. Sci.* 19: 1–14.

Popescu, D.P., Sowa, M.G., Hewko, M.D., Choo-Smith, L.-P. 2008. Assessment of early demineralization in teeth using the signal attenuation in optical coherence tomography images. *J. Biomed. Opt.* 13: 054053.

Popescu, M., Scrieciu, M., Osiac, E. et al. 2022. Applications of optical coherence tomography in the diagnosis of enamel defects. *Diagnostics* 12: 636.

Schmitt, J.M., Knuttel, A., Yadlowsky, M., Eckhaus, M.A. 1994. Optical-coherence tomography of a dense tissue: Statistics of attenuation and backscattering. *Phys. Med. Biol.* 39: 1705–1720.

Schneider, H., Park, K.J., Häfer, M. et al. 2017. Dental applications of optical coherence tomography (OCT) in cariology. *Appl. Sci.* 7: 472.

Serban, C., Lungeanu, D., Bota, S.D. et al. 2022. Emerging technologies for dentin caries detection – a systematic review and meta-analysis. *J. Clin. Med.* 11: 674.

Shimada, Y., Nakagawa, H., Sadr, A. et al. 2014. Noninvasive cross-sectional imaging of proximal caries using swept-source optical coherence tomography (SS-OCT) in vivo. *J. Biophotonics* 7: 506–513.

Smith, B.G., Knight, J.K. 1984. An index for measuring the wear of teeth. *Br. Dent. J.* 156: 435–438.

Sowa, M.G., Popescu, D.P., Friesen, J.R., Hewko, M.D., Choo-Smith, L.P. in. 2011. A comparison of methods using optical coherence tomography to detect demineralized regions in teeth. *J. Biophotonics* 4: 814–823.

Stoica, E.T., Marcauteanu, C., Bradu, A. et al. 2014. Imaging of noncarious cervical lesions by means of a fast swept source optical coherence tomography system. *Fifth Int. Conf. Lasers Med. Biotechnol. Integr. Dly. Med.* 8925: 89250Y.

Sugita, I., Nakashima, S., Ikeda, A. et al. 2017. A pilot study to assess the morphology and progression of non-carious cervical lesions. *J. Dent.* 57: 51–56.

Sugiura, M., Kitasako, Y., Sadr, A., Shimada, Y., Sumi, Y., Tagami, J. 2016. White spot lesion remineralization by sugar-free chewing gum containing bio-available calcium and fluoride: A double-blind randomized controlled trial. *J. Dent.* 54: 86–91.

Tenuta, L.M.A., Cury, J.A. 2010. Fluoride: Its role in dentistry. *Braz. Oral Res.* 24: 9–17.

Wada, I., Shimada, Y., Ikeda, M. et al. 2015. Clinical assessment of non carious cervical lesion using swept-source optical coherence tomography. *J. Biophotonics* 8: 846–854.

Walther, J., Golde, J., Koch, E. et al. 2017. In vivo imaging of human oral hard and soft tissues by polarization-sensitive optical coherence tomography. *J. Biomed. Opt.* 22: 1.

Warren, J.A., Gelikonov, G. V., Gelikonov, V.M. et al. 1998. Imaging and characterization of dental structure using optical coherence tomography. *Conf. Lasers Electro-Optics Eur. Tech. Dig.* 128.

Wijesinghe, R.E., Cho, N.H., Park, K., Jeon, A., Kim, J. 2016. Bio-photonic detection and quantitative evaluation method for the progression of dental caries using optical frequency-domain imaging method. *Sensors (Switzerland)* 16. 16: 1–12.

Wilder-Smith, C.H., Wilder-Smith, P., Kawakami-Wong, H., Voronets, J., Osann, K., Lussi, A. 2009. Quantification of dental erosions in patients with GERD using optical coherence tomography before and after double-blind, randomized treatment with esomeprazole or placebo. *Am. J. Gastroenterol.* 104: 2788–2795.

Yang, V.B., Curtis, D.A., Fried, D. 2019. Use of optical clearing agents for imaging root surfaces with optical coherence tomography. *IEEE J. Sel. Top. Quantum Electron.* 25: 7100507.

Zain, E., Zakian, C.M., Chew, H.P. 2018. Influence of the loci of non-cavitated fissure caries on its detection with optical coherence tomography. *J. Dent.* 71: 31–37.

Zhou, Y., Shimada, Y., Matin, K. et al. 2018. Assessment of root caries under wet and dry conditions using swept-source optical coherence tomography (SS-OCT). *Dent. Mater. J.* 37: 880–888.

4

OCT in Restorative Dentistry: Towards Clinical Applications

Patrícia Makishi,[1] Alireza Sadr,[2] Yasushi Shimada,[3] Junji Tagami[3] and Marcelo Giannini[4]

[1]DDS, PhD, Department of Restorative Dentistry, Piracicaba Dental School, University of Campinas, Brazil

[2]DDS, PhD, Department of Restorative Dentistry, School of Dentistry, University of Washington, USA

[3]DDS, PhD, Department of Cariology and Operative Dentistry, Faculty of Dentistry, Tokyo Medical and Dental University, Japan

[4]DDS, MS, PhD, Department of Restorative Dentistry, Piracicaba Dental School, State University of Campinas, Brazil

CONTENTS

4.1 Introduction

The restorative dental materials based on composite resins have often been used in operative dentistry, prosthodontics, pediatric and endodontic fields of dentistry. These materials have changed the clinical practice of dentists because the new technology of metal-free, polymeric materials and bonding agents, which allow preserving intact/sound tooth structures, bonding to mineralized dental tissues and offering an esthetic treatment modality to the patient.

DOI: 10.1201/9781351104562-4

Composite restorative materials have been investigated by several clinical trials and in vitro methods, however the advances in digital dentistry are reshaping the methods in which dental research and clinical practice are performed. The use of digital imaging for diagnosis and treatment in restorative dentistry requires an entirely new set of professional skills, experience and technology. The evolution of imaging together with restorative materials and dental adhesive developments can allow more conservation of natural tissues, as well as effective and faster dental procedures, resulting in greater patient satisfaction and reliability regarding the quality of dental treatment.

4.2 Evaluation of Restorative Materials Using OCT

Among the array of revolutionary non-invasive imaging techniques, swept-source optical coherence tomography (SS-OCT) uses rapid, high-resolution, volumetric and cross-sectional tomographic imaging of internal restorative material microstructure based on depth-resolved optical reflectivity (Huang et al. 1991; Fujimoto et al. 2008). The principles of SS-OCT technique are based on low-coherence interferometry where light backscattered from inside the specimen is measured by correlation with light that has traveled through a known reference path (Bista et al. 2013). Therefore, SS-OCT imaging is based on differences in light-scattering properties, refractive indices, and composition of various mediums and structures.

Despite the imaging depth limitations of composite restorations (approximately 1.5 mm) (Bakhsh et al. 2011) due to optical attenuation involving absorption and scattering, SS-OCT can detect and quantify underlying defects in an adhesive restoration over a small distance (Bakhsh et al. 2011; Makishi et al. 2011; Bista et al. 2013). When light passes through different mediums with different refractive indices, some of the light is reflected and refracted. This is primarily observed at the interface between different structures, resulting in increased brightness at gaps or defects due to the presence of air (Makishi et al. 2011, 2015b) (Figure 4.1). Several studies have confirmed that these bright features are gaps by performing SS-OCT imaging in conjunction with conventional confocal laser scanner microscopy (CLSM) on a single cross-section (Bakhsh et al. 2011; Makishi et al. 2011; Bista et al. 2013; Shimada et al. 2014; Makishi et al. 2015a, 2015b).

Conventional microscopic observation of marginal adaptation tests often requires multiple sectioning of the samples, followed by immersion into a staining solution and surface polishing. In contrast, SS-OCT provides important information regarding the biomechanical properties of dental materials via non-destructive two-dimensional (2D) and three-dimensional (3D) imaging (Makishi et al. 2011, 2015b). While the optical resolution of

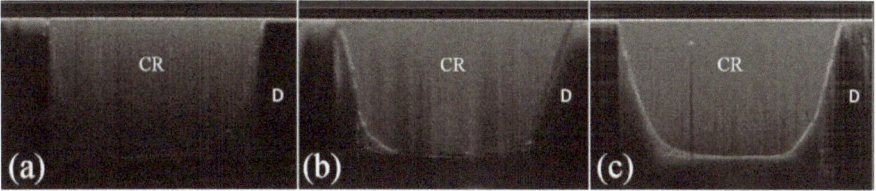

FIGURE 4.1

Three representative stained 2D SS-OCT image slice. (a) High intensity signal was observed only at the surface of composite, showing a good marginal adaptation. (b) High intensity signal was observed at the surface of composite, and between the restorative material and the tooth interface on the left side and part of the bottom, indicating gap presence; an interface with no increased brightness on the right side indicates absence of gap. (c) High intensity signal was observed at the surface of composite, and at the cavity interface with gap. Abbreviations: CR: composite resin; D: dentin. Reprinted with permission from (Makishi. 2015b) © Elsevier Science & Technology Journals.

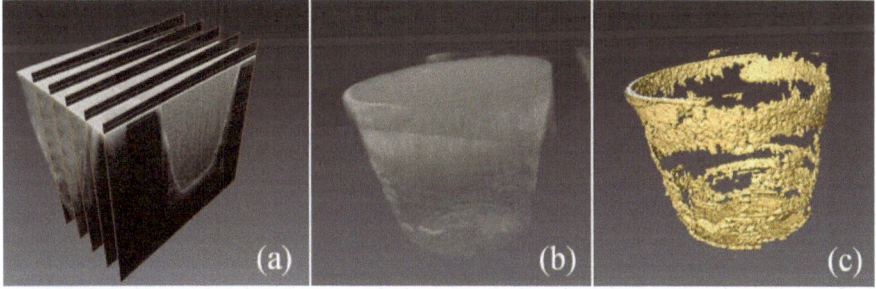

FIGURE 4.2

(a) Representative 3D image and corresponding five 2D images obtained by SS-OCT. (b) Representative 3D image of the same stained restoration in its entirety. (c) Mesial view of the reconstructed 3D image based on the 2D high brightness zones, which are marked in yellow gold color. Reprinted with permission from (Makishi. 2015b) © Elsevier Science & Technology Journals.

SS-OCT remains unchanged regardless of imaging mode, the image resolution of the 2D scans (2001×1019 pixels) and 3D scans (500×500×600 pixels) differ due to current limitations of the digital hardware for the signal conversion and data processing in quasi-realtime (Makishi et al. 2011).

Therefore, most of the reported marginal adaptation studies using SS-OCT are primarily based on 2D scans (Bakhsh et al. 2011; Bista et al. 2013; Makishi et al. 2015a, 2015b; Fronza et al. 2018). For a more detailed analysis, 3D images can be obtained by combining several 2D scans over the volume of interest (Figure 4.2). It is reasonable to assume that defects at an adhesive-tooth interface occur in a 3D-space and a 3D analysis should be ideally considered for their quantification. Although the cross-sectional images of the 3D scans can rapidly provide information regarding the overall restoration, lower image resolution is obtained when compared to the 2D image-scans (Makishi et al. 2011).

4.3 OCT Research Data of Restorative Materials

The marginal adaptation of different adhesive restorations in class I cavities using a silver nitrate solution as an infiltrating agent to enhance the SS-OCT image contrast has been evaluated using 3D OCT scan cross-sectional images (Makishi et al. 2011, 2015b). In these studies, the silver penetrated into the interfacial gap, acting as a metallic contrast agent by efficiently reflecting the incident light. In this way, higher sensitivity for detecting small gaps has been obtained. Different categories of dental adhesives and composite resin were evaluated by OCT and the results showed the best restorative materials regarding the reduction on interfacial gap formation (Makishi et al. 2011, 2015b).

Moreover, 3D images with that contrast agent have revealed that cavity wall gaps can be formed at the base of grooves created by the cutting-bur. This was not visualized in the 2D scan, but only became apparent once 3D imaging was performed (Makishi et al. 2015b) (Figure 4.2). Even though the authors used a finishing bur, their data highlight the importance of creating a smooth dentin finish to improve the bonding performance (Ayad et al. 2011).

A more recent SS-OCT study investigated the real-time gap progress during and after composite polymerization (Hayashi et al. 2017). Hayashi et al. performed real-time cross-sectional imaging using a 2D scan SS-OCT system, and obtained a video at a resolution of 800×600 pixels and 20 frames/ s. In addition, 3D scans were obtained after light curing at different times. The authors observed gap propagation even after composite light curing was completed and the two-step self-etch adhesives tested produced less gap formation compared to one-step self-etch adhesives (Hayashi et al. 2017).

The bonding performance of a restorative system can be evaluated using various parameters, including marginal adaptation, bond strength, and interaction with the tooth substrate (Tagami et al. 2010). Using SS-OCT, it is possible to non-destructively obtain valuable information regarding the restorative material-tooth interface and correlate the obtained data with bond strength tests of the same sample. Generally, SS-OCT studies reported that with the increasing in brightness percentage at the interfacial zone, bond strength values decreased (Bakhsh et al. 2013; Makishi et al. 2015b).

OCT results are highly dependent of the type of restorative material (Makishi at al 2015a; Makishi at al 2015b) and filling technique used (Bakhsh et al. 2013; Fronza et al. 2018). Self-adhesive restorative composites were compared to conventional restoration (based on three-step etch-and-rinse adhesive and hybrid composite) by OCT and dentin bond strength. The results showed that although a self-adhesive presents similar brightness values at the dentin/composite interface to conventional restorative system, lower bond strength was obtained with both self-adhesive materials compared to a conventional system (Makishi et al. 2015a). Confocal laser scanning microscopy images were used to confirm the presence of brightness areas at the interface between the composite and dentin detected by OCT method. The studies have shown that gap formations and debonded areas can be easily observed in confocal microscopy, validating the OCT data and images (Makishi et al. 2011, 2015a).

Regarding filling techniques, another OCT study evaluated the same conventional restorative system and compared to low-viscosity and packable bulk filling composites (Fronza et al. 2018). Considering that the conventional restorative system was the control and the gold standard incremental restorative technique, only one flowable bulk fill composite did not differ from the control, according to the marginal adaptation results by OCT method. However, the bonding efficacy of all restorative materials may decrease over the long-term, according to the dentin bond strength test (Makishi et al. 2011; Fronza et al. 2018).

4.4 Final Considerations

SS-OCT is a promising imaging method that can be used to assess marginal adaptation and gap formation in various composite based restorations (Makishi et al. 2015a; Fronza et al. 2018) and for long-term follow-up studies regarding sealing ability (Makishi et al. 2011, 2015b). As digital technology evolves, the increasing demand for a wider range of dental materials with improved properties must be met. Concurrently, chair-side diagnosis using SS-OCT imaging represents a promising tool for the selection of appropriate dental treatments and preventive measures. Thus, OCT method will allow monitoring the clinical performance of composite restorations and the quality of marginal sealing at composite/tooth interface that is related to the long-term bonding stability of restorations.

References

Ayad, M. F., Maghrabi, A. A., Saif, R. E., García-Godoy, F. 2011. Influence of tooth preparation burs on the roughness and bond strength of adhesives to human dentin surfaces. *American Journal of Dentistry* 24: 176–182.

Bakhsh, T. A., Sadr, A., Shimada, Y. et al. 2013. Concurrent evaluation of composite internal adaptation and bond strength in a class-I cavity. *Journal of Dentistry* 41: 60–70.

Bakhsh, T. A., Sadr, A., Shimada, Y., Tagami, J., Sumi, Y. 2011. Non-invasive quantification of resin-dentin interfacial gaps using optical coherence tomography: Validation against confocal microscopy. *Dental Materials* 27: 915–925.

Bista, B., Sadr, A., Nazari, A., Shimada, Y., Sumi, Y., Tagami, J. 2013. Nondestructive assessment of current one-step self-etch dental adhesives using optical coherence tomography. *Journal of Biomedical Optics.* 18: 076020.

Fronza, B. M., Makishi, P., Sadr, A., Shimada et al. 2018. Evaluation of bulk-fill systems: Microtensile bond strength and non-destructive imaging of marginal adaptation. *Brazilian Oral Research* 32: 1–12.

Fujimoto, J. G., Drexler, W. 2008. *Optical coherence tomography imaging: Technology and applications.* Springer.

Hayashi, J., Shimada, Y., Tagami, J., Sumi, Y., Sadr, A. 2017. Real-time imaging of gap progress during and after composite polymerization. *Journal of Dental Research* 96: 992–998.

Huang, D., Swanson, E., Lin, C. P. et al. 1991. Optical coherence. *Science* 254:1178–81.

Makishi, P., Pacheco, R.R., Sadr, A. et al. 2015a. Assessment of self-adhesive resin composites: nondestructive imaging of resin-dentin interfacial adaptation and shear bond strength. *Microscopy and Microanalysis* 21: 1523–1529.

Makishi, P., Thitthaweerat, S., Sadr, A. et al. 2015b. Assessment of current adhesives in class I cavity: Nondestructive imaging using optical coherence tomography and microtensile bond strength. *Dental Materials* 31: 190–200.

Makishi, P., Shimada, Y., Sadr, A., Tagami, J., Sumi, Y. 2011. Non-destructive 3D imaging of composite restorations using optical coherence tomography: Marginal adaptation of self-etch adhesives. *Journal of Dentistry* 39: 316–325.

Shimada, Y., Nakagawa, H., Sadr, A. et al. 2014. Noninvasive cross-sectional imaging of proximal caries using swept-source optical coherence tomography (SS-OCT) in vivo. *Journal of Biophotonics* 7: 506–513.

Tagami, J., Nikaido, T., Nakajima, M., Shimada, Y. 2010. Relationship between bond strength tests and other in vitro phenomena. *Dental Materials* 26: 1–5.

5

Dental Materials Evaluation by Optical Coherence Tomography

Anderson S. L. Gomes,[1] **Cláudia C. B. O. Mota**[2,3] **and Gabriela Monteiro**[4]

[1]*Universidade Federal de Pernambuco, Physics Department and Graduate Program in Dentistry, Av. Prof. Luis Freire s/n, Recife, Pernambuco, Brazil*

[2]*Faculty of Dentistry, Centro Universitário Tabosa de Almeida, ASCES-UNITA, Brazil*

[3]*School of Dentistry, Universidade de Pernambuco, Campus Arcoverde, UPE, Brazil*

[4]*Universidade de Pernambuco, Dental School, Hospital Universitário Oswaldo Cruz, Faculdade de Odontologia da Universidade de Pernambuco – FOP/UPE, R. Arnóbio Marques, Santo Amaro, Recife-PE, Brazil*

CONTENTS

5.1 Introduction

The subject of dental materials encompasses quite a broad and multidisciplinary range of topics, as recently reviewed in the book by Rezaie and collaborators (Rezaie et al., 2020). Another recent review can also be of interest for broad insight into the subject (Iftikhar et al., 2021). There is a wide variety of dental materials, encompassing all classes of materials: polymers,

DOI: 10.1201/9781351104562-5

metals, ceramics and composites, with each class of material depending on the intended purpose. For instance, resin-based materials, composites and ceramics are used as restorative solutions, enabling bonding to the tooth structure and the tooth restoration itself. Different alloys are used in dental implants, prosthodontics, orthodontics and endodontic instruments. Polymers are used in all areas of dentistry, as impression materials, in prosthetic rehabilitation, implant components, and orthodontic appliances. Nanomaterials and bioceramics have also been recently widely utilized in dentistry. The materials can be employed in various areas, used as instruments, and therapeutic applications for preventive, temporary or final purposes. Therefore, a proper evaluation of dental materials depends on their purpose, and different methods, including invasive and destructive ones, have been employed. Non-invasive imaging methods such as scanning, transmission electron microscopes, or x-rays are generally destructive.

This chapter deals with the use of OCT to evaluate, in a non-invasive and non-destructive way, dental materials, both in the lab environment but also intra-oral evaluations in clinical settings. We shall skip revising OCT technical details, historical content and operational modes, already described in earlier chapters. Also, in Chapters 3, 4, 6, 7, 8 and 9, dental materials were implicitly employed in the related treatments, and OCT applied to those branches of dentistry was exploited in the indicated chapters. In this chapter, we shall review the applications of OCT to characterize dental materials, covering several examples from pioneer work to the recent literature. A search on the homepage of OCTNEWS (octnews.org) with the terms "OCT in dental materials" brings 68 articles. Among those, we highlight the use of OCT to evaluate spiral dental polishing systems (Silva et al., 2023), self-etch adhesives (Bakhsh and Turkistani, 2021), polymeric dental restorations (Bakhsh et al., 2020), pre-heated dental fissure-sealing materials (Borges et al., 2016), nanomaterials (gold and silver nanoparticles, Braz et al., 2012), dental prostheses (Sinescu et al., 2010), dental ceramics (Sinescu et al., 2011), fiber reinforced dental composites (Kyotoku and Gomes, 2007), nanoparticles in endodontic irrigating solutions (Topala et al., 2021), resin composites (Lammeier et al. 2012, Monteiro et al., 2011a, Monteiro et al., 2011b), sealants (Braz et al., 2011). One significance for OCT application related to dental materials is the possibility of evaluation of those materials once placed in the patient's mouth *in vivo*, as reported by Graça et al. (2019) and Castello et al. (2021), for observation of adhesive interface in oral aesthetic rehabilitation and the evaluation of ceramic veneer adaptation, respectively.

In what follows, we describe selected examples from the literature and our group in Brazil, covering some of the applications described above.

5.2 OCT Evaluation of Dental Resin Composites

Dental resin composites are restorative materials based on synthetic resins that can bond to the tooth structure. The bonding strengthens the tooth's structure and effectively restores its physical integrity. Dental resin composites are usually employed as an adhesive or restorative material for direct or indirect applications. The indirect restorations are bonded to the tooth structure using resin-based luting agents. For instance, resin composites are widely used for veneers in aesthetic rehabilitation. As previously mentioned, these veneers may be directly (built-up in the mouth) or indirectly prepared (fabricated in a dental laboratory and later bonded to the tooth). Regardless of how the restorations are made, the bonding process is critical and can be directly evaluated by OCT *in vivo*, as will be discussed.

As a recent example, an evaluation of the internal adaptation of class V resin restorations on dentin using OCT was performed (Abdelaziz et al. 2020). Using a commercially available (Axsun) swept-source OCT operating at 1310 nm with an axial resolution of 6.8 μm in the air, the authors studied 32 extracted posterior teeth, divided into groups, with two groups (eight each) having simulated caries in the dentin restored with Clearfil APX resin composite. Through OCT images, it was possible to visualize air bubbles and defects in the internal and marginal adaptations. An earlier work (Monteiro et al., 2011a) also employed a commercially available OCT system (Spectral radar OCP930SR/Thorlabs) with 930 nm central wavelength for evaluating resin composite restorations marginal integrity. For their study, class I cavities were prepared in 30 extracted human premolars and were randomly divided according to the restorative systems evaluated: Filtek P90™/P90 Adhesive System™, Filtek Z350™, and Filtek Z250™/Single Bond™ (3 M/ESPE). The qualitative analysis of the OCT images of the internal margins did not show noticeable gaps even after an A-scan examination. On the other hand, distinctive patterns were found for each restorative system, whereas penetration of Single Bond and Filtek P90 self-etch primer into dentin was also observed. A thick adhesive layer was found for the Filtek P90 bonding agent. Figure 5.1 shows the OCT image results of a single bond application, and Figure 5.2 shows representative OCT images for a sample restored with a P90 adhesive system.

In analyzing Figure 5.1, the authors described the observation of the interactions between the bonding agents and the tooth's substrates. For the conventional two-step bonding agent, Single Bond, they pointed out the presence of a very thin and diffuse zone on dentin after 35% phosphoric acid etching, corresponding to the structural alterations of the tissues after the procedure. The unpolymerized Single Bond layer initial penetration into the substrate could be observed. After polymerization, very few changes were visualized. On the other hand, for the P90 Adhesive System, the interaction of the primer with dental substrates could be observed, as well as the

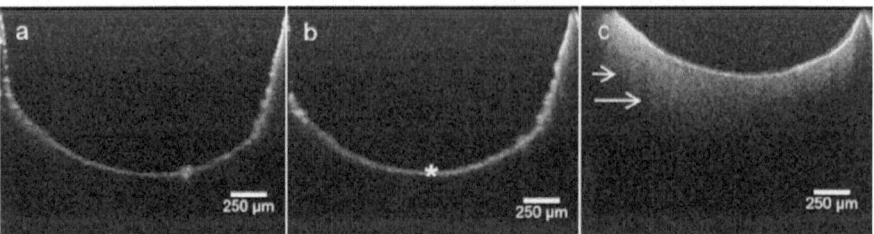

FIGURE 5.1

Single Bond application: (a) prepared cavity and (b) after 35% phosphoric acid etching. Note that the interface line (asterisk) is now thicker than in (a); (c) after a Single Bond application. Note the diffusion of the bonding agent into the dentin substrate (arrows). Reprinted with permission from (Monteiro et al., 2011a) © Elsevier Science & Technology Journals.

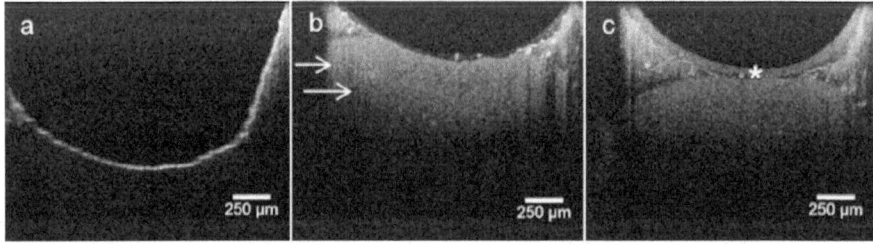

FIGURE 5.2

The P90 adhesive system: (a) prepared cavity and (b) after self-etching primer application. Note the diffusion of the primer into the dentin substrate (arrows); (c) after bond application. Note the presence of another distinct layer (asterisk). Reprinted with permission from (Monteiro et al., 2011a) © Elsevier Science & Technology Journals.

application of a second layer (bond) could also be distinguished by OCT imaging, as identified in Figure 5.2.

Other examples of OCT studies in composite resins include the determination, in a non-invasive way, of the shrinkage of restorative resin composites from different brands (Monteiro et al. 2011b). The results showed that polymerization shrinkage values vary with the method used, and the authors could determine the material that suffered the least shrinkage.

Under clinical service, resin composite restorations are constantly submitted to mechanical, chemical and biological challenges. Regarding some detrimental effects, the material undergoes fatigue and can lead to fractures within the material. Early failures can be visualized through the observation of initial crack propagation. In the work of Kyotoku and Gomes (2007) and Braz *et at.* (2009), a homebuilt OCT operating in the spectral domain was used to evaluate crack propagation artificially induced in rectangular bar specimens of composite resin (Suprafill®, SSWHITE) reinforced by different dental fibers (Superfiber®, Superdont, and Interlig®, Angelus). The OCT scanning was carried out before and after the thermal/mechanical cycling of specimens and, through the images, it was possible to observe the features of crack propagation, which could be qualitatively compared to theoretical patterns predicted in the literature.

5.3 OCT as a Tool to Assess the Integrity of Dental Sealants

It is widely recognized that dental sealants are important in providing mechanical protection against caries by sealing pits and fissures, although somewhat overlooked regarding applications, particularly in developing countries (Kassebaun et al., 2015). A recent study by (Balian et al., 2022) entitled "long-term caries prevention of dental sealants and fluoride varnish in children with autism spectrum disorders: a retrospective cohort study" reported an 11-year data analysis. Although the example given here was for children with disability, children without and in an unfavorable condition of buccal hygiene should also be taken care of regarding caries prevention.

In 2011, we demonstrated the ability of OCT to evaluate the integrity of dental sealants (Braz et al., 2011). For evaluation of the structure of pit and fissure sealants, a home-built spectral OCT system, see diagram in Figure 5.3,

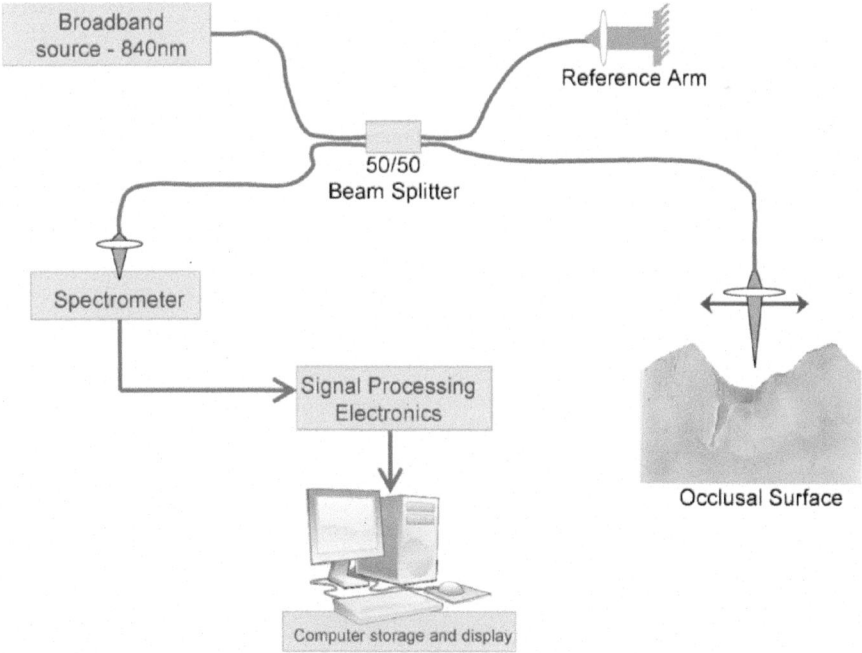

FIGURE 5.3

Schematic setup of SD-OCT used to evaluate sealant integrity. Reprinted with permission from (Braz et al., 2011) © Elsevier Science & Technology Journals.

operating in the spectral domain (SD-OCT) at 840 nm and a measured spatial resolution of 10 µm, was employed.

Five human third molars were employed for the sealant integrity evaluation, and the light-cured resin-based sealant Alpha Seal Light (DFL) was applied following the manufacturer's instructions.

The occlusal surfaces of the teeth were scanned in a buccolingual direction, and tomographic images parallel to the long axis of the tooth were obtained. The crowns were sectioned in the occlusal-gingival direction, and new images from each section were obtained and evaluated by an optical microscope for comparison. The representative images provided by the OCT system clearly showed the surface and the internal structure of dental sealant applied over the tooth, and the subjacent enamel, as seen in Figures 5.4–5.6. Sealant and enamel were very well distinguished, and failures at the interior and at the surface were well detected.

It can be seen in Figure 5.4 A, a shallow and wide fissure, whereas Figure 5.4B shows a deep and narrow fissure. Following the application of the dental sealant, the superficial limit of the material is delineated by a high-intensity homogenous and high-intensity white line due to the difference

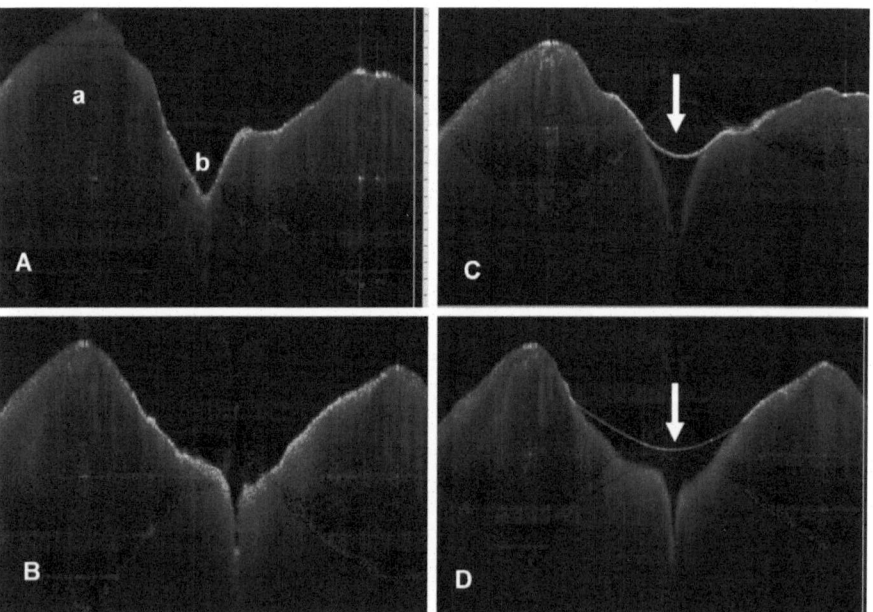

FIGURE 5.4

OCT images showing the comparison between the fissures before (A and B) and after (C and D) the sealant application. Small letters (a) and (b) indicate the tooth enamel and pit region, respectively. The arrow indicates the sealant–air interface. No defects can be observed in the sealant region. Reprinted with permission from (Braz et al., 2011) © Elsevier Science & Technology Journals.

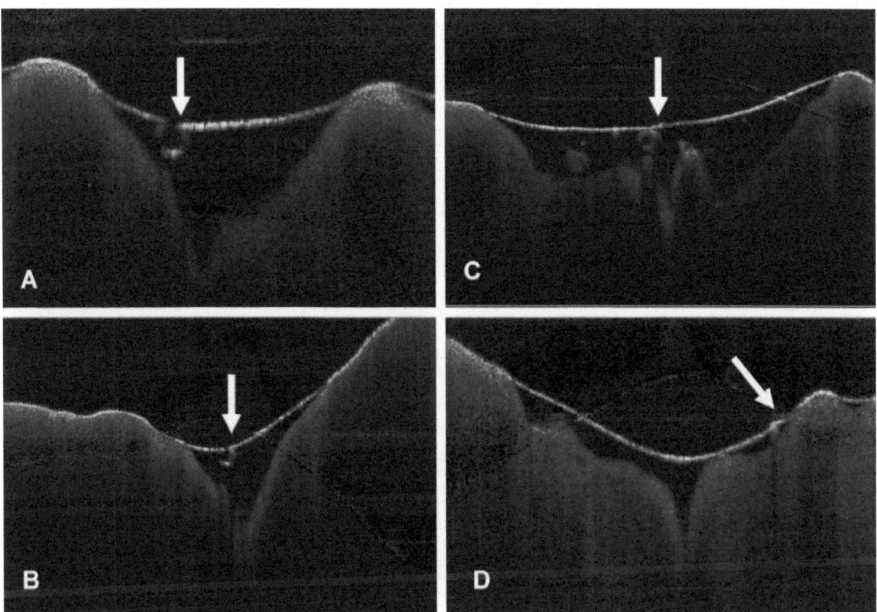

FIGURE 5.5
OCT images after sealant application. The arrows indicate the presence of bubbles (A–C) in the sealant region and gap (D) in the sealant–tooth interface. Reprinted with permission from (Braz et al., 2011) © Elsevier Science & Technology Journals.

in the refractive index compared to air. In that example, no defects were detected.

Conversely to the results of Figure 5.4, Figure 5.5 shows unwanted defects after the sealant application. The bubbles on the surface or internally in the sealant region are seen in Figures 5.5A–C. In contrast, Figure 5.5D shows a gap between the sealant and the tooth structure (indicated by the arrow).

Finally, Figure 5.6 shows that sealant penetration is incomplete, and a direct comparison with a stereomicroscopic image (Figure 5.6A), is shown, where a bubble located at the tooth–sealant interface, into the fissure, can be observed. This feature was also clearly observed in the OCT image of Figure 5.6B. The comparison with the stereomicroscopic demonstrates the ability of OCT in detecting sealant defects, so an OCT handpiece device could be a valuable tool for clinical imaging of posterior teeth.

The results in this section showed how the OCT is a powerful imaging tool for analyzing the structure of pit-and-fissure sealants and the subjacent enamel substrate, able to provide images of fissures, bubbles and failures in the adaptation of sealants. Its use can undoubtedly aid in monitoring sealant application and long-term retention. More recent research on this subject has been published by Oancea et al. (2015). Further *in vivo* studies are still required to potentialize the technique for clinical application.

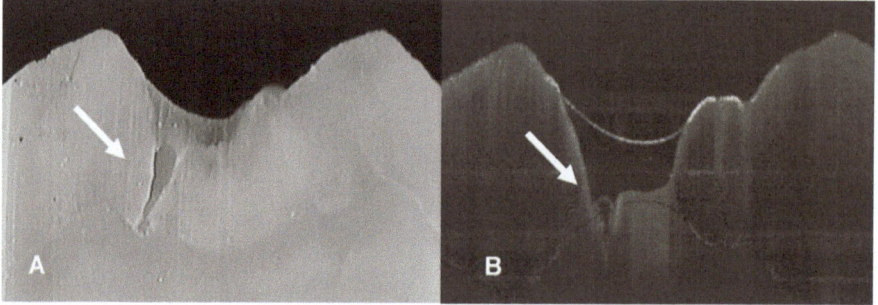

FIGURE 5.6
Optical microscope (A) and OCT (B) images of a tooth with incomplete sealant penetration.
The arrows in A and B indicate the region where the sealant failed to adapt to the tooth.
Reprinted with permission from (Braz et al., 2011) © Elsevier Science & Technology Journals.

5.4 OCT to Evaluate Dental Polishing Systems

In restorative dentistry, besides the restorative materials themselves, finishing and polishing procedures, essential for improving aesthetics and increasing the longevity of dental restorations, also require special instruments. Nowadays, these instruments are made of different materials, including diamond or carbide burs, diamond-impregnated rubber wheels, polishing discs and cups, as some examples. Different shapes and sizes are manufactured within the same polisher to fit the adaptation to the surface best to be polished.

Spiral-shaped polishers were introduced not so long ago for use as reduced-step polishers. They contain diamond particles impregnated in rubber and have unique shapes provided to be adaptable to all tooth surfaces. However, some instruments have a limited lifetime and are discarded based on manufacturer instruction or operator experience. Therefore, a means of evaluating the instrument wear is desirable. We recently demonstrated that OCT could provide a valuable measurement tool to evaluate the performance of spiral polishers associated with resin composites and ceramics (Silva et al., 2023). Two aspects were evaluated: the smoothness pattern achieved in the polished materials and the structural wear suffered by the polisher, which was the study's primary aim. Two two-step spiral polishing systems were evaluated on resin composite (Tetric N-Ceram, Ivoclar Vivadent, Schaan, Liechtenstein), feldspathic ceramics (Cerec Blocs, Dentsply Sirona, Bensheim, Germany) and nanohybrid glass-ceramic composite (Brava Block, FGM Dental Products, Joinvile, Brazil). A polishing protocol was employed to ensure reproducibility (see Silva et al., 2023, for further details and specimen preparation and polishing protocol).

TABLE 5.1

Specimens and Polishers Evaluated with OCT

Polisher	Restorative Material		Acronym
MR	Composite resin (R)	Medium-grit resin polisher X composite resin	MR-R
FR		Fine-grit resin polisher X composite resin	FR-R
MC	Ceramic (C)	Medium-grit ceramic polisher X ceramic	MC-C
EFC		Extra-fine grit ceramic polisher X ceramic	EFC-C
MR	Composite glass-ceramic (GC)	Medium-grit resin polisher X composite glass-ceramic	MR-GC
FR		Fine-grit resin polisher X composite glass-ceramic	FR-GC
MC	Composite glass-ceramic (GC)	Medium-grit ceramic polisher X composite glass-ceramic	MC-GC
EFC		Extra-fine grit ceramic polisher X composite glass-ceramic	EFC-GC

Source: From Silva et al., 2023, with permission.

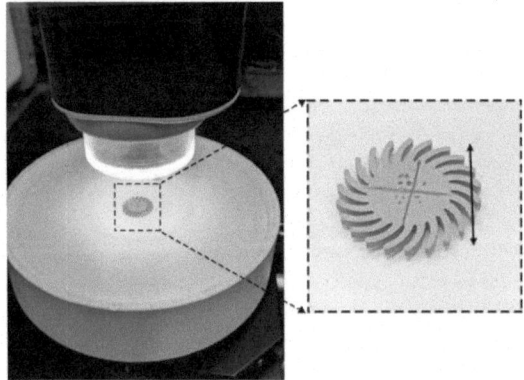

FIGURE 5.7
OCT head with polisher in place and an enlarged view of the polisher under illumination. Arrows indicate the direction of the scan, with the beam coming from the top of the sample. The sample can be rotated to scan all four quadrants. Reprinted with permission from (Silva et al., 2023) © The Optical Society.

For this work, a commercial OCT system (Ganymede, Thorlabs Inc., New Jersey, USA), operating in the spectral domain (SDOCT), with a super luminescent diode as a light source, with 930 nm of the central wavelength, 100 nm of spectral bandwidth, and a maximum output power of 5 mW and axial resolution of 7.5 μm was employed.

The specimens and polishers evaluated are shown in Table 5.1, and Figure 5.7 shows the OCT head with the polisher in place.

The surface roughness of restorative materials was measured, and images of the polishers were acquired by OCT and stereomicroscope, as shown in Figures 5.8 and 5.9.

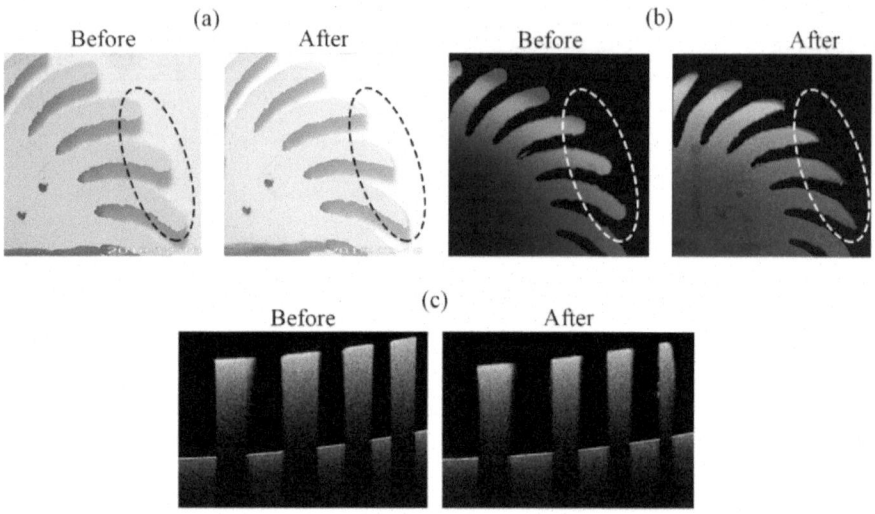

FIGURE 5.8

(a) Stereomicroscope; (b) and (c) OCT en face and B-scan, respectively, images for EFC-C obtained before (T0) and after (T10) polishing. Image (b) shows the surface of the polisher, providing information equivalent to the stereomicroscope image (a). In the region demarcated by the ellipse, the alteration of the bristle tip of the polisher can be observed. Figure (c) shows OCT 2D in which the thickness of each polish bristle can observe lateral wear. This image was taken in the same region as (b). Reprinted with permission from (Silva et al., 2023) © The Optical Society.

The images of the polishers were obtained and compared at 03 different times: before use (T0), after five uses (T5), and after ten uses (T10). 2D images acquired with OCT were processed and evaluated using ImageJ Software (National Institutes of Health, Bethesda, MD), and also used to generate the 3D images.

In Figure 5.8(a), the images acquired by the stereomicroscope are shown, while in Figures 5.8(b) and 5.8(c), images were obtained from the 3D and 2D OCT scan, respectively, after using ImageJ software. The en face of 3D scan images give us information equivalent to the stereomicroscope image. In contrast, considering the shape and thickness, the 2D scan enhances the lateral wear, which can be seen for each polish bristle, particularly in the external region. The swept region in Figure 5.8(b) (identified by the dashed ellipse) indicates changes in the extremity of the polishing bristles before and after its use. As the OCT beam sweeps different regions of the polisher bristles, it is possible to observe wear in different regions of the structure. The OCT images readily confirm these findings in Figure 5.9.

The main conclusion for this section is that spiral polishers performed well in promoting surface smoothness in ceramic and glass-ceramic composites. After ten uses, surface area variation was observed on all polishing

Before   After

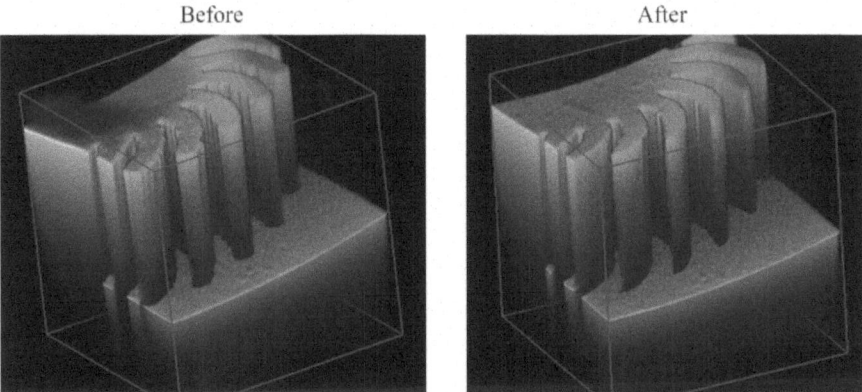

FIGURE 5.9
OCT 3D image in *over* mode in time (T0) and after (T10). The reduction of bristle thickness after 10 polishing cycles (the image shows a quadrant) can be observed. This image can be obtained throughout the polisher. Reprinted with permission from (Silva et al., 2023) © The Optical Society.

instruments except for one combination: the medium-grit polisher tested in ceramic. OCT proved to be a tool capable of evaluating qualitative and quantitative (see quantitative results in Silva et al. 2023) wear areas in the polishing systems. Therefore, from the data shown, OCT finds another application as an important alternative tool for evaluating polishers, filling this information gap regarding these dental materials.

5.5 OCT in Clinical Evaluation for the Performance of Dental Materials

In modern days, the oral aesthetic is a social demand for different reasons, and follow-up of oral aesthetic rehabilitation is generally performed through visual inspection and radiographic examinations. However, both methods may not suffice for properly evaluating treatment success. In this section, we describe the use of OCT as a follow-up method for evaluating the adhesive interface of ceramic laminate in a clinical environment (Castello et al., 2021). It is worth mentioning that the gingival recovery was also followed up in one of the case reports (Graça et al., 2019), which was performed prior to the laminate placement. OCT provides a unique way to evaluate *in vivo* the placement of laminates in a patient, identifying if there are any immediate failures.

The use of ceramic veneers has increased in recent years, mainly due to their aesthetic appeal and biocompatibility, besides abiding by the principles

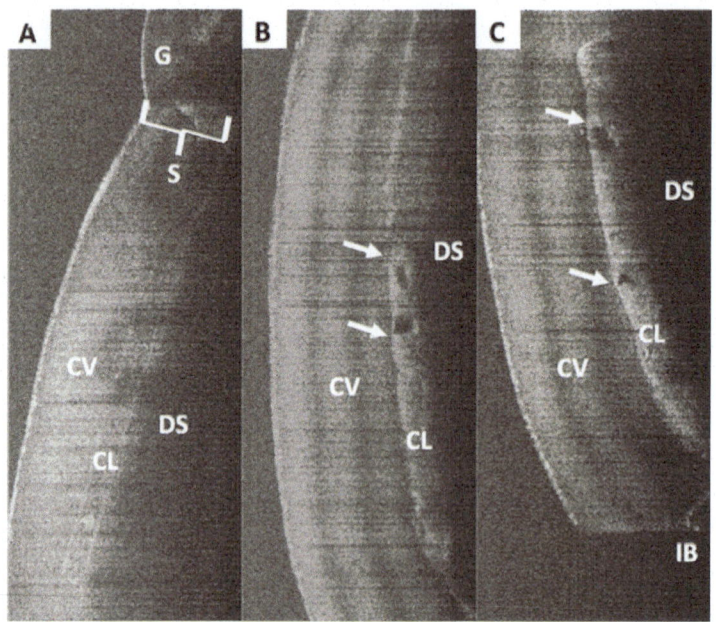

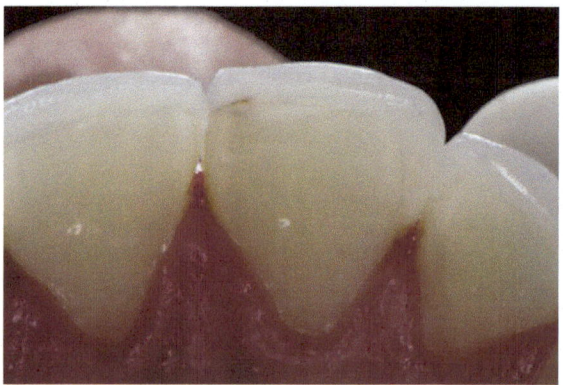

FIGURE 5.10

(Bottom) Palatal view of the right maxillary central incisor. (Top) Initial sagittal OCT images of the right maxillary central incisor. The cervical (A), middle (B) and incisal (C) thirds of the right maxillary central incisor show the dental substrate (DS), gingiva (G), gingival sulcus (S) and incisal border (IB), as well as the presence of the ceramic veneer (CV) and cementation line (CL). Arrows show the presence of bubbles and gaps in the cementation line. (Castello et al., 2021, with permission).

of minimal-invasive dentistry. They are a restoration procedure of choice to correct tooth forms/position, close diastemas, restore tooth fracture, or even mask tooth discolorations. They have high compressive strength, surface smoothness and gloss and present low or almost no plaque accumulation.

However, the most frequent failures reported in ceramic veneers are marginal discoloration, debonding, fracture/chipping, and secondary caries. In two earlier studies (de Andrade Borges et al., 2015; Fernandes et al., 2016), OCT has been employed to evaluate *in vitro* ceramic laminate's performance regarding adhesion to a tooth surface. The reported work showed the feasibility of OCT use in the clinical environment, as recently reported by (Graça et al., 2019; Castello et al., 2021). In the case report work of (Castello et al., 2021), a 24-year-old female patient was unsatisfied with the observation of a color change in the ceramic veneer placed on the right maxillary central incisor. The OCT system used was the SS-OCT 1325 nm (Thorlabs, New Jersey USA), operating in Fourier Domain (spectral bandwidth ~100 nm, axial scan rate of 16 kHz/25 fps, lateral resolution ~25 μm and axial resolution of 12 μm in air). Figure 5.10 (left) shows a photograph of the tooth, whereas Figure 5.10 (right) shows the OCT sagittal images showing the presence of gaps or bubbles, suggesting the cause for the color change.

With the patient signed informed consent, a proposed treatment consisting of repair of the restoration by infiltration of a resin composite was carried out. Visual inspection gave satisfactory results, but the OCT system still showed failures, not detected by the naked eye, as seen in Figure 5.11.

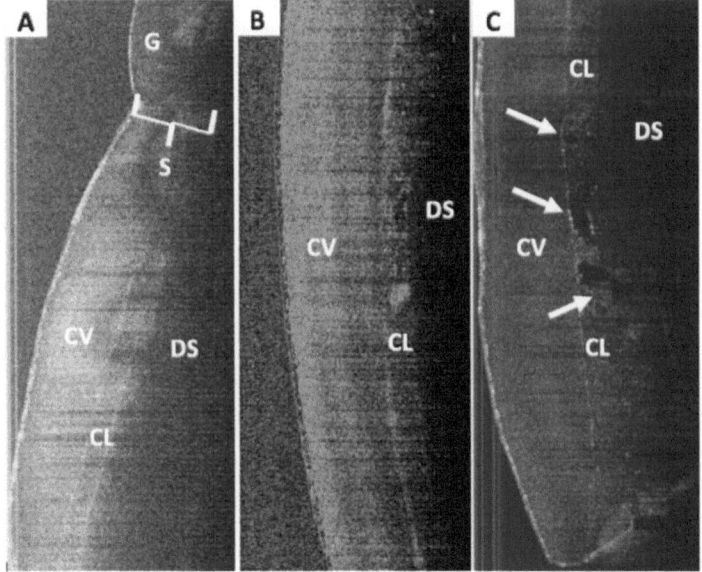

FIGURE 5.11
Sagittal OCT images of the right maxillary central incisor after repair. The cervical (A), middle (B) and incisal (C) thirds of the right maxillary central incisor show the dental substrate (DS), gingiva (G), gingival sulcus (S) and incisal border (IB) as well as the presence of the ceramic veneer (CV) and cementation line (CL). Arrows show the presence of bubbles and gaps in the cementation line. (Castello et al. 2021, with permission).

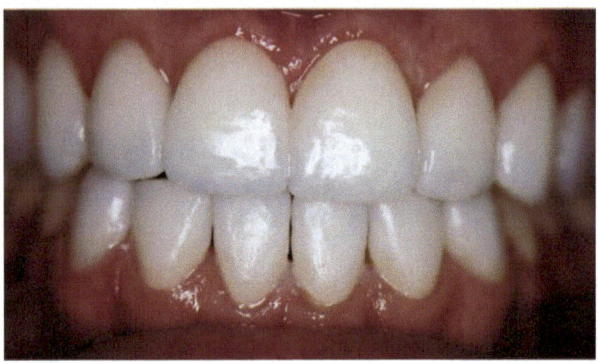

FIGURE 5.12
Immediate clinical view after the cementation of the veneers. (Graça et al., 2019, with
permission).

In a related work using the same OCT system as in Castello's (2021) work,
Graça et al. (2019) attended a 23-year-old woman reporting dissatisfaction
with the visual appearance of her smile, which was related to the presence of
yellowish teeth, a generalized anterior diastema, and a gummy smile. With
the patient's signed consent, treatment consisted of periodontal plastic surgery, tooth whitening, and cementation of ceramic veneers. Figure 5.12 shows
the patient's result immediately after the cementation of veneers (for further
details, see Graça et al., 2019).

Figure 5.13 shows a sagittal OCT set of images of the right maxillary central
incisor showing a normal tooth and its surrounding periodontal structures of
the patient, including follow-up images after the periodontal plastic surgery
and veneer placement.

5.6 Conclusion

This chapter dealt with using OCT to evaluate different aspects of dental
materials. The knowledge of dental materials is essential to understand the
materials' clinical performance in all areas of dentistry, being an extensive
area of research and applications.

Besides the given references, OCT applied to dental materials covers
much more than this chapter has covered. We highlighted applications in
dental composites, sealants and spiral dental polishing systems. We showed
how OCT has been used to evaluate dental materials once placed in the
patient's mouth.

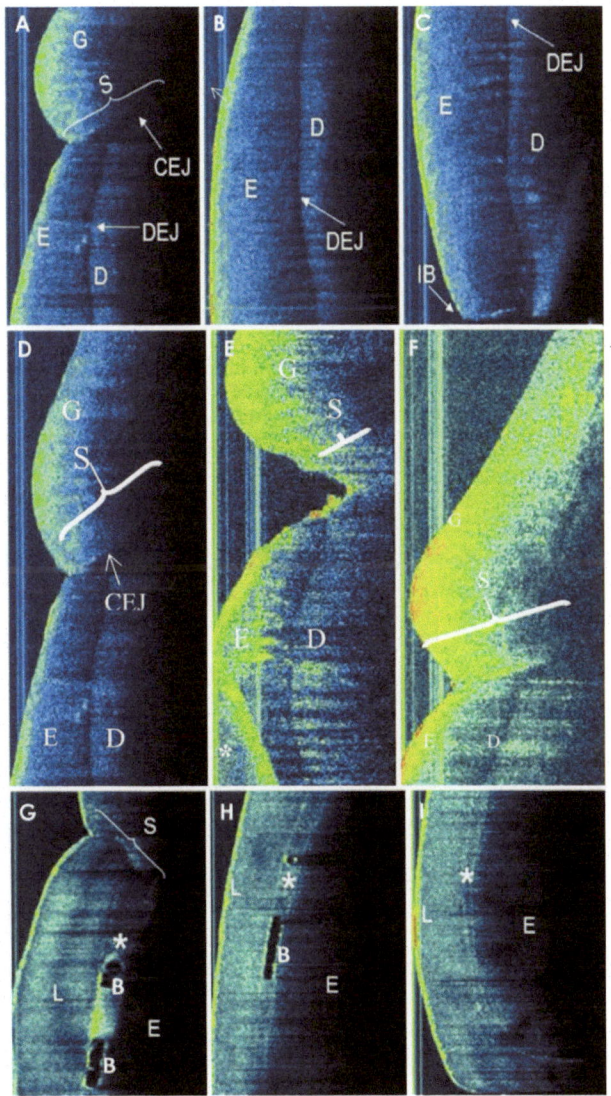

FIGURE 5.13

Sagittal optical coherence tomography images. The cervical (A), middle (B) and incisal (C) thirds of the right maxillary central incisor show a normal tooth and its surrounding periodontal structures, such as enamel (E), dentin (D), the dentin-enamel junction (DEJ), the cementoenamel junction (CEJ), gingiva (G), gingival sulcus (S) and incisal border (IB). (D) Cervical third of the tooth at 15 days (E) and 60 days (F) after the periodontal plastic surgery demonstrating gingival recovery, given the formation of a new gingival sulcus around the teeth and close contact of the gingiva with the tooth, as shown before surgery. The cervical (G), middle (H) and incisal (I) thirds of the right maxillary central incisor after cementation of the ceramic veneers showing the tooth and its surrounding periodontal structures, as well as the presence of the cementation line (*), bubbles (B) and the laminate veneer (L). (Graça et al., 2019, with permission).

Furthermore, several other studies have been reported on subsurface defect detections (Duncan et al., 1998), evaluation of single ceramic crowns (Gabor, 2016), fiber-reinforced dentures (Negrutiu et al., 2008a), complete denture analysis (Negrutiu et al., 2008b), temperature effects during sintering of metal-ceramic tooth prostheses (Sinescu et al., 2017).

The use of OCT in dental materials' evaluation is undoubtedly one of the most promising niches of OCT applications in dentistry, which deserves further assessment and worldwide-scale dissemination.

References

Abdelaziz, M., Zuluaga, A.F., Betancourt, F., Fried, D., Krejci, I., Bortolotto, T. 2020. Optical coherence tomography (OCT) for the evaluation of internal adaptation of class V resin restorations on dentin. *Proc SPIE Int Soc Opt Eng.*

Bakhsh, T.A., Tagami, J., Sadr, A., Luong, M.N. et al. 2020. Effect of light irradiation condition on gap formation under polymeric dental restoration; OCT study. *Zeitschrift für Medizinische Physik* 30: 194–200.

Bakhsh, T. A., Turkistani, A. 2021. The effect of thermocycling on interfacial bonding stability of self-etch adhesives: OCT study. *BioMed Research International* Vol. 2021, Article ID 5578539: 9 pages.

Balian, A., Campus, G., Bontà, G. et al. 2022. Long-term caries prevention of dental sealants and fluoride varnish in children with autism spectrum disorders: a retrospective cohort study. *Sci Rep.* 12: 8478.

Borges, B.C.D., de Assunção, I.V., de Aquino, C.A., Monteiro, G.Q.M., Gomes, A.S.L. 2016. Marginal and internal analysis of pre-heated dental fissure-sealing materials using optical coherence tomography. *International Dental Journal* 66: 23–28.

Braz, A.K.S., Kyotoku, B.B.C., Braz, R., Gomes, A.S.L. 2009. Optical coherence tomography evaluation of crack propagation in dental composites *Dental Materials* 25: 74–79.

Braz, A.K.S., Aguiar, C.M., Gomes, A.S.L. 2011. Evaluation of the integrity of dental sealants by optical coherence tomography. *Dental Materials* 27: e60–e64.

Braz, A.K.S., de Araujo, R.E., Ohulchanskyy, T.Y. et al. 2012. In situ gold nanoparticles formation: contrast agent for dental optical coherence tomography. *J. Biomed. Opt.* 17: 066003/1-5.

Castello, L.F., Osorio, L., Pedrosa, M., Heliomar, C., Gomes, A.S.L. 2021. Evaluation of ceramic veneer adaptation by optical coherence tomography: a clinical report, *Braz. Dent. Sci.* 24(2): 1–7.

de Andrade Borges, E., Cassimiro-Silva P.F., Fernandes L.O., Gomes A.S.L. 2015. Study of lumineers' interfaces by means of optical coherence tomography. *Proc. SPIE Biophotonics South America* 9531: 953147.

Duncan, M.D., Bashkansky, M., Reintjes, J. 1998. Subsurface defect detection in materials using optical coherence tomography. *Opt. Express 2*: 540.

Fernandes, L.O., Graça, N.D.R.L., Melo, L.S.A., Silva, C.H.V., Gomes, A.S.L. 2016. Optical coherence tomography investigations of ceramic lumineers. *Proc. SPIE* 9692: Lasers in Dentistry XXII: 96920P.

Gabor, A., Jivanescu, A., Zaharia, C. et al. 2016. OCT evaluation of single ceramic crowns: comparison between conventional and chair-side CAD/CAM technologies. *Sixth Int. Conf. Lasers Med.* 9670: 96700Z.

Graça, N.D.R.L., Palmeira, A.R.B.L.S., Fernandes, L.O et al. 2019. In vivo optical coherence tomographic imaging to monitor gingival recovery and the adhesive interface in aesthetic oral rehabilitation: A case report, *Imaging Science in Dentistry* 49: 171–176.

Iftikhar, S., Jahanzeb, N., Saleem, M., Ur Rehman, S., Matinlinna, J.P., Khan, A.S. 2021. The trends of dental biomaterials research and future directions: A mapping review. *Saudi Dent. J.* 33(5): 229–238.

Kassebaum, N. J., Barnabé, E., Dahiya, M., Bhandari, B., Murray, C.J.L., Marcenes, W. 2015. Global burden of untreated caries: a systematic review and metaregression. *J. Dent. Res.* 94: 650–658.

Kyotoku, B.B.C., Gomes, A.S.L. 2007. Dental fiber-reinforced composite analysis using optical coherence tomography, *Opt. Commun.* 279: 403–407.

Lammeier, C., Li, Y.P., Lunos, S., Fok, A., Rudney, J., Jones, R.S. 2012. Influence of dental resin material composition on cross-polarization-optical coherence tomography imaging. *J. Biomed. Opt.* 17(10): 106002.

Monteiro, G.Q.M., Montes, M.A.J.R., Gomes, A.S.L., Mota, C.C.B.O., Campello, S.L., Anderson Z. Freitas, A.Z. 2011a. Marginal analysis of resin composite restorative systems using optical coherence tomography. *Dental Materials* 27: e213–e223.

Monteiro, G.Q.M., Monte, M.A.J.R., Rolim, T.V. et al. 2011b. Alternative methods for determining shrinkage in restorative resin composites. *Dental Materials* 27: e176–e185.

Negrutiu, M.L., Sinescu, C., Hughes, M. et al. 2008a. Fibres reinforced dentures investigated with en-face optical coherence tomography. *Biophotonics Photonic Solut. Better Heal. Care* 6991: 69911U.

Negrutiu, M.L., Sinescu, C., Todea, C., Podoleanu, A.G. 2008b. Complete denture analyzed by optical coherence tomography. *Lasers Dent.* XIV 6843: 68430R.

Oancea, R., Bradu, A., Sinescu, C. et al. 2015. Assessment of the sealant/tooth interface using optical coherence tomography. *J. Adhes. Sci. Technol.* 29: 49–58.

Rezaie, H.R., Rizi, H.B., Khamseh, M.M.R., Öchsner, A. 2020. *A Review on Dental Materials*, Springer Cham.

Sinescu, C., Negrutiu, M.L., Ionita, C et al. 2010. Morphological characterization of dental prostheses interfaces using optical coherence tomography, *Proc. SPIE* 7626, *Medical Imaging 2010: Biomedical Applications in Molecular, Structural, and Functional Imaging*, 76261P.

Sinescu, C., Negrutiu, M.L., Ionita, C. et al. 2011. Biomedical implications of dental-ceramic defects investigated by numerical simulation, radiographic, microcomputer tomography, and time-domain optical coherence tomography *Proc. SPIE* 8172, *Optical Complex Systems*. OCS11: 817207.

Silva, K.Y.S., Falcão, C.M.C., Fernandes, L.O., and Gomes, A.S.L. 2023. Exploiting optical coherence tomography to evaluate wear in spiral dental polishing systems. *Appl. Opt.* 62: C8–C13.

Sinescu, C., Bradu, A., Duma, V.F., Topala, F., Negrutiu, M. 2017. Effects of temperature variations during sintering of metal-ceramic tooth prostheses investigated non-destructively with optical coherence tomography. *Appl. Sci.* 7: 1–14.

Topala, F., Nica, L., Boariu, M. et al. 2021. Optical coherence tomography analysis of gold and silver nanoparticles in endodontic irrigating solutions: An in vitro study. *Exp. Ther. Med.* 22: 992.

6

Optical Coherence Tomography in Endodontics

Carlos Menezes Aguiar[1] and Anderson S. L. Gomes[2]

[1]*Universidade Federal de Pernambuco, Graduate Program in Dentistry, Av. Prof. Luis Freire s/n, Recife, Pernambuco, Brazil*

[2]*Universidade Federal de Pernambuco, Physics Department and Graduate Program in Dentistry, Av. Prof. Luis Freire s/n, Recife, Pernambuco, Brazil*

CONTENTS

6.1 Introduction

Imaging exams are an essential component of the diagnosis of endodontic problems. It supports all procedures of endodontic treatment from diagnosis and treatment planning to assessing outcome. The amount of information acquired from analogic X-ray film or digitally captured periapical radiographs are limited by the fact that the three-dimensional anatomy of the area being radiographed is compressed into a two-dimensional image. These problems may be solved using imaging techniques that can produce three-dimensional images of individual teeth and the surrounding tissues.

DOI: 10.1201/9781351104562-6

Optical coherence tomography (OCT) was developed in medical imaging technology that was first introduced in 1991 (Huang et al. 1991). Since then, it has become a standard tool in ophthalmology and the chosen imaging method for a diversity of other pathologies, as revised in Drexler and Fujimoto (Drexler et al. 2015).

OCT potential in endodontics is already well documented. OCT images of hard and soft tissues in the oral cavity were compared with histology images as a gold standard using animal models, or *in vitro* studies using human natural teeth showing an excellent match, as will be reviewed in this chapter.

6.2 Basics on Pulp-Dentin Complex

The dental pulp is an ectomesenchymal differentiated tissue that produces the dentin component of teeth. The intimate anatomic and physiologic relationships between both tissues have encouraged dentists to refer to these tissues as the pulp-dentin complex (Sloan 2014). The odontoblast process and nerves of the pulp that reside within the dentinal tubules make dentin a living tissue. Consequently, when carrying out clinical operative procedures, the operator must view dentin in the same way as other living tissue. The pulp and dentin are integrally connected in the sense that physiologic and pathologic reactions in one of the tissues will also affect the other. Figure 6.1(a) shows a typical tooth structure, while in Figure 6.1(b) a histologic section with more details of the dentine-pulp region can be seen.

6.3 Root Canal Morphology Studies

The knowledge and a detailed understanding of the root canal anatomy and its variations is imperative to ensure successful root canal therapy. Shemesh & cols (Shemesh et al. 2007) evaluated the ability of an optical coherence tomography (OCT) system in imaging root canal walls after endodontic preparation and correlated the images to histologic sections. They presented a qualitative discussion of the intensity distribution in OCT images, compared to the micrographs, and what information these provide about the dentin. They concluded that the OCT proves to be a reliable method to image root canals and root dentin in a nondestructive way (van Soest et al. 2008). To obtain the endodontic imaging Shemesh & cols (Shemesh et al. 2007), employed an optical fiber probe whose tip was placed inside the root canal so that the distal end is inserted through the apex. The apical constriction was

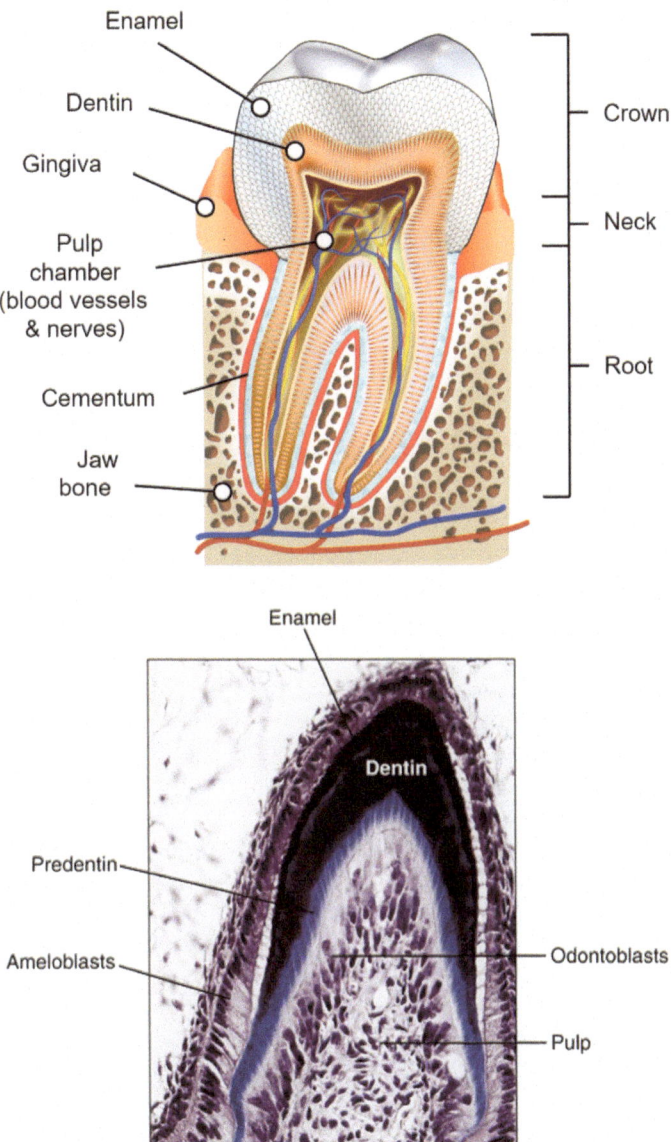

FIGURE 6.1

(Top) Illustrative parts of a tooth, showing the pulp-dentin complex (Human tooth diagram. By K. D. Schroeder, reprinted with permission from National Library of Medicine, Mesh ID D003804 – 2001, NIH). (Bottom) In histologic sections, predentin stains distinctively from dentin. (Reprinted with permission from Dentin-Pulp Complex, © Pocket Dentistry.)

opened thus with #45 K-file to allow the optical fiber to penetrate through the canal. OCT pullback scans were performed by using a commercially available OCT system (LightLab Imaging M2-CV system in combination with an ImageWire 2 catheter) employed for intracoronary imaging in atherosclerotic plaque diagnosis. The tooths were single-rooted mandibular incisors, and further details can be seen in (Shemesh et al. 2007).

The works of Shemesh & cols and van Soest & cols (Shemesh et al. 2007; van Soest et al. 2008) were pioneer in the application of OCT in endodontics, where they presented the first data of an experiment investigating the potential of OCT to identify vertical root fracture and showed the promise of the technique for full *in vivo* endodontic imaging.

6.4 Detection of Vertical Root Fracture

A vertical root fracture (VRF) is a root fracture extending along the longitudinal axis of roots and is often noted in endodontically treatment (Chan et al. 1999). VRF is a considerable threat to the prognosis of a tooth during and after root canal treatment (Shemesh et al. 2007; van Soest et al. 2008). VRFs present a challenge to the clinician in that the diagnosis is often difficult and is based on subjective parameters. The current available methods to clinically diagnose VRF include illumination, X-ray, periodontal probing, staining, surgical exploration, bite test, direct visual examination and operative-microscope examination. All of these have limited success (Morfis 1990; Fuss et al. 1999; Tamse et al. 1999). Radiographic images could reveal VRF only if the X-ray beam is parallel to the fracture line (Rud et al. 1970). The cone-beam computed tomography (CBCT) is a three-dimensional imaging modality and its use for the diagnosis of endodontic alterations and treatment plans is increasing, with significant potential for VRF diagnosis (Gaêta-Araujo et al. 2017). For teeth with gutta-percha, fiber glass and metal into the root canal the CBCT seems to influence the detection of VRF in a significant manner (Salineiro et al. 2019; Iikubo et al. 2020).

Shemesh et al. presented an *in vitro* study where OCT was employed for evaluating VRF (Shemesh et al. 2008). In their study, the authors describe a methodology for detection of VRF. All teeth (pre-molars) were pooled and scanned with an M2-CV OCT system (LightLab Imaging Inc, Westford, MA) in combination with an ImageWire 2 catheter that had a diameter of 0.3 mm at its thinnest part with a "pullback" technique starting at the apex, same system as used in the work of Shemesh & cols (Shemesh et al. 2007). Figures 6.2 and 6.3 show the main results.

In analyzing the data in Figures 6.2 and 6.3, the authors concluded that, because the values of sensitivity and specificity, which were measured and reported in Shemesh & cols (Shemesh et al. 2008), fell inside the 95%

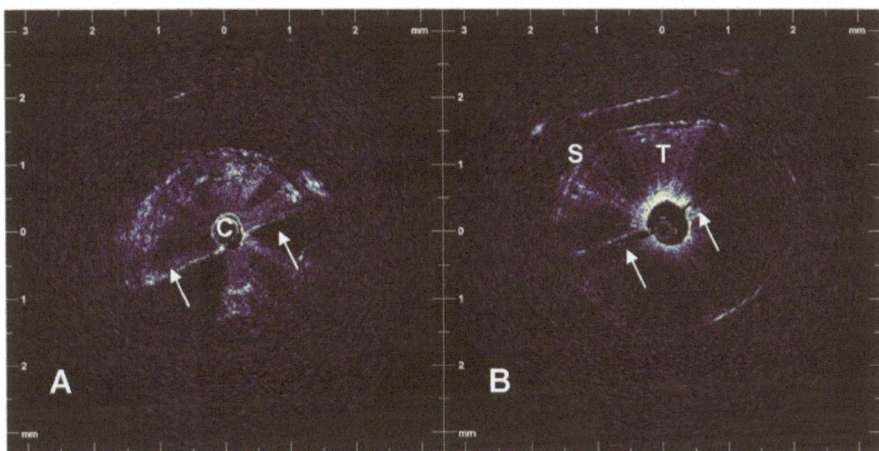

FIGURE 6.2
Appearance of VRF through an OCT scan. (A) VRF extends through the root 2.5 mm from the apex on 2 opposing sides of the canal; it appears as a bright line. The OCT catheter (C) is inside the canal. (B) VRF that has separated the dentin, 8 mm from the apex; the crack can be traced to the external root surface (S), and dentinal tubules can also be identified (T). Reprinted with permission from (Shemesh et al. 2008) © Elsevier Science & Technology Journals.

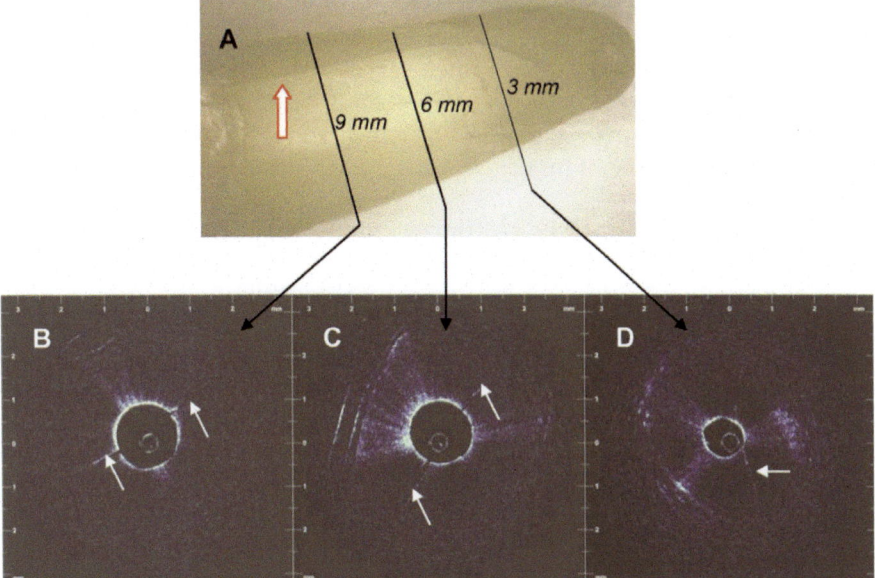

FIGURE 6.3
Root sample (A) where the fracture is marked by an arrow, and the corresponding OCT images at 9 mm (B), 6 mm (C) and 3 mm (D) from the apex. OCT visualization of the VRF is marked by arrows. Reprinted with permission from (Shemesh et al. 2008) © Elsevier Science & Technology Journals.

confidence interval from one of the measured groups to the other group, the groups did not differ regarding of these parameters. Therefore, specifity and sensitivity measured by three different observers in two groups proved that OCT can be a reliable method. Besides, no statistical differences were measured between the groups.

It is worth pointing out that the research of Shemesh & cols (Shemesh et al. 2008) was carried out using an OCT probe designed for intracoronary imaging in atherosclerotic plaque diagnosis and is commercially available for clinical use in cardiac catheterization laboratories. An appropriate similar probe designed for dental applications, not yet available, could perform even better regarding imaging generation.

6.5 Viewing the Pulp-Dentin Interface

The pulp-dentin interface is a sensitive region and extreme care must be taken when treating the dentin to avoid invading the pulp chamber. Braz & cols (Braz et al. 2009) showed that OCT images of human pulp-dentin complex were able to provide information in a very clear way compared with histology as the gold standard, thus providing a powerful tool for noninvasive and nondestructive procedures in particular situations in which the healthy pulp should not be unnecessarily exposed. Furthermore, OCT at two different wavelengths were evaluated in (Fonsêca et al. 2009) by the same group, aiming to identifying which should be more appropriate from the point of view of image contrast, and further compared the results with CBCT.

The OCT system employed in (Braz et al. 2009b) was a SD-OCT home-built system, based on a femtosecond Ti:sapphire mode-locked laser operating at 800 nm. To obtain an improved axial resolution, the output beam of the femtosecond laser was further broadened by self-phase modulation in an optical fiber, to provide image resolution of $6\,\mu$m in depth and 30 μm laterally. The typical SD-OCT scheme is reproduced in Figure 6.4(a), which employs a fiber-based beam-splitter. Other experimental details can be found in (Braz et al. 2009b).

The images of pulp-dentin complex were taken by scanning the occlusal surface in a mesiodistal direction. The laser penetrated into the teeth structure, and a tomographic image of pulp-dentin complex, parallel to long axis of teeth, was obtained. The whole system was controlled by a LabVIEW supported software (National Instruments Corporation, Austin, TX) that collected and processed the data generating the tomography image. The pulp-dentin complex is clearly seen in Figure 6.4, and well delineated, as observed in 6.4(b, c). As indicated in Figure 6.4(c) the pulp exposition site is

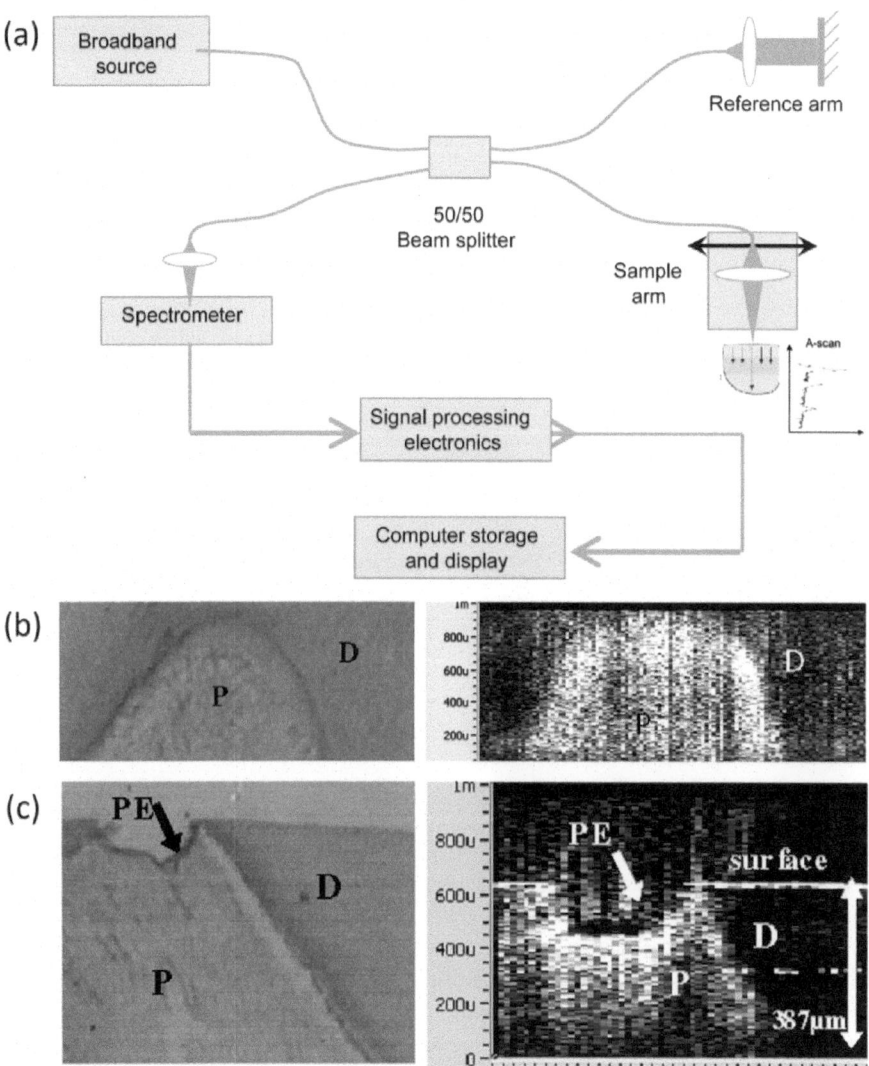

FIGURE 6.4

(A) Diagram of home-built spectral OCT. (B) Left, histologic image of dentin-pulp interface. Right, OCT image. (C) Site of pulpal exposure. Left, histologic cross-section. Right, OCT image. (P, pulp; D, dentin). Adapted with permission from (Braz et al. 2009b) © Elsevier Science & Technology Journals.

shown in the OCT image as a discontinuity at the dentin surface as a homogenous white line of high intensity, well reproducing the histologic image.

Further evaluation of the pulp-dentin complex was performed by comparing two different OCT systems (SD-OCT and TD-OCT), also operating at two different wavelengths (850 nm and 1280 nm, which allow different penetration depths due to the different extinction coefficients), besides comparing with CBCT. The experimental setup and main results are shown in Figure 6.5.

The basics and technical details on the two schemes depicted in Figure 6.5(A) can be seen in (Fonsêca et al. 2009) and in chapter 2. The results of Figure 6.5(B) show the CBCT images, where the important point to be raised is its limited resolution of 120 µm. Figure 6.5(C) shows the OCT images obtained with both systems, where the gap between dentin and pulp chamber is well resolved, particularly with the 850 nm SD-OCT system. One can envisage this kind of system being used as a niche application when dentin treatment is being carried out and OCT can be exploited on-site to allow controlling the dentin-pulp distance to a safe margin.

6.6 SS-OCT Applications

SS-OCT, as an alternative to FD-OCT, has been widely employed in dentistry studies. This section highlights some recent results, although in the other topics in this chapter SS-OCT may also have been employed. In 2014, Iino & cols (Iino et al. 2014), reported a study investigating the ability of swept-source optical coherence tomographic (SS-OCT) imaging to detect a second mesiobuccal canal (MB2) in maxillary molars compared with visual inspection and dental operating microscopy.

A SS-OCT system (Prototype 2; Panasonic Health Care Co Ltd, Tokyo, Japan; 1330 nm center wavelength; 30 kHz sweep rate; 10 mW output power) had an axial resolution of 12 µm in air (8 µm in tissue). Other technical information can be seen in (Iino et al. 2014). Figure 6.6 shows the cross-sectional images of the sample showing (a) micro-CT image and (b) OCT image. MB2 is indicated by the arrows in both images.

In the work reported in (Nakajima et al. 2014), cracks were created in 30 porcine premolars subject to impact. SS-OCT images and direct comparison with stereomicroscopic photographs of the surface were acquired for each specimen before and after impaction. Histological sections were also prepared after impaction. The length and width of cracks and lamellae were then evaluated and compared to the corresponding SS-OCT image. As a result, cracks and lamellae were clearly detected, as seen by intensified scattering signals on corresponding positions obtained by microphotographs and histological sections. Significant correlations regarding line length and width were observed between SS-OCT and histological sections (length: $r = 0.65$, $P < 0.001$; width: $r = 0.60$, $P < 0.001$).

In yet another work described in (de Oliveira et al. 2017), the authors evaluated and compared the ability of SD-OCT and SS-OCT systems to detect

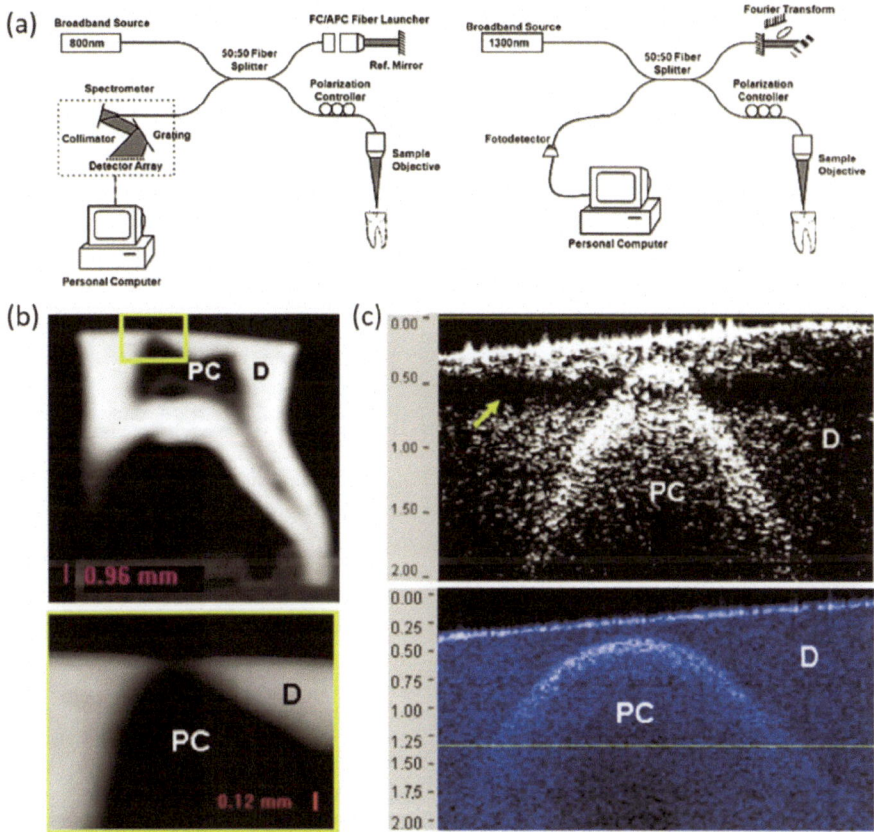

FIGURE 6.5

(A) Schematic diagram of the two optical coherence tomography systems employed: (left) SD-OCT operating at 850 nm and TD-OCT operating at 1280 nm with a Fourier domain delay line. (B) i-CAT cone beam volumetric tomography image of the dentin and pulp chamber studied: (top) 0.12 mm slice longitudinal of the tooth and (bottom) zoom 400% at the dentin-pulp interface. (C) OCT images of the dentin D and pulp chamber PC corresponding to the i-CAT CBVT image of (B): (top) OCT at 1280 nm and (bottom) OCT at 850 nm. (The black transversal region indicated by the arrow is an artifact.) Reprinted with permission from Fonseca, Deborah DD, *et al.* "In vitro imaging of remaining dentin and pulp chamber by optical coherence tomography: comparison between 850 and 1280 nm". *Journal of Biomedical Optics* 14.2 (2009): 024009.

apical dentinal microcracks. The gold standard for comparison was a micro-CT system. Human single-rooted (mandibular) incisors were employed, which had the root canal appropriately prepared with R40 Reciproc file. The results of their research showed that, according to micro-CT measurements, 60% of the roots (for $N=20$) presented dentinal microcracks in the apical region. The images generated by the OCT systems showed microcrack lines located at

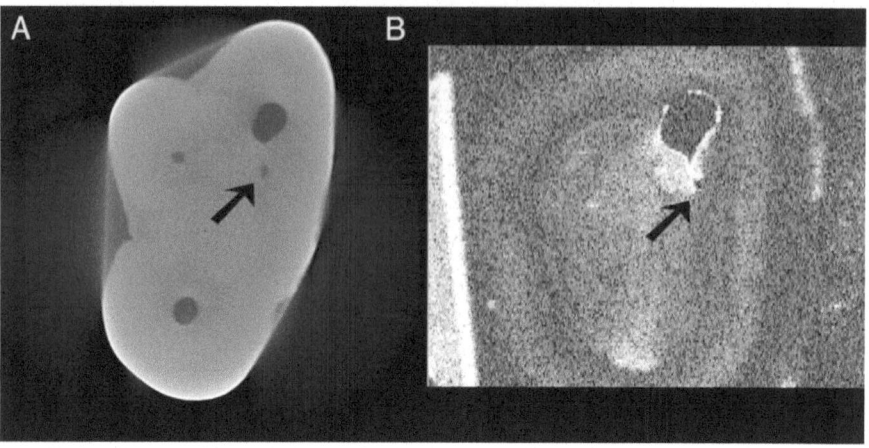

FIGURE 6.6
Cross-sectional images of the samples studied in (Iino et al. 2014), showing (A) micro-CT image and (B) OCT image. MB2 is indicated by the arrows in both images. Reprinted with permission from (Lino et al. 2014) © Elsevier Science & Technology Journals.

the same position as the corresponding micro-CT cross sections. As for the comparison between the two OCT systems, there were no statistically significant differences between the two OCT devices ($P > 0.05$). Inter-examiner (03 independent examiners) agreement was substantial to almost perfect for the SD-OCT system and moderate to almost perfect for the SS-OCT system, whereas intra-examiner agreement was substantial to almost perfect for both OCT devices. The main conclusion of de Oliveira & cols (de Oliveira et al. 2017) was that the detection ability was verified for both OCT systems, which makes them promising tools for the imaging diagnostics of apical microcracks. In (Suassuna et al. 2018), the authors analyzed the use of OCT on apical endodontic filling, and compared the results with micro-CT. The *in vitro* work compared the differences in the apical filling regarding working length (WL) change and presence (or absence) of voids, besides validating the use of OCT in comparison with micro-CT for the detection of failures in the apical filling. Both the micro-CT (parameters: 80 kV, 222 µA) and SS-OCT (1300 nm) had very close axial resolutions (11 µm and 12 µm, respectively). The studied group was composed of 45 inferior premolars, and preparation followed protocols described in (Suassuna et al. 2018). The images were analyzed by two blind and calibrated observers using ImageJ software to measure the boundary of the obturation WL and voids' presence. Quantitatively, the WL average remained constant for all obturation techniques and image methods. OCT showed adequate sensitivity and specificity to detect voids in the WL of apical obturations *in vitro* in comparison with µCT. Both image methods found a higher number of voids for LC technique (µCT $p = 0.011$/OCT $p = 0.002$).

More recently, and evaluation of apical root defects when two different nickel-titanium (NiTi) are used for canal instrumentation, using a SS-OCT with axial and transverse image resolutions of 16 μm and 25 μm, respectively, was reported by Chen & cols (Chen et al. 2022). They were motivated by the fact that advances in rotary NiTi instruments have opened the way to new designs and techniques for root canal preparation. Two of the most commonly used are Pro-Taper Universal (Dentsply Maillefer, Ballaigues,Switzerland) and HyFlex CM (Coltene-Whaledent, Allstetten, Switzerland). Their findings, according with the procedures and limitations of the experiments performed in (Chen et al. 2022), were that when the canals of mandibular incisors were instrumented with apical files (size #30 and #40), the Pro-Taper Universal system would create more defects than the HyFlex CM system. The use of OCT was only limited by its penetration depth.

6.7 Crack Formation and Propagation

Crack formation and propagation in hard tissue can arise from different causes and can occur in dental composites (Braz et al. 2009a) as well as from dentinal defects during microsurgical endodontics (Rashed et al. 2019). In both cases, OCT has been a reliable method to observe the detrimental effect.

In the work reported in (Braz et al. 2009a), 2 mm × 3 mm × 25 mm bar specimens of fiber reinforced composite were employed after mechanical and thermal cycling to emulate oral conditions. These samples had their inner parts imaged by OCT prior to and after loading. The SD-OCT used was a home-built system working at 800 nm with 6 μm axial resolution. As a result, it was clearly seen that OCT images provide an insight into crack propagation, which is not naturally seen by the naked eye.

More recently, the study reported in (Rashed et al. 2019) had as the objective the determination of the effect of root-end resection, ultrasonic root-end preparation, and root-end filling on the incidence of crack formation and propagation by using three different optical methods: a digital microscope (DM), optical coherence tomography (OCT) and micro-CT as a reference standard. The aim was to evaluate the performance of OCT on the detection of cracks when compared with microcomputed tomography. The samples were extracted human mandibular incisors, without the existence of caries, restoration and root canal treatments. Proper preparation procedures are described in detail in (Rashed et al. 2019). The micro-CT employed (inspeXio SMX-100CT, Shimadzu, Kyoto, Japan) was used twice: before any treatment (to exclude existing fractures or cracks) and after 60 days of the root-end resection filling. Exposure parameters were set at 80 kV and 130 μA with a voxel size of 20 μm. The OCT device was a commercially available SS-OCT

(Santec OCT-2000, Santec Co., Komaki, Japan), used immediately following the root-end resection, ultrasonic preparation and root-end filling. Follow-up scanning was performed at 15 days, 30 days and 60 days. The axial resolution of this system in air is 11 µm, which is equal to 7 µm in dental tissue (considering the refractive ~1.5). Each sample was also evaluated using a digital microscope (DM; VH-8000, Keyence, Osaka, Japan) with 40× magnification. Figure 6.7 shows the representative results of the research carried out in (Rashed et al. 2019). The samples employed in the measurements were randomly divided into three groups ($n = 10$). This division was made according to the material for root-end filling: group MTA was filled with ProRoot MTA (Dentsply Sirona) and group EBA was filled with and super-EBA fast set (Harry J. Bosworth, Skokie, IL, USA). No obturation was done in the control group.

The capital A in Figure 6.7 is used to identify the DM images, showing crack formation after root-end resection (indicated by the arrows). DM observation detected crack formation in 47% and 87% of samples after the root-end resection and ultrasonic root-end cavity preparation, respectively, as described in (Rashed et al. 2019). Forty percent of the resected surfaces had new dentinal cracks after the ultrasonic preparation, while only 3% had dental cracks that propagated from a partial crack to a complete crack.

The capital B indicates the representative OCT images, which corresponds to the DM images (capital A). The differences in contrast in the dentin are clear and the crack line is visualized as a white line caused by the high backscattered intensities. OCT detected crack formation in 40% of the samples after the root-end resection and in 30% of the samples after the ultrasonic root-end cavity preparation, according to Rashed & cols (Rashed et al. 2019). However, an important outcome of Rashed & cols (Rashed et al. 2019) was that, under their experimental condition, OCT showed an overall lower performance in detecting dentin crack lines compared with DM. Several reasons are pointed out by the authors and this point deserves further research.

More recent work exploited en-face OCT (efOCT) to evaluate endodontic fillings (Țogoe et al. 2021), and to analyze, *in vitro*, the use of gold and silver nanoparticles in endodontic irrigating solutions (Topala et al. 2021).

In the work of Togoe & cols (Țogoe et al. 2021), an *in vitro* study was carried out to assess the quality of endodontic fillings by using efOCT, micro-CT and SEM (scanning electron microscopy). 14 freshly extracted human teeth (caries free) were selected and used. For the endodontic filling, the employed technique was the continuous wave of compaction.

An OCT system operating at 1300 nm with a depth resolution of 10 µm in air was employed, with a confocal channel operating at 970 nm to guide the OCT investigation. The system operated in time domain efOCT mode and provided real-time images in two orthogonal planes (B- and C-scans).

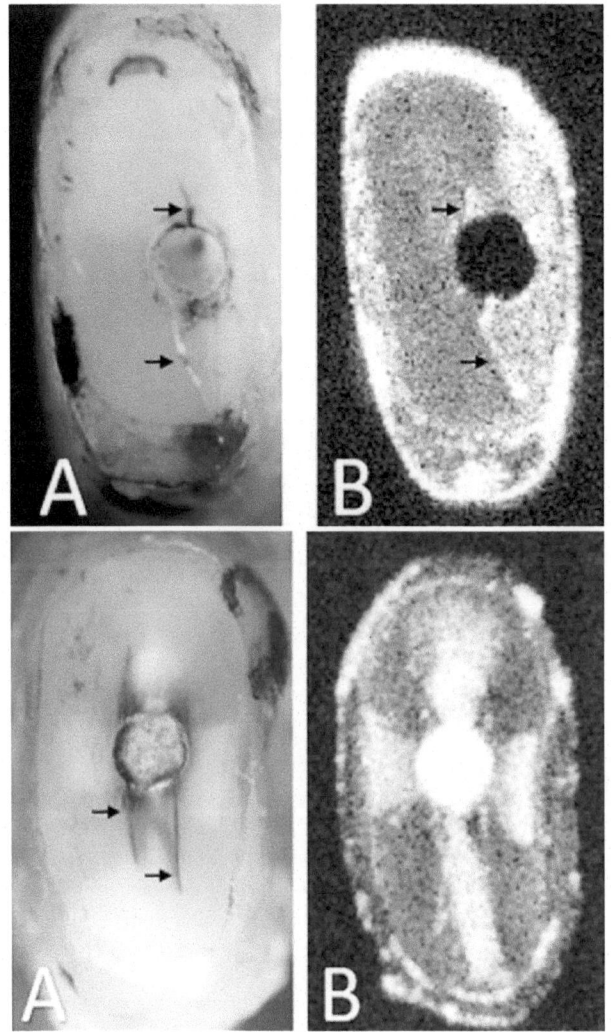

FIGURE 6.7
Representative images showing the same surface by DM (A) and OCT (B). (top) MTA
group after two months of obturation. (bottom) Control group immediately after ultrasonic
preparation. The crack lines are indicated by the arrows. Reproduced from (Rashed et al. 2019).

Figure 6.8 shows the clinical aspects of the endodontic filling technique and
a radiographic evaluation.

Examples of the results obtained in (Ţogoe et al. 2021) are shown in
Figure 6.9. efOCT shows defects at the interface formed by the root canal
wall and endodontic filling material. For some investigated samples, the
defects are inside the endodontic filling material, such as representative

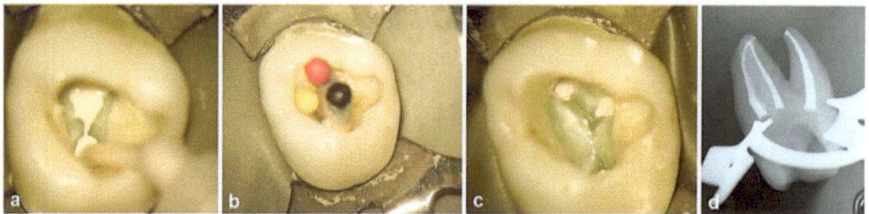

FIGURE 6.8
(a–c) Clinical aspects of the endodontic filling technique. (d) Radiographic evaluation of one of the prepared samples. Reprinted with permission from (Țogoe et al. 2021) © Romanian Academy Publishing House.

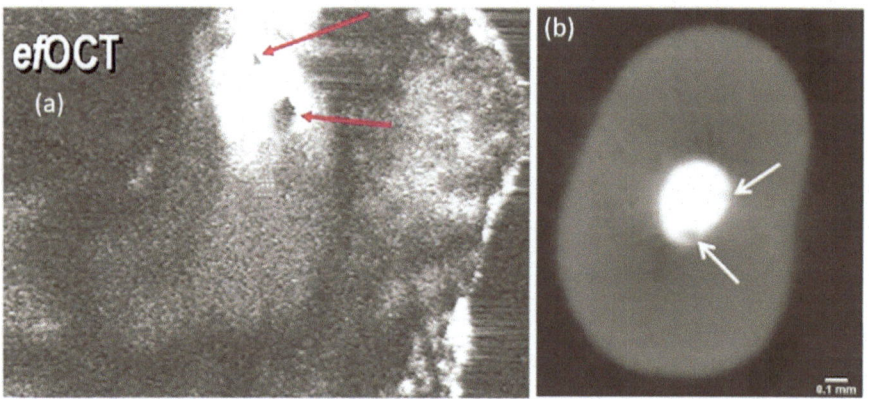

FIGURE 6.9
(a) C scan image (0.95 Å~0.95 mm), approximately 0.975 mm inside the apical root measured in depth, 18° lateral scanning size. (b) µCT investigation of the same sample presented in (a). µCT: microcomputed tomography. Reprinted with permission from (Țogoe et al. 2021) © Romanian Academy Publishing House.

images in Figure 6.9, which compares efOC and microCT for the same sample.

Two gaps in the apical end can be seen in Figure 6.9(a), laterally positioned toward the dentin walls of the root canal. The high contrast between the filling material and dentin is clearly defined. The efOCT image was validated by µCT investigation. The 2D cross-sectional image of the apical end filling demonstrates the two defects of different diameters, Figure 6.9(b), which are marked by arrows.

The main conclusion of this work, which also used SEM to add to the comparison, was the ability of OCT to image gaps as small as 50 µm, whose resolution can be improved by using a wider band source. Another advantage is, of course, the invasiveness of the technique. Further experimental details and discussion can be found in (Țogoe et al. 2021).

6.8 Conclusion

OCT in dentistry has indeed found applications in many subareas, and this is not different for endodontics. All comparison with gold standard shown in this chapter confirm the potential of OCT for clinical environment. In particular, the FD-OCT, both SD-OCT and SS-OCT, are reliable chairside imaging tools for visualizing the boundaries of underlying bone lesions in endodontic. The FD-OCT can provide thickness and distance measurements of bone covering the lesions. OCT system renders them promising tools for diagnosis of apical microcracks. SD-OCT and SS-OCT allows for visualization of the lesion boundaries via intact bone surfaces and may be a promising practical and noninvasing adjunct tools for chairside localization of periradicular lesions in bone.

References

Braz, A.K.S., Kyotoku, B.B.C., Braz, R., Gomes, A.S.L. 2009a. Evaluation of crack propagation in dental composites by optical coherence tomography. *Dent. Mater.* 25: 74–79.

Braz, A.K.S., Kyotoku, B.B.C., Gomes, A.S.L. 2009b. In vitro tomographic image of human pulp-dentin complex: optical coherence tomography and histology. *J. Endod.* 35: 1218–1221.

Chan, C.P., Lin, C.P., Tseng, S.C., Jeng, J.H. 1999. Vertical root fracture in endodontically versus nonendodontically treated teeth: A survey of 315 cases in Chinese patients. *Oral Surg. Oral Med. Oral Pathol. Oral Radiol. Endod.* 87: 504–507.

Chen, C., Zhang, W., Liang, Y. 2022. Evaluation of apical root defects during canal instrumentation with two different nickel-titanium (NiTi) systems by optical coherence tomography (OCT) scan. *J. Dent. Sci.* 17: 763–770.

de Oliveira, B.P., Câmara, A.C., Duarte, D.A. et al. 2017. Detection of apical root cracks using spectral domain and swept-source optical coherence tomography. *J. Endod.* 43: 1148–1151.

Drexler, W., Fujimoto, J.G. 2015. *Optical Coherence Tomography: Technology and Applications*, 2nd Edition. ed. Springer.

Fonsêca, D.D.D., Kyotoku, B.B.C., Maia, A.M.A., Gomes, A.S.L. 2009. In vitro imaging of remaining dentin and pulp chamber by optical coherence tomography: comparison between 850 and 1280 nm. *J. Biomed. Opt.* 14: 024009.

Fuss, Z., Lustig, J., Tamse, A. 1999. Prevalence of vertical root fractures in extracted endodontically treated teeth. *Int. Endod. J.* 32: 283–286.

Gaêta-Araujo, H., Silva de Souza, G.Q., Freitas, D.Q., de Oliveira-Santos, C. 2017. Optimization of tube current in cone-beam computed tomography for the detection of vertical root fractures with different intracanal materials. *J. Endod.* 43: 1668–1673.

Huang, D., Swanson, E.A., Lin, C.P. et al. 1991. Optical coherence tomography. *Science Reports* 254: 1178–1181.

Iikubo, M., Kagawa, T., Fujisawa, J. et al. 2020. Effect of exposure parameters and gutta-percha cone size on fracture-like artifacts in endodontically treated teeth on cone-beam computed tomography images. *Oral Radiol.* 36: 344–348.

Iino, Y., Ebihara, A., Yoshioka, T. et al. 2014. Detection of a second mesiobuccal canal in maxillary molars by swept-source optical coherence tomography. *J. Endod.* 40: 1865–1868.

Morfis, A.S. 1990. The vertical root fracture. *Oral Surg Oral Med Oral Pathol* 69: 631–635.

Nakajima, Y., Shimada, Y., Miyashin, M., Takagi, Y., Tagami, J., Sumi, Y. 2014. Noninvasive cross-sectional imaging of proximal caries using swept-source optical coherence tomography (SS-OCT) in vivo. *J. Biophotonics* 7: 506–513.

Rashed, B., Iino, Y., Ebihara, A., Okiji, T. 2019. Evaluation of crack formation and propagation with ultrasonic root-end preparation and obturation using a digital microscope and optical coherence tomography. *Scanning 2019.* 2019: 1–6.

Rud, J., Omnell, K. A. 1970. Root fractures due to corrosion diagnostic aspects. *Eur. J. Oral Sci.* 78: 397–403.

Salineiro, F.C.S., Talamoni, I.P., Velasco, S.K., Barros, F.M., Cavalcanti, M.D.G.P. 2019. Artifact induction by endodontic materials. *Clin. Lab. Res. Dent.* 1–10.

Shemesh, H., van Soest, G., Wu, M.K., van der Sluis, L.W.M., Wesselink, P.R. 2007. The ability of optical coherence tomography to characterize the root canal walls. *J. Endod.* 33: 1369–1373.

Shemesh, H., van Soest, G., Wu, M.K., Wesselink, P.R. 2008. Diagnosis of vertical root fractures with optical coherence tomography. *J. Endod.* 34: 739–742.

Sloan, A.J. 2014. Biology of the Dentin-Pulp Complex. In: Vishwakarma, A., Sharpe, P., Songtao, S., Ramalingam, M. (Eds.), Stem Cell Biology and Tissue Engineering in Dental Sciences. *Academic Press Inc.*, pp. 371–378.

Suassuna, F.C.M., Maia, A.M.A., Melo, D.P., Antonino, A.C.D., Gomes, A.S.L., Bento, P.M. 2018. Comparison of microtomography and optical coherence tomography on apical endodontic filling analysis. *Dentomaxillofacial Radiol.* 47: 2017–20174.

Tamse, A., Fuss, Z., Lustig, J., Kaplavi, J. 1999. An evaluation of endodontically treated vertically fractured teeth. *J. Endod.* 25: 506–508.

Țogoe, M.M., Crăciunescu, E.L., Topală, F.I. et al. 2021. Endodontic fillings evaluated using en face OCT, microCT and SEM. *Rom. J. Morphol. Embryol.* 62: 793–800.

Topala, F., Nica, L.M., Boariu, M. et al. 2021. En-face optical coherence tomography analysis of gold and silver nanoparticles in endodontic irrigating solutions: An in vitro study. *Exp. Ther. Med.* 22: 1–6.

van Soest, G., Shemesh, H., Wu, M.K., van der Sluis, L.W.M., Wesselink, P.R. 2008. Optical coherence tomography for endodontic imaging. *Lasers Dent.* XIV 6843: 68430F.

7

OCT in Pediatric Dentistry

Ana Marly Araújo Maia Amorim,[1,*] Cecília Maria de Sá Barreto Cruz Falcão[2,†] and Anderson S. L. Gomes[3,‡]

[1]*Universidade Estadual da Paraíba, Dentistry Department and Post Graduate Program in Dentistry, Brazil*

[2]*Universidade Federal of Pernambuco, Graduate Program in Dentistry, Brazil*

[3]*Universidade Federal of Pernambuco, Physics Department and Graduate Program in Dentistry, Brazil*

[*]*anamarlyamaia@gmail.com*

[†]*ceciliaodonto@gmail.com*

[‡]*anderson@df.ufpe.br*

CONTENTS

7.1 Introduction

Pediatric dentistry involves preventive measures, early diagnosis and treatment of the multitude of oral diseases and conditions found in the child's and the adolescent's mouth, including caries, periodontal disease, mineralization disturbances, disturbances in tooth development and tooth eruption, and traumatic injuries (Koch et al. 2009).

The first aim consists of prevention and interception of oral diseases and soft tissue alterations to avoid complications that could increase resistance and fear of children to go to dentists. In this context, to optimize and include

DOI: 10.1201/9781351104562-7

prevention protocols to pediatric dentistry routine, the use of technology seems to be essential. In pediatric dentistry – as well as in dentistry as a whole – the most widely used non-destructive evaluation is the X-ray technique. The 2-D radiographs and also 3-D tomographs are valuable aids for the oral health care of infants, children and adolescents, allowing dentists to diagnose and treat oral diseases that cannot be detected during a visual clinical examination. However, due to ionizing radiation, there are researches focused on optimizing the X-ray dose protocols of children and adolescents.

To solve this problem, optical techniques that consist of the use of different light sources operating in a non-ionizing spectral region, such as visible-near infrared light emitting diodes (LEDs) or LASERS, applied to different system devices have been demonstrated as an excellent option to enhance chances of early diagnoses of minimal mineral loss of hard tissue, due to dental caries or erosion, and also to detect and monitor soft tissues lesions.

Considering the use of an optical technique applied to dentistry diagnostic in general, optical coherence tomography (OCT) is a non-invasive and non-destructive emerging imaging technology with a wide range of dentomaxillofacial applications, including pediatric dentistry. And is also important to emphasize the technique generate high definition 2-D and 3-D images, without ionizing radiation doses, which could be an efficient method of diagnosis in pediatric patients. OCT has already been proven to be a feasible method to detect and determine the dimensions and severity of caries by measuring the loss of penetration depth caused by the increased attenuation due to demineralization (Amaechi et al. 2003).

Owing to the differences in structure and composition between permanent and primary teeth, and also the fact that caries progresses more rapidly in primary enamel than in permanent enamel, new methods of caries diagnosis need to be tested on primary teeth (Ando et al. 2001). A full characterization by OCT of the sound enamel surface in primary teeth is also very important, because it allows that early lesions can be appropriately detected (Maia et al. 2010). SS-OCT images have shown better sensibility than visual inspection (Nakajima et al. 2014). In addition, the technique has demonstrated great potential to be used in pediatric dentistry on early caries detection with no pain (Maia et al. 2010).

It is also important to mention that the primary dentition is exposed to the physiological process in which the hard root tissues of the primary teeth are lost, allowing their replacement with permanent teeth. This process is called external root resorption. Popescu & cols (Popescu et al. 2017) were the first to use OCT to describe and compare pathological external root resorption in permanent teeth with a control group of primary teeth with physiological root resorption. The OCT analysis confirms the macroscopic aspect of the resorption lesion and distinguishes the pathological resorption lesion from physiological resorption lesion. The aspect of the OCT signal is

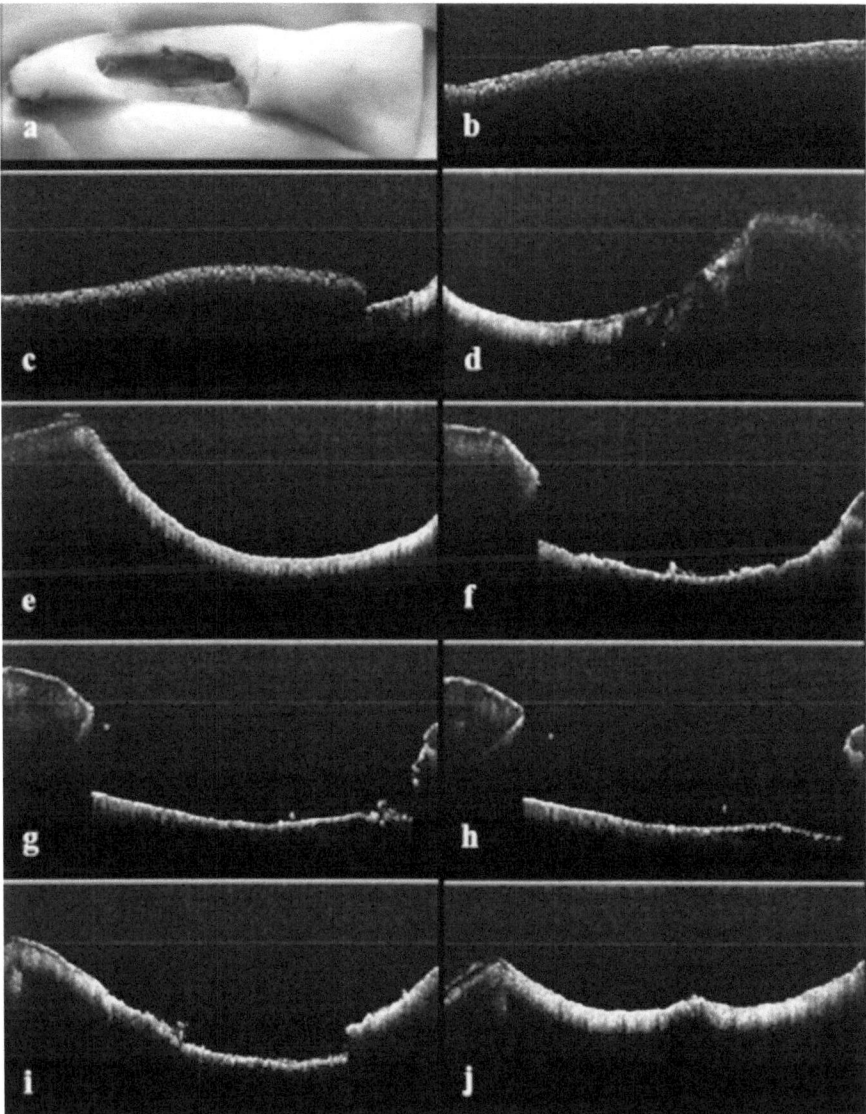

FIGURE 7.1

OCT-images (b–j) present physiological root resorption process of a primary incisor (a). Root cement (b) was observed as a well contoured OCT signal on exterior and diffuse in interior, but on (c) the exterior contour is diffused showing the root resorption advance. Root dentin exposed (d,e), pulp chamber (f–h) and root dentin (i–j) could be observed. Reprinted with permission from (Popescu et al. 2017) © Romanian Journal of Morphology and Embryology.

different in the cement comparative with dentin, being stronger in teeth with pathological resorption than physiological resorption. The morphology of OCT signal is also different between the two types of resorption, pathological resorption having a wavy form compared with smooth form in physiological resorption (Popescu et al. 2017).

Most of the OCT studies in pediatric dentistry so far focused mainly on the topics of pediatric research that have been applied to dental caries and dental restorations. In this chapter, we shall review the work beyond these two topics to include erosion monitoring evaluation and also periodontal disease. We shall consider that the readers are acquainted with the basics of OCT or can be deferred to Chapter 2.

7.2 Dental Caries in Primary Teeth

As with any optical diagnosis technique for caries, it is necessary to understand the optical properties of dental hard tissue inherent to the complex, inhomogeneous biological structure. Dental enamel is an ordered array of inorganic apatitelike crystals surrounded by a protein/lipid/water matrix (Welborn 2020). The crystals are clustered together and roughly perpendicular to the tooth surface, see Figure 7.2. Due to this structure, scattering distributions are generally anisotropic and depend on tissue orientation relative to the irradiating light source (Zijp et al. 1993; Fried et al. 1995; Darling et al. 2006) in addition to the polarization of the incident light.

The near-IR region from 780 to 1550 nm offers the greatest potential for new optical imaging modalities due to the weak scattering and absorption in dental hard tissue (Qian et al. 2022). Maia & cols (Maia et al. 2010), demonstrated the efficacy of the OCT technique in generating images to characterize the enamel layer in order to measure its depth, whose result was statistically compared with histology. It was possible to see a better resolution at 840 nm in the spectral domain-OCT (due to the shorter wavelength) but a deeper penetration of light in the time domain-OCT image operating at 1280 nm (mainly due to reduced scattering and absorption). Thinner enamel layer in primary teeth may cause less attenuation of laser scanning light of SS-OCT resulting in the higher sensitivity for the detection of dentin caries (Nakajima et al. 2014).

By analyzing the optical properties of carious enamel one can establish a method for characterizing the severity of the carious lesion. Demineralized regions present higher porosity, which in turn increases light backscattering, thus making the lesion appear brighter (Angmar-Månsson et al. 1987). It is estimated that there is an increase in backscattered intensity of the order of two to three times (Maia et al. 2010)

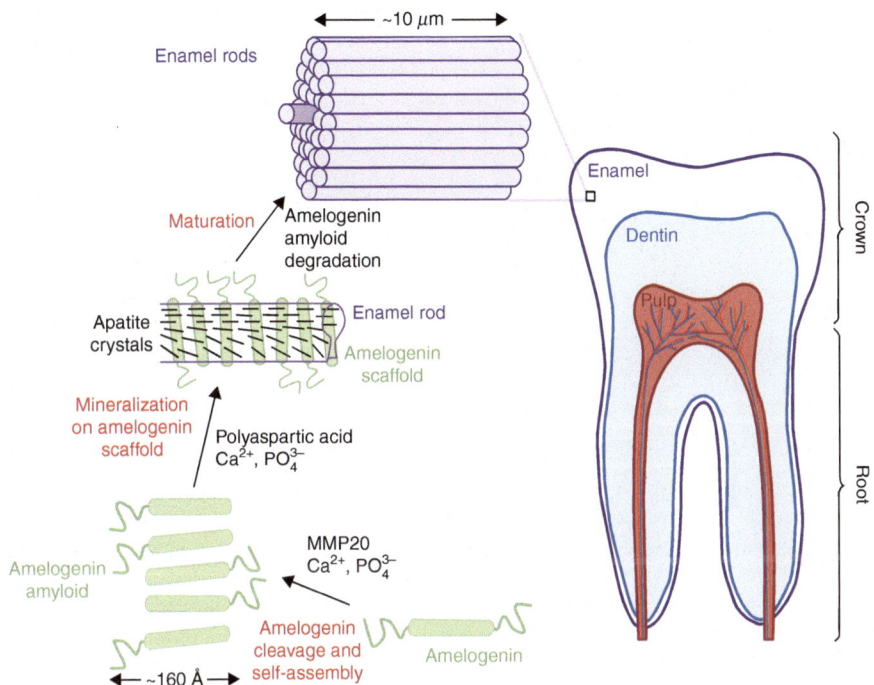

FIGURE 7.2

In a commentary paper, Welborn (Welborn 2020) commented that the work of Bai & cols (Bai et al. 2020) unveiled the molecular mechanisms responsible for the oriented growth of apatite crystals in enamel tissues. The product of the enzyme MMP20 self-assembles into amyloid-like structures that guide the growth of apatite minerals along one direction. The packing of the resulting rods gives enamel its unique microstructure and therefore its mechanical properties. Reprinted with permission from (Welborn 2020).

OCT is clearly a promising method for the quantification of mineral loss from dental caries but has not been widely exploited on deciduous dentition. Presence of cavitated and non-cavitated occlusal caries lesions in deciduous teeth were demonstrated by SS-OCT and confirmed by CLSM (Nakajima et al. 2014). Furthermore, it is particularly important to implement the method to evaluate caries development in the proximal surfaces, since as already mentioned, caries evolution in primary teeth is faster than in permanent teeth, and therefore a fast and non-invasive evaluation is imperative. As the evaluation of carious processes in clinic is often initiated by visual inspection and may be followed by X-ray imaging, a non-invasive method such as OCT can prove very valuable.

SS-OCT provided a clear image of lesions ranging from early enamel to deep dentin caries at occlusal pits and fissures, with comparatively high specificity caries. However, imaging depth of OCT is limited due to technical obstacles such as light attenuation through the tissue. SS-OCT laser beam

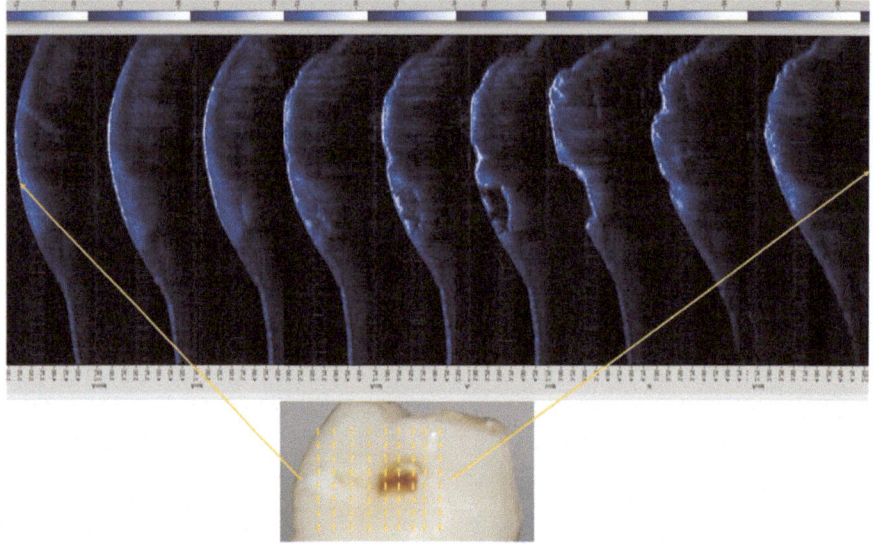

FIGURE 7.3
Series of 2D OCT-images, named B-scans, from left to right, showing details of different mineral loss of a natural caries lesion development referent to the deciduous tooth shown in the bottom. The scanned regions are indicated by the dashed lines. Source: the authors.

undergoes significant attenuation in dentin; therefore, in the case of very deep penetration of caries into dentin, estimation of lesion extent may be challenging. Though, cross-sectional images generated by SS-OCT provided useful information for the detection of dentin caries (Nakajima et al. 2014). As a general example and proof-of-concept of OCT application to characterize the evolution of a natural caries process performed on a deciduous extracted tooth, Figure 7.3 shows a set of 2D OCT images ranging from sub-surface carious changes through to more advanced regions.

The extracted tooth photograph is shown in the bottom part of Figure 7.3, and the scanned region is indicated by the yellow dashed lines. The region of interest was analyzed perpendicularly to the enamel surface by a home-built SDOCT (λ = 850 nm, $\Delta\lambda$ = 49,9 nm, axial resolution = 6 μm).

Although the visual inspection in this case would naturally indicate the main carious region, it is clear from the picture the white lesions appeared over a great extension. However, one of the greatest advantages of OCT is its penetration in tissue, and in this case for a thin (1 mm or less) enamel in primary teeth, the whole internal extension up to the dentin can be imaged. The results of Figure 7.3 clearly demonstrate the capacity of quantitative assessment and penetration of OCT, which can quantify not only the lateral extension but also its depth. Using this method, enamel lesions with high porosity and excavations under the intact surface can also be identified. One way

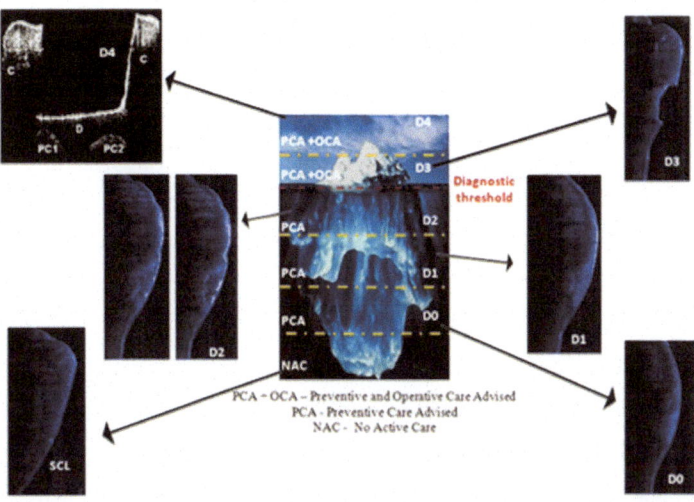

FIGURE 7.4

The scheme shows different stages of caries lesions on deciduous tooth by OCT images in correlation with the "iceberg of dental caries" proposed by Pitts (2004). From top to bottom: D4, lesions into pulp (reprinted with permission from Fonsêca (2009)); D3, clinically detectable cavities limited to enamel; D2, clinically detectable lesions in dentine; D1, clinically detectable enamel lesions with "intact" surfaces; D0, lesions detectable only with traditional diagnostic aids; SCL, sub-clinical initial lesions in dynamic state of progression.

to classify carious regions on the different levels can be done using the Pitts concepts of the Iceberg (Pitts 2004), as didactically illustrated in Figure 7.4.

The OCT system possesses great potential to be used routinely in pediatric dentistry clinical practice to evaluate early caries detection in a non-invasive way, therefore with no pain, allowing an in-depth view of the enamel. For practical use, a hand-piece, optical probe that can be used intraorally or an appropriate head for the imaging acquisition is required, which is a technologically solvable issue, as already reported (Wang et al. 2016; Eom et al. 2019; Li et al. 2020). In Wang & cols (Wang et al. 2016), an optical probe for oral cavity has been demonstrated for simultaneous OCT and Raman acquisition data (see also Chapter 2). Lenton & cols (Lenton et al. 2012) obtained CP-OCT (cross polarization) images under intraoral conditions and on pediatric subjects. This frame rate not only was efficient at sampling multiple sections of the tooth but also allowed for freehanded acquisition with minimal motion artifact on pediatric subjects as young as 4 years old.

Regarding non-invasive methods for diagnosing carious lesions, Macey & cols (Macey et al. 2021), displayed fair evidence of the accuracy of ECM (electric conductivity measurement) for detecting non-cavitated caries lesions. Poor evidence was found for all other methods, such as traditional visible inspection, bitewing radiography or other radiographic technologies and adjunct methods such as FOTI (fibre-optic transillumination), LF (laser fluorescence) and QLF (quantitative light-induced fluorescence) and lesion activity assessment (based on visual inspection).

There are studies monitoring incipient carious lesions at the interface of restorations with resin composite and it is recognized that incipient carious lesions in smooth surfaces under fluoride therapy can be monitored by optical methods (Maia et al. 2010; Lenton et al. 2014). Optical coherence tomography possesses great potential to be used routinely in clinical practice for the complex diagnosis of early enamel caries, promoting possible remineralized preventive measures (Maia et al. 2010).

Lenton & cols (Lenton et al. 2012) brought an important finding: CP-OCT proved to be efficient to evaluate the interface enamel/composite restoration, and even an interface of composite restoration that seems to be clinically sound, showed and increased dispersion before cavitation. The CP-OCT image differentiates the composite resin material from the dental enamel based on the degree of scattering and depolarization (Lenton et al. 2014).

CP-OCT can detect demineralization by measuring the increase in scattering and depolarization of the NIR light by underlying enamel. Differences of backscattered intensity between recently and cavitated restoration interface, which means that the CP-OCT image could be applied to confirm the marginal integrity of composite resins (Lenton et al. 2012, 2014). CP-OCT images of the underlying enamel (below the composite) commonly show a dark or almost "ghost-like" outline of the tooth. This is a common phenomenon due to the birefringence (Lenton et al. 2014). Some B-scans demonstrated diffuse interrupted backscattered reflection (bright cluster of pixels) at the cavity floor in some areas, which was an indication of interfacial microleakage and gap existence, while other areas were showing continuous smooth dark pixels at the cavity floor that were referred to as no loss of interfacial adaptation (Bakhsh et al. 2011).

Intact enamel–composite interfaces and sound underlying enamel show minimal scattering and depolarization. Composite dental fillings create various index of refraction mismatch boundaries that can be a source of a strong back reflected signal. These back reflected signals can potentially confound clinical evaluation in OCT imaging. Dental composites are not birefringent and cause uniform scattering in depth, which allowed the material to be differentiated from the birefringent dental enamel (Lenton et al. 2012).

Al Tuwirqi & cols (Al Tuwirqi et al. 2021) showed in laboratorial study with primary teeth that OCT has great potential for direct evaluation of dental restoration when used in combination with pulp capping materials. For this reason, OCT can be beneficial in clinical settings and allow dentists to screen and evaluate restorations during follow-up.

Summarized in Table 7.1 are the identified literature references on the use of OCT for caries evaluation in primary teeth.

TABLE 7.1

Studies Using OCT-images in Primary Teeth

Study	Clinical or laboratorial	Aim	OCT	Results
Maia et al. 2010	Laboratory evaluation of six primary teeth	Characterization of sound dental structure and detect natural caries	TD-OCT system (1280 nm, axial resolution 11 μm) and SD-OCT (840 nm, axial resolution 6 μm)	The efficacy of the OCT technique was demonstrated to measure the depth of the enamel layer and increase in backscattered intensity between sound and caries regions.
Lenton et al. 2012	Clinical evaluation of more than 200 images from 27 children	Dental caries detection	CP-OCT (1310 nm, axial resolution 11 μm)	CP-OCT was efficient to evaluate interface enamel/composite restauration, as even interface of composite restauration that seems to be clinical sound showed and increase of dispersion before cavitation. CP-OCT was also enable to visualize *ex vivo* biofilms on dental composites and measure thickness
Nakajima 2014	Laboratory evaluation of 38 images scanned from 26 deciduous teeth with alterations on occlusal fissures (with or without cavitation)	Dental caries detection by six examiners	SS-OCT (1330 nm, axial resolution 12 μm)	Evaluation of SS-OCT images shows better sensibility than visual inspection and the presence of cavitated and non-cavitated occlusal caries lesions in deciduous teeth were demonstrated by SS-OCT and confirmed by CLSM
Lenton et al. 2014	Clinical evaluation of 84 images from 62 pediatric patients	Dental caries detection and preservation after restorative treatment	CP-OCT (1310 nm, axial resolution 8,5 μm)	Differences of backscattered intensity between recently and cavitated restoration interface was shown, which means that the CP-OCT image could be applied to confirm the marginal integrity of composite resins with limitation

(continued)

TABLE 7.1 (Continued)
Studies Using OCT-images in Primary Teeth

Study	Clinical or laboratorial	Aim	OCT	Results
Murayama et al. 2018	Laboratory evaluation of 18 primary teeth	Examination of the effects of a coating filler on changes in the structure of artificially demineralized tooth enamel	TD-OCT (1310 nm)	OCT was successfully used to track remineralization and test the ability of a coating material to inhibit demineralization
Thomas et al. 2021	Laboratory evaluation of 36 primary teeth	Identification of remineralizing efficacy of Fluoride Varnish	SS-OCT (1325 nm, axial resolution 12 μm)	SS-OCT images showed demineralization and an outer growth layer in post-remineralization
Bakhsk et al. 2021	Laboratory evaluation of 40 primary teeth. Class-V cavities were prepared on the buccal and lingual surfaces of each tooth	Assessing microleakage upon composite restorations in primary teeth	CP-OCT (1310 nm, axial resolution 12 μm)	OCT was able to demonstrate interfacial microleakage and no loss of interfacial adaptation
Al Tuwirqi et al. 2021	Laboratory evaluation of 30 primary molars with a standardized round class-V cavity on the buccal surface	Evaluating of the internal adaptation of pulp capping materials when used as indirect pulp capping	CP-OCT (1310 nm, axial resolution 12 μm)	OCT showed the internal adaptation of the tested dental pulp capping materials non-destructively

7.3 Dental Erosion

Dental erosion is defined as the loss of tooth substance, which is chemically removed from the tooth surface by acid or chelating substances without bacterial involvement. This mineral tissue loss may be caused by intrinsic sources (decrease in saliva flow and gastrointestinal disorders) and extrinsic sources (dietary, and use of medications) or by idiopathic factors (no established cause) (Lussi et al. 2008; Moazzez et al. 2014).

In vitro models should be the primary method for assessing new products or new techniques for reducing the erosive effects of acid exposure, although with some disadvantages over real tooth in a proper environment. One of the main advantages of *in vitro* models is the potential to analyze these effects using a range of techniques, each providing specific information. Surface hardness, surface profilometry, longitudinal or transversal microradiography, and scanning electron microscopy associated with energy-dispersive X-rays are some of the techniques used previously (Schlueter et al. 2011), besides the use of confocal scanning microscopy (Maia et al. 2014).

The potential of OCT to qualitatively and quantitatively evaluate mineral loss on a controllable manner has been well demonstrated (Freitas et al. 2009), and its effective use for measuring mineral loss due to erosive challenges in *in vitro* studies opens avenues to clinical erosion studies in terms of detection and lesion preservation (Chan et al. 2013; Habib et al. 2018).

According to published studies, there is evidence that the prevalence of dental erosion in deciduous teeth is steadily increasing (Kreulen et al. 2010; Moimaz et al. 2013; Corica et al. 2014). The consumption growth of acidic foods and soft drinks seems to be a relevant factor for the development of this erosive wear (Wang et al. 2012, 2014). Due to the structural differences, the deciduous teeth are more susceptible to erosive wear as permanent, since they have a thinner layer of enamel, a lower degree of mineralization, higher permeability (Hunter et al. 2000; Nahás Pires Corrêa et al. 2011). Therefore, given the difficulty to get away potentially erosive eating habits, preventive mechanisms that promise to act on erosion control appear to be a valid strategy.

Because of their widespread daily use, toothpastes could be an ideal mode by which protection against dental erosion could be provided. Fluoride compounds have been widely used to prevent caries and dental erosion (Wiegand et al. 2003; Huysmans et al. 2011). However, the inadequate ingestion of high concentrations of fluoride can cause fluorosis, especially in young children (World Health Organization (WHO 2019)).

The prevalence of erosion in the primary dentition of young children increased with age, with clinically detectable lesions forming between 24 and 36 months of age (Huang et al. 2015). Therefore, as soon as there is the detection of erosive lesions, preventive and therapeutic procedures can be implemented more effectively. An optimal clinical method for monitoring would permit longitudinal quantification of early mineral loss. It is recognized that incipient carious lesions in smooth surfaces under fluoride therapy can be monitored by optical methods (Maia et al. 2010). Non-invasive analysis methods are required for this to be achieved. It is with this in mind that we propose the use of OCT, which has great potential in dentistry. OCT could be considered as an efficient and accurate quantitative method for evaluating mineral loss.

Considering the high incidence of dental mineral loss caused by enamel erosion· in primary teeth, studies on preventive methods are important. Techniques that can perform quantitative *in vivo* evaluations, such as optical coherence tomography, can be used not only for diagnosis but also for clinical follow-up and monitoring treatment. CP-OCT imaging along the material interface clearly demonstrates strong contrast between sound versus demineralized tooth enamel (Lenton et al. 2012). Demineralization increases the roughness of enamel surfaces, thereby increasing light scattering by two to three orders. Therefore, a strong increase in the signal visible in B-scans indicates severe demineralization and roughening of the enamel surface (Murayama et al. 2018).

Different stages of remineralization could be observed in SS-OCT images. Active lesions, visually as rough surface, depicted more uptake of minerals in SS-OCT (Thomas et al. 2020). As an example of OCT application to erosion, Figures 7.5 and 7.6 show results reported by Habib & cols (Habib et al. 2018). The authors conducted a pilot study and investigated the erosion through the attenuation coefficient obtained from OCT A-scan data. The samples consisted of human premolar roots subjected to citric acid treatment. Details of the erosion protocols employed for sample preparation can be seen in Habib et al. (2018), and were designed in a way to reproduce dental erosion in initial clinical stages. A commercial SSOCT system (OCS1300SS, Thorlabs Ltd., United Kingdom, central wavelength 1325 nm, manufacturer-specified axial and transverse resolutions of 9 and 15 µm in free space, respectively). The B-scan (set of 1024 A-scans) frequency was 19.7 frames/s, which were also employed to generate 2D images.

In Figure 7.5, part (a) shows a B-scan image of a treated tooth containing both varnished and eroded region. Part (b) shows the surface detected by using a Canny edge detector for surface detection. In part (c) the tooth sur-face is shown flattened by aligning the A-scans. Then, in part (d) the varnish region was covered, to leave only the eroded region for the curve fitting process. In part (e) an A-scan from the eroded region is shown and fitted with the Lambert–Beer equation. In Figure 7.6, an *en-face* map of the attenu-ation coefficient at different erosion time points is shown on a false color scale, where red represents the greater extent of scattering (greater extent of erosion).

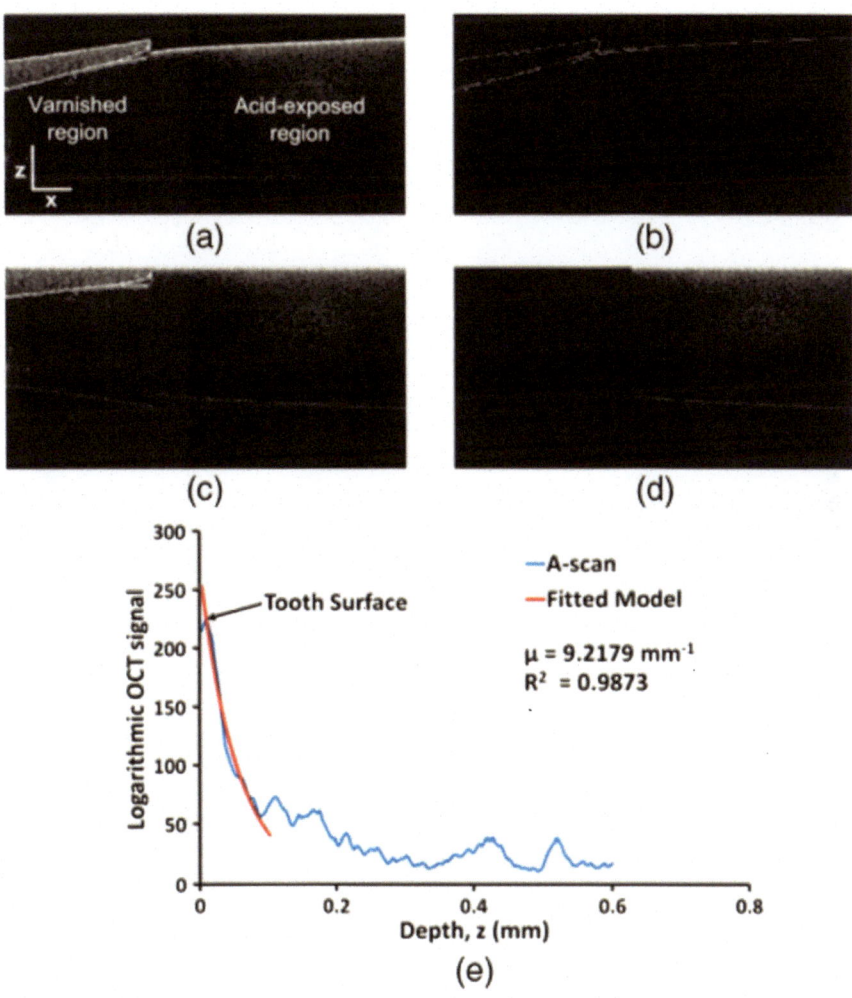

FIGURE 7.5

(a) B-scan of a citric acid treated tooth containing both varnished and acid exposed region.
(b) Tooth surface was detected using a Canny edge detector. (c) Tooth surface was flattened by aligning the A-scans. (d) Varnish region was masked, leaving the acid exposed (eroded) region for the curve fitting process. (e) An A-scan from the eroded region is fitted with the Lambert–Beer equation. Fitting takes place from the surface to 100 μm in depth. Scale bar in (a) represents a physical distance of 500 μm. Reprinted with permission from (Habib 2018) © The Optical Society.

An important finding of that study was the increasing trend of a normalized attenuation coefficient with the duration of acid challenge. Such measurement was validated against morphological characteristics and the microwear features on scanning electron microscope scans. The potential of OCT is then clear, once again, since it can be used *in vivo* for such measurements.

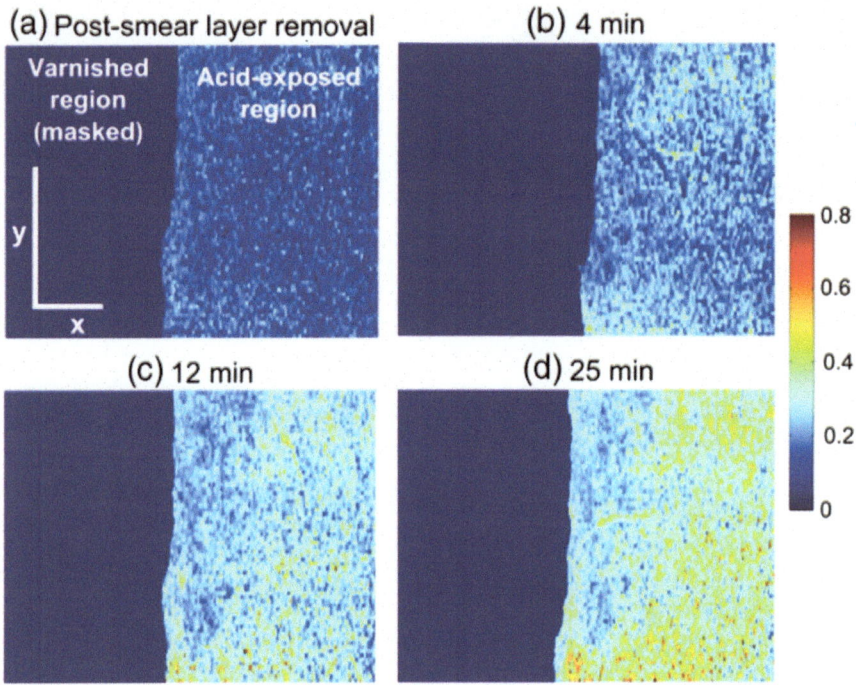

FIGURE 7.6

En face attenuation coefficient map at different erosion time points. Red indicates greater extent of scattering, i.e., greater extent of erosion. Color bar represents normalized attenuation coefficient value. Reprinted with permission from (Habib 2018) © The Optical Society.

7.4 Periodontal Aspects of Children Oral Health

It is evident from historical and more recent research that the oral health of children mirrors their general health and that is also a strong predictor of their oral health in adolescence and adulthood. Oral health care for children is often delivered with a focus on dental caries and is usually isolated from children's general health care; accordingly, oral signs and symptoms do not always alert oral health practitioners to think of their signficance beyond the mouth. Therefore, it is becoming even more important to understand the health and disease of oral tissues, in particular periodontal tissues, to promote good long term oral health in adulthood.

According to the American Academy of Pediatric Dentistry (American Academy of Pediatric Dentistry 2018), children and adolescents should have periodontal assessment and recording as part of their routine dental visits. This includes observing the shape of the gingival margins and their color, and the height of interproximal crestal bone on radiographs. Plaque should be recorded using disclosing agents, thus allowing identification of sites where it may be contributing to gingivitis and/or caries. A routine screen (the Community Periodontal Index or periodontal screening and recording) (Ainamo et al. 1982; Bassani et al. 2006) is recommended for the mixed and early permanent dentitions of children and adolescents.

Such screens help to identify early signs of periodontal destruction, as research has indicated that clinical signs of gingivitis and plaque may be less obvious in younger mouths, even when there is bone loss. This applies especially to the permanent incisors and first permanent molars.

The guidelines are less clear about the need for probing in younger children who may not tolerate this comfortably. What has been established is the importance of following up early loss of primary teeth and/or obvious bone loss visible on posterior bitewing radiographs, which may be indicators of periodontal disease.

At this point, it is very important to notice that OCT has been already employed for evaluation of periodontal diseases *in vitro* and also in clinical practice (Mota et al. 2015; Fernandes et al. 2017, 2019; Lai et al. 2019). This aspect of OCT in periodontics is dealt with in Chapter 9 of this book. To date, no study of OCT to periodontics in children has been reported.

References

Ainamo, J., Barnes, D., Cutress, T., Martin, J., Sado-Infirri, J. 1982. Development of the World Health Organization (WHO) community periodontal index of treatment needs (CPITN). *Int. Dent. J.* 32: 281–291.

Al Tuwirqi, A.A., El Ashiry, E.A., Alzahrani, A.Y., Bamashmous, N., Bakhsh, T.A. 2021. Tomographic evaluation of the internal adaptation for recent calcium silicate-based pulp capping materials in primary teeth. *Biomed Res. Int.* 2021: 5523145.

Amaechi, B.T., Podoleanu, A., Higham, S.M., Jackson, D.A. 2003. Correlation of quantitative light-induced fluorescence and optical coherence tomography applied for detection and quantification of early dental caries. *J. Biomed. Opt.* 8: 642.

American Academy of Pediatric Dentistry. 2018. Periodicity of examination, preventive dental services, anticipatory guidance/counseling, and oral treatment for infants, children and adolescents, *The Reference Manual of Pediatric Dentistry*. Chicago.

Ando, M., Van Der Veen, M.H., Schemehorn, B.R., Stookey, G.K. 2001. Comparative study to quantify demineralized enamel in deciduous and permanent teeth using laser- and light-induced fluorescence techniques. *Caries Res.* 35: 464–470.

Angmar-Månsson, B., ten Bosch, J.J. 1987. Optical methods for the detection and quantification of caries. *Adv. Dent. Res.* 1: 14–20.

Bai, Y., Yu, Z., Ackerman, L. et al. 2020. Protein nanoribbons template enamel mineralization. *PNAS* 117: 22

Bakhsh, T.A., Sadr, A., Shimada, Y., Tagami, J., Sumi, Y. 2011. Non-invasive quantification of resin-dentin interfacial gaps using optical coherence tomography: Validation against confocal microscopy. *Dent. Mater.* 27: 915–925.

Bassani, D.G., Da Silva, C.M., Oppermann, R.V. 2006. Validity of the "Community Periodontal Index of Treatment Needs" (CPITN) for population periodontitis screening. *Cad. Saude Publica* 22: 277–283.

Chan, K.H., Chan, A.C., Darling, C.L., Fried, D. 2013. Methods for monitoring erosion using optical coherence tomography. *Lasers Dent. XIX 8566*: 856606.

Corica, A., Caprioglio, A. 2014. Meta-analysis of the prevalence of tooth wear in primary dentition. *Eur. J. Paediatr. Dent.* 15: 385–388.

Darling, C.L., Huynh, G.D., Fried, D. 2006. Light scattering properties of natural and artificially demineralized dental enamel at 1310 nm. *J. Biomed. Opt.* 11: 034023.

Eom, J.B., Eom, J., Park, A., Ahn, J.C. 2019. Optical coherence tomography-based 3D intraoral scanner. *Opt. InfoBase Conf. Pap.* Part F142: 3–6.

Fernandes, L.O., Mota, C.C.B. d. O., Oliveira, H.O., Neves, J.K., Santiago, L.M., Gomes, A.S.L. 2019. Optical coherence tomography follow-up of patients treated from periodontal disease. *J. Biophotonics* 12.

Fernandes, L.O., Mota, C.C.B.O., de Melo, L.S.A., da Costa Soares, M.U.S., da Silva Feitosa, D., Gomes, A.S.L. 2017. In vivo assessment of periodontal structures and measurement of gingival sulcus with optical coherence tomography: a pilot study. *J. Biophotonics* 10: 862–869.

Fonsêca, D.D.D., Kyotoku, B.B.C., Maia, A.M.A., Gomes, A.S.L. 2009. In vitro imaging of remaining dentin and pulp chamver by optical coherence tomography: comparison between 850 nm and 1280 nm. *J. Biomed. Opt.* 14: 024009.

Freitas, A.Z., Zezell, D.M., Mayer, M.P.A., Ribeiro, A.C., Gomes, A.S.L., Vieira, N.D. 2009. Determination of dental decay rates with optical coherence tomography. *Laser Phys. Lett.* 6: 896–900.

Fried, D., Glena, R.E., Featherstone, J.D.B., Seka, W. 1995. Nature of light scattering in dental enamel and dentin at visible and near-infrared wavelengths. *Appl. Opt.* 34: 1278.

Habib, M., Lee, K.M., Liew, Y.M., Zakian, C., Ung, N.M., Chew, H.P. 2018. Assessing surface characteristics of eroded dentine with optical coherence tomography: a preliminary in vitro validation study. *Appl. Opt.* 57: 8673.

Huang, L.L., Leishman, S., Newman, B., Seow, W.K. 2015. Association of erosion with timing of detection and selected risk factors in primary dentition: A longitudinal study. *Int. J. Paediatr. Dent.* 25: 165–173.

Hunter, M.L., West, N.X., Hughes, J.A., Newcombe, R.G., Addy, M. 2000. Erosion of deciduous and permanent dental hard tissue in the oral environment. *J. Dent.* 28: 257–263.

Huysmans, M.C.D.N.J.M., Jager, D.H.J., Ruben, J.L., Unk, D.E.M.F., Klijn, C.P.A.H., Vieira, A.M. 2011. Reduction of erosive wear in situ by stannous fluoride-containing toothpaste. *Caries Res.* 45: 518–523.

Koch, G., Poulsen, S. 2009. *Pediatric Dentistry: A Clinical Approach.* Chichester: Wiley-Blackwell.

Kreulen, C.M., Van'T Spijker, A., Rodriguez, J.M., Bronkhorst, E.M., Creugers, N.H.J., Bartlett, D.W. 2010. Systematic review of the prevalence of tooth wear in children and adolescents. *Caries Res.* 44: 151–159.

Lai, Y.C., Chiu, C.H., Cai, Z.Q. et al. 2019. OCT-based periodontal inspection framework. *Sensors (Switzerland)* 19: 1–18.

Lenton, P., Rudney, J., Chen, R., Fok, A., Aparicio, C., Jones, R.S. 2012. Imaging in vivo secondary caries and ex vivo dental biofilms using cross-polarization optical coherence tomography. *Dent. Mater.* 28: 792–800.

Lenton, P., Rudney, J., Fok, A., Jones, R.S. 2014. Clinical cross-polarization optical coherence tomography assessment of subsurface enamel below dental resin composite restorations. *J. Med. Imaging* 1: 016001.

Li, K., Yang, Z., Liang, W., Shang, J., Liang, Y., Wan, S. 2020. Low-cost, ultracompact handheld optical coherence tomography probe for in vivo oral maxillofacial tissue imaging. *J. Biomed. Opt.* 25: 1.

Lussi, A., Jaeggi, T. 2008. Erosion – Diagnosis and risk factors. *Clin. Oral Investig.* 12: 5–13.

Macey, R., Walsh, T., Riley, P. et al. 2021. Electrical conductance for the detection of dental caries. *Cochrane Database Syst. Rev.* 2021.

Maia, A.M.A., Fonsêca, D.D.D., Kyotoku, B.B.C., Gomes, A.S.L. 2010. Characterization of enamel in primary teeth by optical coherence tomography for assessment of dental caries. *Int. J. Paediatr. Dent.* 20: 158–164.

Maia, A.M.A., Longbottom, C., Gomes, A.S.L., Girkin, J.M. 2014. Enamel erosion and prevention efficacy characterized by confocal laser scanning microscope. *Microsc. Res. Tech.* 77: 439–445.

Moazzez, R., Bartlett, D. 2014. Intrinsic causes of dental erosion. *Erosive Tooth Wear – From Diagnosis to Ther.* 20: 180–196.

Moimaz, S., Araújo, P., Chiba, F., Garbín, C., Saliba, N. 2013. Prevalence of deciduous tooth erosion in childhood. *Int. J. Dent. Hyg.* 11: 226–230.

Mota, C.C.B.O., Fernandes, L.O., Cimões, R., Gomes, A.S.L. 2015. Non-invasive periodontal probing through Fourier-domain optical coherence tomography. *J. Periodontol.* 86: 1087–1094.

Murayama, R., Nagura, Y., Yamauchi, K. et al. 2018. Effect of a coating material containing surface reaction-type pre-reacted glass-ionomer filler on prevention of primary enamel demineralization detected by optical coherence tomography. *J. Oral Sci.* 60: 367–373.

Nahás Pires Corrêa, M.S., NahNahás, M.S., Nahás Pires Corrêa, F., Nahás Pires Corrêa, J.P., Murakami, C., Mendes, F.M. 2011. Prevalence and associated factors of dental erosion in children and adolescents of a private dental practice. *Int. J. Paediatr. Dent.* 21: 451–458.

Nakajima, Y., Shimada, Y., Sadr, A. et al. 2014. Detection of occlusal caries in primary teeth using swept source optical coherence tomography. *J. Biomed. Opt.* 19: 016020.

Pitts, N.B. 2004. Modern concepts of caries measurement. *J. Dent. Res.* 83: 39–48.

Popescu, S.M., Mercuţ, V., Scrieciu, M. et al. 2017. Radiological and optical coherence tomography aspects in external root resorption. *Rom. J. Morphol. Embryol.* 58: 131–137.

Qian, J., Feng, Z., Fan, X., Kuzmin, A., Gomes, A.S.L., Prasad, P.N. 2022. High contrast 3-D optical bioimaging using molecular and nanoprobes optically responsive to IR light. *Phys. Rep.* 962: 1–107.

Schlueter, N., Hara, A., Shellis, R.P., Ganss, C. 2011. Methods for the measurement and characterization of erosion in enamel and dentine. *Caries Res.* 45: 13–23.

Thomas, C.S., Sharma, D.S., Sheet, D., Mukhopadhyay, A., Sharma, S. 2020. Cross-sectional visual comparison of remineralization efficacy of various agents on early smooth surface caries of primary teeth with swept source optical coherence tomography. *J Oral Biol Craniofac Res.* 11: 628–637.

Wang, J., Zheng, W., Lin, K., Huang, Z. 2016. Development of a hybrid Raman spectroscopy and optical coherence tomography technique for real-time in vivo tissue measurements. *Opt. Lett.* 41: 3045.

Wang, X., Lussi, A. 2012. Functional foods/ingredients on dental erosion. *Eur. J. Nutr.* 51.

Wang, Y.L., Chang, C.C., Chi, C.W. et al 2014. Erosive potential of soft drinks on human enamel: An invitro study. *J. Formos. Med. Assoc.* 113: 850–856.

Welborn, V.V. 2020. Enamel synthesis explained. *Proc. Natl. Acad. Sci. U. S. A.* 117: 21847–21848.

Wiegand, A., Attin, T. 2003. Influence of fluoride on the prevention of erosive lesions-- a review. *Oral Health Prev. Dent.* 1: 245–253.

World Health Organization (WHO) 2019. Preventing Disease Through Healthy Environments Inadequate or Excess Fluoride: A Major Public Health Concern. Geneva, Switzerland.

Zijp, J.R., ten Bosch, J.J. 1993. Theoretical model for the scattering of light by dentin and comparison with measurements. *Appl. Opt.* 32: 411.

8

OCT in Orthodontics

Mônica Schäffer Lopes,[1] Vanda Sanderana Macêdo Carneiro[2],
Cláudia C. B. O. Mota[3,4] and Anderson S. L. Gomes[5]

[1]Graduate Program in Dentistry, Universidade Federal de Pernambuco, UFPE, Brazil

[2]Faculty of Dentistry, Universidade de Pernambuco, UPE, Brazil

[3]Faculty of Dentistry, Centro Universitário Tabosa de Almeida, ASCES-UNITA, Brazil

[4]School of Dentistry, Universidade de Pernambuco, Campus Arcoverde, UPE, Brazil

[5]Physics Department and Graduate Program in Dentistry, Universidade Federal de Pernambuco, UFPE, Brazil

CONTENTS

8.1 Introduction

Optical coherence tomography (OCT) is a noninvasive and nondestructive imaging technique that uses low-coherence interferometry to collect the reflected and backscattered light from a sample. Depending on the characteristics of the material – e.g. density, particle sizes and water

DOI: 10.1201/9781351104562-8

content – and the light source characteristics, such as the central wavelength, it will present different scattering and reflection intensities. The intensity of reflected and backscattered light is measured as a function of its axial position in the tissue. The low-coherence interferometry principle is used to selectively remove or gate out the component of the backscattered signal that has undergone multiple scattering events, resulting in high-resolution images of reflectivity versus depth (1.5–3.0 mm, depending on the analyzed tissues) (Leitgeb et al. 2021). OCT has been widely used to study bio-tissues, to characterize and detect changes of the optical properties with axial resolution reaching the submicron regime (Harper et al. 2018).

Technical support information related to OCT systems involving optical instrumentation, software, data acquisition and processing, is well exploited in Chapter 2. This chapter will discuss the possibilities of OCT application in orthodontics, from the initial enamel analysis up to the bonding protocol, demineralization close to orthodontic fixed appliances, monitoring of remnant resin layer after debonding, cracks related to microimplants' insertion, and periodontal changes associated to tooth movement during orthodontic treatment. It is important to register that, for orthodontic purposes, axial resolution is the most important characteristic in OCT systems. The changes related to orthodontic treatment are, in general (except those related to periodontics and microimplants), limited to the surface and subsurface of enamel; in this way, the evolution in optical instrumentation could increase the benefits of OCT technique in orthodontics.

8.2 OCT for Orthodontic Bonding Protocols

Most of the orthodontics treatments primarily involve the bonding of the brackets to the enamel surface, with different types of bracket attachment methods currently practiced in dentistry (Ravichandran et al. 2021). Despite years of research, there still are concerns about the irreversible changes promoted by fixed orthodontic appliances on enamel tissue (Koprowski et al. 2014; Machoy et al. 2020). These changes are potentially harmful, since the etching, debonding or cleanup procedures always lead to alterations on its initial sound condition.

Adhesive methods are continuously adapted, and new approaches are proposed for effective and efficient adhesive application techniques to aid orthodontic treatment without damaging the tooth surface or bracket integrity (Ravichandran et al. 2021). Even with cautious diagnosis and treatment planning, orthodontic treatment can fail if bonding fails or can last much longer depending on bonding quality (Sinescu et al. 2008). As an undesired side effect, it could decrease patient trust and compliance (Rominu et al.

2011). To minimize failures, the brackets should be considered as a funda-mental part of orthodontic treatment (Leão Filho et al. 2016).

One of the primary goals of the orthodontic treatment is to achieve a stable interface between orthodontic brackets and tooth enamel with low suscepti-bility to degradation over treatment time (Abbassy et al. 2021). Though, the adhesion of the brackets should be strong enough to prevent bond failure during the treatment, supporting mechanical and thermal effects of the oral environment, but weak enough to minimize enamel damages during the bracket removal at the end of the treatment (Shinya et al. 2008; Leão Filho et al. 2015, 2016). Superficial enamel must be maintained intact as it contains the highest degree of mineral and mechanical properties to minimize the enamel damage during bracket debonding phase (Abbassy et al. 2021).

The success of the bracket-tooth strength involves a combination of mech-anical or chemical retention of a surface considering the etching protocols, the correct choice and manipulation of adhesive material and the retentive potential of the accessories or the bracket to be used (Leão Filho et al. 2016; Machoy et al. 2020). For the best stability, the bracket and bonding material (type and thickness) need to match the tooth shape (Sinescu et al. 2008b). Before starting the treatment, the initial condition of teeth, sound or non-sound, and the enamel thickness should be considered in order to select the appropriate orthodontic bonding, debonding and cleanup methods (Koprowski et al. 2014; Machoy et al. 2019).

In this context, optical coherence tomography (OCT) was proposed as an optical tool for analyzing the enamel and its alterations before, during and after orthodontic treatment, as well as the presence of remnant resin over the surface after bracket debonding and/or cleanup protocols. It is possible to evaluate surface and subsurface alterations in tissue scanned through the light interactions captured by these scans, as shown qualitatively in Figure 8.1:

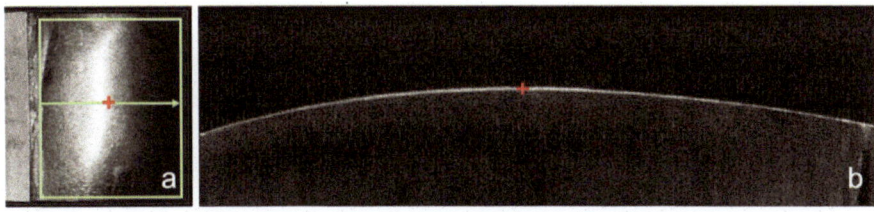

FIGURE 8.1

The OCT analysis is divided into a coronal view (a) and axial plane view (b) of the sample. The selected point of interest can be identified also in the coronal view (red cross). The material thickness was measured perpendicular to the labial surface. The three-dimensional image of surface (a) was acquired with Ganymed Spectral Radar SR-OCT: OCP930SR and resolution of < 5.8 μm, and axial (cross-sectional) image (b) with Callisto Spectral Radar SR-OCT: OCP930SR (both from Thorlabs, USA). Image courtesy of Lopes (Lopes et al. 2012).

Regarding Figure 8.1, it is important to consider that, in 2D images, the reflection is more evident at interface lines, as already pointed out by other studies that evidenced a more reflective thin layer outer enamel boundary (Ravichandran et al. 2021).

The scattering happens into each medium in which light propagates. It explains why the enamel superficial line is usually more evident than the area into the tooth – where the light propagation has a natural exponential decay, represented in gray scales (as shown in Figure 8.1). The 2D scanning evaluates up to 2 mm of depth into the enamel tissue, depending on the central wavelength of the light source. It is favorable to evaluate the initial morphology with the ability to identify even specific aspects of enamel evolution (Leão Filho et al. 2013).

OCT was validated as a tool for *in vitro* studies to assess the initial morphology of enamel, the superficial enamel defects, and its thickness before orthodontic treatments (Rominu et al. 2011; Şen et al. 2018; Machoy et al. 2019).

Through OCT analysis it is possible to access the enamel thickness measurement, evaluate bracket debonding and complementary quantify the enamel structural changes during the orthodontic treatment, supported by a dedicated auto detection algorithm for enamel (Şen et al. 2018; Machoy et al. 2019; Ravichandran et al. 2021). Initially, the literature indicates an enamel loss about 80 μm after polishing with orthodontic paste (Koprowski et al. 2014). Clinical steps adopted before bracket bonding, such as pumice and enamel surface etching, promote demineralization involving loss of superficial hydroxyapatite and also porosities in the deep subsequent layers (Jumanca et al. 2018).

In OCT images the enamel etched is characterized by an increase of reflection of the superficial line and high intensity of light scattering in deep layers of the demineralized area of the sample. It is evidenced as the white band under the enamel superficial line (Figure 8.2).

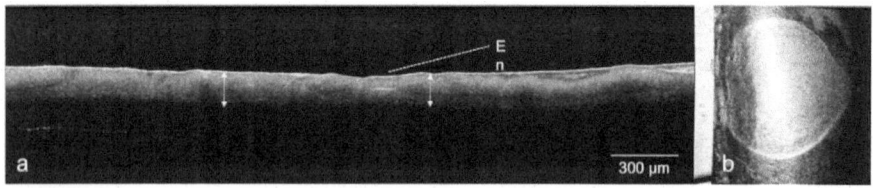

FIGURE 8.2

(a) 2D-OCT image representing the demineralization depth promoted by the acid etching. (b) 3D-OCT aspect after acid etching with 37% phosphoric acid. *En*, enamel superficial line. Both images were acquired with Ganymede Spectral Domain SD-OCT (Thorlabs, USA): cross-sectional image (a) presents axial and lateral resolution lower than 6.0 μm and 8.0 μm, respectively, whilst for the three-dimensional image (b), the volume scanned was an area of 8.0 mm × 8.0 mm and image depth of 1.6 mm. Image courtesy of Lopes (Lopes et al. 2012).

When using self-etching adhesive systems, the enamel loss pattern is similar to that observed after the acid etching, but with shallower deep penetration of the adhesive and resin (Sundfeld et al. 2005; Iijima et al. 2008) due to mild etching effect. Despite this, Machoy & co-authors (Machoy et al. 2020) did not find a significant difference between classic etching or self-etching adhesives for enamel loss. After the phosphoric acid etching, the enamel loss varies between 435 µm and 472.75 µm, whilst using self-etching adhesive is around 469.03 µm. In this way, the shallower depth penetration could be considered an advantage of self-etching adhesive systems, since it implies a reduced risk of damage to the enamel in debonding procedure (Koprowski et al. 2014; Machoy et al. 2020).

The literature brings alternatives to the conventional acid-etching procedures previously to bracket adhesion or the use of self-etching adhesive systems, such as the high-power laser irradiation (Jumanca et al. 2018; Lopes et al. 2019, 2020, 2021). The Er:YAG (2940 nm; 120 mJ, 10 Hz and 1.2 W) laser irradiation was proposed as a substitute of phosphoric acid-etching promoting lower, but enough, strength union bracket-enamel if compared to the conventional acid etching (Leão Filho et al. 2016). Despite the mechanism of action, the laser etching alters the calcium-to-phosphorus ratio on enamel, reducing the carbonate to phosphate ratio. The changes promoted by erbium laser irradiation usually can be seen on the 2D-OCT images as a set of dense points (white points in the enamel surface line that may even continue like straps as the depth of penetration increases, evidenced in Figure 8.3). Currently the Er,Cr:YSGG laser is widely used for dental applications, due to its strong absorption in hard tissues when it interacts with water and OH- from hydroxyapatite at the tissue interface (Lopes et al. 2020).

Lopes & cols (Lopes et al. 2020) evaluated enamel preparation for bonding protocols using the Er,Cr:YSGG laser emitting at 2.78 µm with 20 Hz repetition rate and the pulse width was approximately 140 µs, varying the output power (1.1 W, 1.7 W, 2.41 W) and observed the morphologic changes in enamel. The authors concluded that erbium laser irradiation is better than the conventional acid etching protocol, since laser irradiation

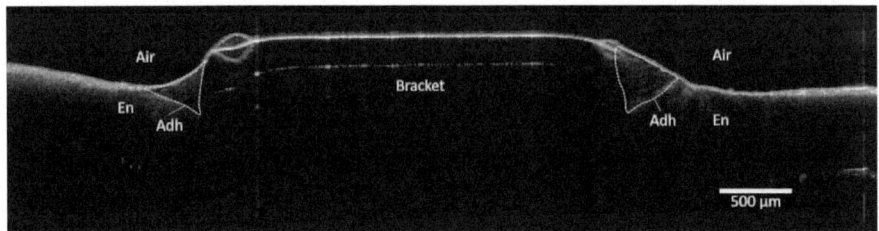

FIGURE 8.3
Two-dimensional OCT image obtained from a metallic bracket bonded on the lingual enamel surface. *Adh*, the adhesive that extrapolated around the bracket during the bonding procedure. *En*, Enamel. Image courtesy of Dr. Monica Lopes.

presents similar results of shear bond strength and, in addition, prevents the enamel demineralization around orthodontic brackets. 2D-OCT images allowed them to observe irregularities on the surface and subsurface, which were more intense with the increase of laser energy density. The irregularities in the backscattered signal from the subsurface of the lased samples decreased after debonding, in which a decrease in bright areas is observed when compared with samples after irradiation, as demonstrated in their publication.

Still, Nd:YAG laser promotes fluoride uptake and prolongs its releasing time in an oral environment (Lopes et al. 2021). It is especially interesting due to the potential of the inhibitory effect of caries on the irradiated enamel (Harazaki et al. 2001; Üşümez et al. 2002; Zezell et al. 2009). As a side effect, the high-power lasers interaction promotes an ablation process that makes the tissue more resistant to demineralization, reducing secondary caries, which is essential for the prevention of the white spot lesions that may occur around the brackets during the orthodontic treatment (Lopes et al. 2020, 2021).

8.3 OCT Evaluation during the Orthodontic Treatment

During the orthodontic treatment, OCT can be used to evaluate the bracket-enamel interface regarding the occurrence of microleakage (Sinescu et al. 2008b; Abbassy et al. 2021), air bubble inclusion on adhesive-resin layer (Rominu et al. 2011), the thickness of the adhesive-resin layer (Sinescu et al. 2008a), the incongruences between the bracket base and the tooth surface (Sinescu et al. 2008b; Rominu et al. 2011), characterization of orthodontic bracket debonding (Ravichandran et al. 2021) and also relevant complementary interventions of the orthodontic treatment, such as the durability of surface sealants (Louie et al. 2005; Şen et al. 2018), and monitoring white spot lesions (WSL) (Şen et al. 2018).

To analyze these topics, 2D image (B-scan) is the most used OCT scan method. Additionally, polymeric or ceramic brackets are preferable for OCT studies, since metallic ones totally reflect the incident light at the surface, and there is no backscattering signal from the subjacent layers (Figure 8.3).

Previous studies proposed another sectional view of OCT images, the en-face (Sinescu et al. 2008a, 2008b) format. This format allows the comparison of the quality of bonding between ceramic or polymeric brackets and the enamel, considering the presence or absence of voids in the adhesive-resin interface (Figure 8.4). The polymeric brackets showed slightly larger gaps than the ceramic ones. These defects were mainly located at the inner part

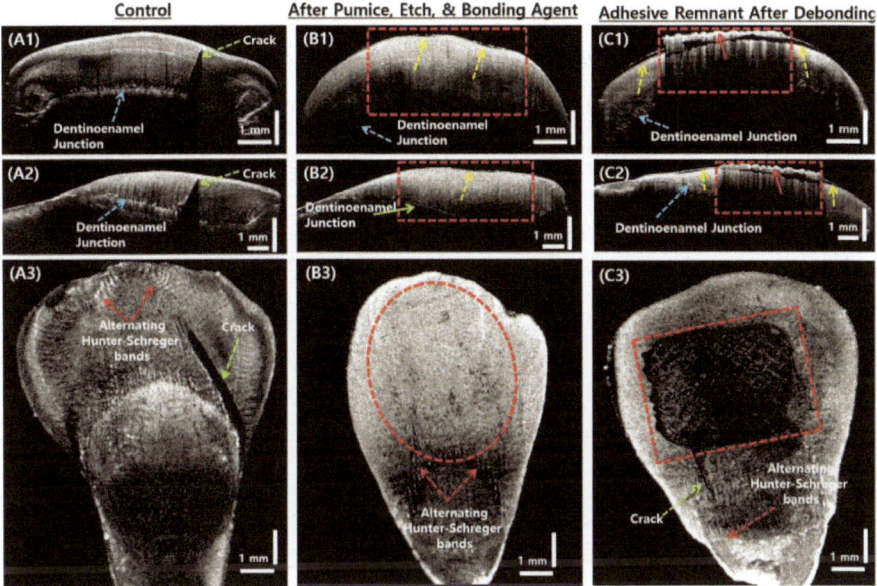

FIGURE 8.4

Two-dimensional (lines 1 and 2) and *en-face* (line 3) OCT images obtained from tooth samples in three different moments: (A) control, without treatment, (B) after pumice etching and bonding agent application, (C) after bracket debonding, in which it is possible to visualize the remnant adhesive. Rectangular and circular dashed areas indicate the regions of tooth surface submitted to the treatment. Reprinted from (Ravichandran et al. 2021).

of the interface, which was attributed as a consequence of wrong bracket placement or to the shrinkage occurring during the curing process. These *en-face* images allow the improvement in bonding protocols since it can both investigate the bracket bonding technique and assess the material defects inside the used composite resin. The advantages of the *en-face* visualization are the versatile orientation and the instant and easy comparison with microscopy images. It also allows control of the dynamic focus, easy identification of defects, and their volume measurement. Based on this, the *en-face* can also three-dimensionally reconstruct the adhesive-resin layer interface in order to characterize and quantify them more accurately (Rominu et al. 2011). The 3D reconstruction has the great advantage that it leaves the sample intact and ready for further testing.

Traditionally, orthodontic appliances are mostly bonded with composite resins (Leão Filho et al. 2013, 2015), but it can also be performed using glass ionomer or resin cements (Sinescu et al. 2008a) – and different bonding materials have distinct responses of thickness and presence of voids, which could be easily investigated by OCT.

8.4 Debonding Protocols Evaluated by OCT

Bracket debonding is an orthodontic procedure with an increased risk of damage to the enamel in the form of scratches, cracks or tissue loss (Petrescu et al. 2021). When a debracket occurs, accidentally or not, it is necessary to completely remove the remaining composite. It can ensure the formation of resin tags in the exposed enamel to guarantee adequate adhesion of the replacement composite (Louie et al. 2005), or to restore the initial aspect at the end of the treatment.

Enamel breakouts after debonding were detectable in 27% of the cases (Koprowski et al. 2014). It is estimated that 150 to 160 μm of enamel loss occurs after debonding, among fractures and cracks (Diedrich 1981), being considered the most critical step in orthodontic treatment (Leão Filho et al. 2013). It also compromises the aesthetic results achieved by the orthodontic treatment.

Debonding of ceramic and polycrystalline brackets is usually considered more dangerous than metallic ones (Leão Filho et al. 2013; Machoy et al. 2019) due to the strong chemical interaction between those materials and the adhesive-resin system, and their friability if compared to the metallic material. For this reason, fractures of ceramic brackets commonly occur in the debonding step and leave their fragments bonded on the tooth surface. It hampers the removal of the remnant resin and polishing of the enamel (Petrescu et al. 2021). Also, when comparing the debonding of ceramic and metallic brackets with different techniques, it was observed that the metallic ones generated a larger amount of remaining adhesive on enamel surfaces. Meanwhile the surfaces bonded with ceramic ones presented enamel damage, such as cracks, whose incidence and extension were not dependent of the debonding technique.

After bracket debonding, OCT is able to measure the remaining resin, the enamel loss after debonding, to monitor the cleanup procedure, and to evaluate the general final enamel morphology, such as fractures and scratches (Diedrich 1981; Leão Filho et al. 2013, 2015; Machoy et al. 2019).

8.4.1 Remaining Resin Measurements before Cleanup

The most used techniques for debonding brackets include the use of pliers that rely on a combination of tensile and shear forces, producing three types of failures: adhesive failure between the adhesive and the base of the bracket (Figure 8.5), adhesive failure between the adhesive and the enamel, and cohesive failure between the molecules of the adhesive layer (Pont et al. 2010).

The key to enamel tissue preservation may be the use of techniques that prevent the development of adhesive failures at the enamel-adhesive interface, leaving larger quantities of remnant resin on the tooth surface as possible, as shown in Figure 8.6, aiming to prevent cohesive failures (Knösel et al. 2010). It allows its cautious removal of cleanup procedures. Despite

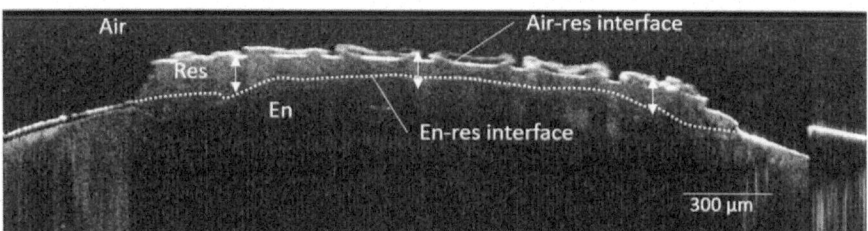

FIGURE 8.5

Two-dimensional OCT image showing the remnant resin layer (double arrows) after the bracket debonding, corresponding to an adhesive failure between the bracket-resin interface. Dotted line delimits the enamel-resin interface. *En*, enamel. *Res*, remnant resin layer. Image courtesy of Lopes (Lopes et al. 2012).

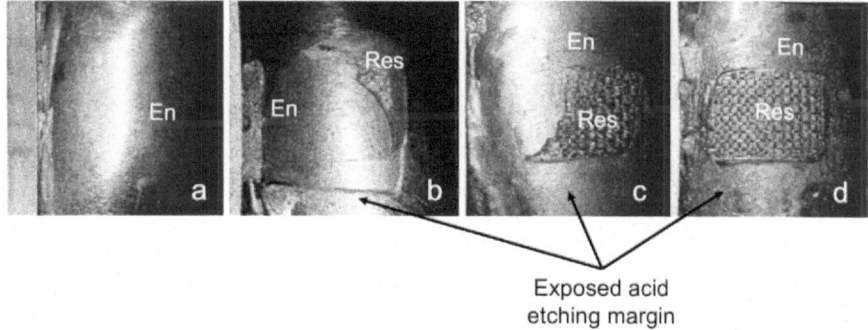

Exposed acid
etching margin

FIGURE 8.6

ARI scores represented by 3D OCT images. (a) Score 0, (b) score 1, (c) score 2 and (d) score 3. Image courtesy of Lopes (Lopes et al. 2012).

this, some authors believe that adhesive failures are an advantage because there will be less adhesive remnant and, consequently, less time will be spent to remove it, and also reduce the risk of excessive wear (Leão Filho et al. 2016; Petrescu et al. 2021).

It is important to observe the contrast between the scanned interfaces. Every time the surface changes, there is a peak of reflection represented by a whiter aspect. The reflection promoted by the air-resin interface is higher than the enamel-resin interface, due to the greater difference of refractive indexes between these surfaces. Due to the similarity between the refractive indexes, the enamel-resin interface is less evident than the air-resin interface, once the air has a very different refractive index. In this way, Koprowski & cols (Koprowski et al. 2014) estimated the remnant resin layer around 265 μm according to two-dimensional Fourier domain OCT images.

After bracket debonding, the remnant resin is commonly classified according to the Adhesive Remnant Index (ARI) (Kinch et al. 1989), with scores from 0 to 3:

- Score 0 = no adhesive remnant left on the tooth.
- Score 1 = less than 50% adhesive remnant left on the tooth.
- Score 2 = more than 50% adhesive remnant left on the tooth.
- Score 3 = 100% adhesive remnant left on the tooth.

This classification was initially performed by visual and stereomicroscopy observations, and currently can also be seen by 3D-OCT images, as shown in Figure 8.6.

The presence of remnant adhesive on enamel depends on the etching protocol employed, the used material, the type of plier, the operator experience and the applied force for bracket removal. Considering the etching procedure of *in vitro* samples, and subsequent debonding by a universal test machine, independent of the samples etching preparation (acid etching or laser irradiation), there was a prevalence of scores 0 and 1 (Leão Filho et al. 2016). It indicates fractures mainly occurred between the enamel-adhesive interface. When the debonding occurs manually with pliers, 2D- and 3D-OCT images indicate a higher incidence of failure at the adhesive-bracket interface for different types of brackets, with no difference between the pliers. But the authors did not classify samples as ARI scores (Leão Filho et al. 2013).

Distinct debonding procedures of ceramic and metallic brackets were evaluated by OCT. Petrescu & cols (Petrescu et al. 2021) compared the use of pliers and side cutters for brackets debonding and found that side cutter generated fractures of the ceramic brackets more frequently than the anterior bracket removal pliers. The debonding procedure generated marked detachment forces, causing enamel cracks, and only fragments of ceramic brackets remained on the enamel surface. Both pliers used in the present experiment generate variable amounts of remaining adhesive on the enamel surface.

There is a lack of studies of ARI determination through optical methods, besides optical microscopy. The other efficient way to assess the enamel surface after debonding is the atomic force microscopy (AFM), but it does not analyze the whole tissue as the OCT does (Machoy et al. 2019), and is not possible for application in a clinical setting. Additionally, the measurements of the remnant resin thickness are not possible by using other imaging techniques (Leão Filho et al. 2015). Otherwise, OCT studies are limited by system resolution and the depth penetration may not allow observation of structural changes (Petrescu et al. 2021).

8.4.2 Remaining Resin and Enamel Thickness After Cleanup

After the cleanup procedure of the remnant resin, the visual examination cannot be precise enough to confirm the presence and the depth of the adhesive layer (Leão Filho et al. 2013). It can be assumed that remnants after polishing may stay unrecognized and may be confused with enamel damage.

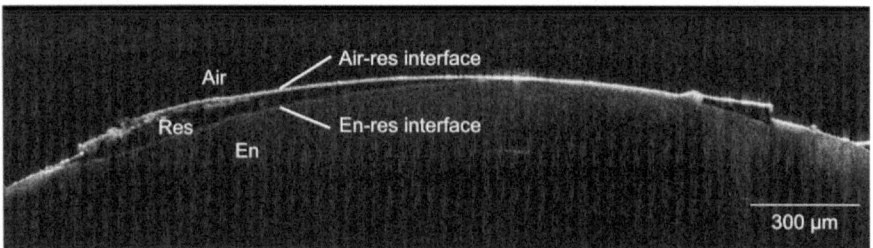

FIGURE 8.7

2D-OCT (930 nm) image of resin layer on the enamel surface after cleanup; *Res*, resin; *En*, enamel; the white contours indicate the thickness of the remnant resin; *arrow* delimit the resin-enamel interface. Image courtesy of Lopes (Lopes et al. 2012).

Such phenomena have a major impact on the results of the examination (Machoy et al. 2019).

The real-time 2D-OCT images allow the monitoring and quantification of any remnants during the cleanup, increasing the efficiency of this procedure. Furthermore, OCT can be used to identify the location of adhesive remnants on the enamel since it is easily possible to differentiate remnant resin and enamel, as shown in Figure 8.7. This is possible due to the high scattering of light at the boundary of each medium inside the sample, then an increasing brightness is observed at the enamel-adhesive interface (Leão Filho et al. 2013; Koprowski et al. 2014).

The most used technique for the cleanup procedure in the literature includes the use of carbide tungsten finishing burs (Leão Filho et al. 2013; Koprowski et al. 2014; Leão Filho et al. 2015; Machoy et al. 2020). When comparing the damage in enamel structure by cleanup with high- or low-speed carbide tungsten burs, OCT images showed better results for the low-speed procedure, which presented both depth and remnant resin layer area significantly lower after polishing than in the high-speed ones. The 3D-OCT surface analysis allows the comparison of the effects of different cleanup methods after debonding (Figure 8.8), evidencing that high-speed burs promoted more scratches on enamel surface, if compared to the low-speed ones (Leão Filho et al. 2013, 2015).

Few studies (Koprowski et al. 2014; Machoy et al. 2019, 2020) measured the enamel thickness after the cleanup procedure. To allow precise measurements they have associated a Fourier domain OCT to a 3D camera for data acquisition, and data was processed through mathematical algorithms to identify the enamel boundary and quantify its thickness layer before and after orthodontic treatments. In general, the remnant resin after debonding is around 105 µm, and after cleanup, there is an enamel loss of approximately 125 µm. The enamel loss depends on the type of bracket (metallic, polymeric or ceramic); even using the same cleanup method (low-speed carbide burs, for example), the type of failure that occurs could be different, and also enamel surface

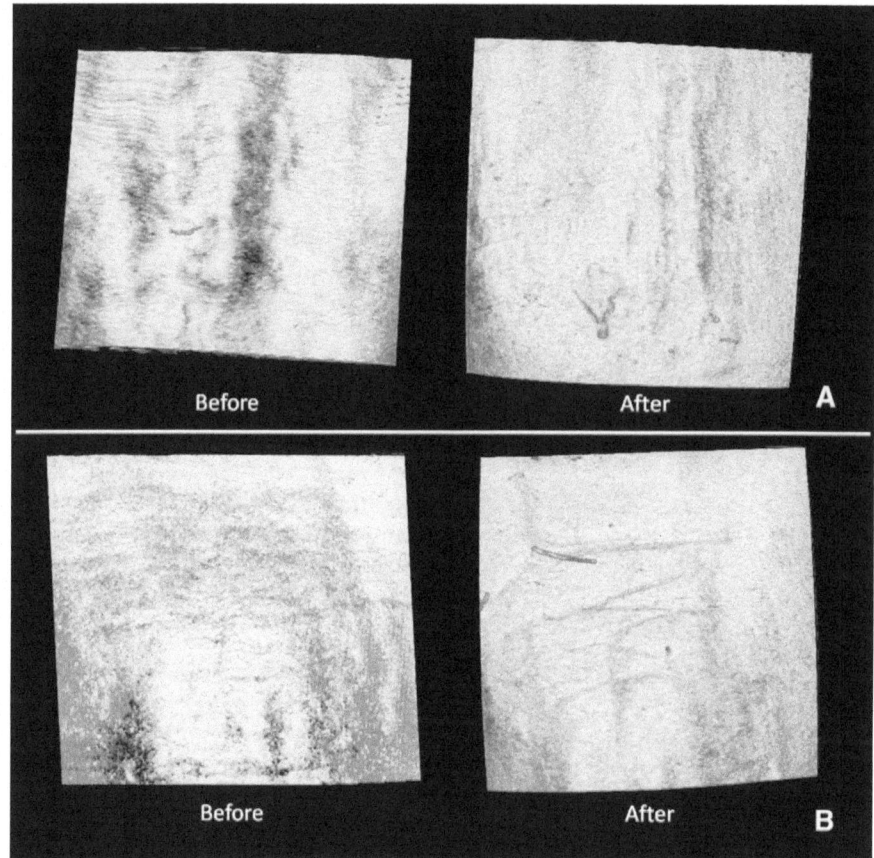

FIGURE 8.8
Three-dimensional OCT images of enamel surface before and after removal of residual
adhesive with high (A) and low (B) speed burs. Scans, 10 × 8 mm. Reprinted with permission
from (Leão Filho et al. 2013) © Elsevier Science & Technology Journals.

fractures can be more prevalent, as observed at different studies. In this way,
the metallic bracket removal is more conservative for enamel, since the resin
debonds of metal surface; whilst in ceramic brackets there is a higher strength
bonding resistance between the resin-bracket interface, increasing the risk of
enamel fractures (Machoy et al. 2019; Petrescu et al. 2021).

8.5 White Spot Lesions and Caries Adjacent to Brackets

Fixed orthodontic appliances (FOAs) may interfere with oral hygiene, due to
the difficulty in removing the biofilm around them (Bakhsh et al. 2017) – as a

result, enamel demineralization may occur in these areas. White spot lesions (WSLs) around brackets and bands are considered one of the most clinical side deficits associated with FOAs (Pithon et al. 2015).

WSLs are the first clinical sign of caries disease and occur as a result of repeated episodes of mineral loss from enamel surface caused by dental bio-film and saliva (Pithon et al. 2015). They comprehend areas usually located at tooth smooth surfaces that have subsurface enamel porosity due to the demineralization. These early incipient subsurface lesions present no cavi-tation and maintain the enamel surface intact, making the diagnostic of the WSLs difficult during their initial stages (Velusamy et al. 2019).

Initial lesions also present "a milky white opacity" appearance, resulting in porosity and low translucency of the affected area. The noncavitated surface layer has ~40–50 mm thickness and exhibits less than 20% demineralization, and the subsurface layers can be up to 70% demineralized. These decalcified lesions result not only in unfavorable esthetics, but they may also demand additional restorative treatment for advanced cases (Chong et al. 2007; Pithon et al. 2015).

WSLs can appear within approximately four weeks from the start of fixed appliance therapy and thereabout up to 96% of the patients with FOA may develop WSLs after prolonged period of orthodontic treatment. Early detection of WSLs followed by efforts to arrest or remineralize enamel sur-face lesions is a critical step during orthodontic therapy (Bakhsh et al. 2017; Velusamy et al. 2019).

Some methods have already been used in clinical studies to diagnose and monitor the WSLs, and the visual inspection associated with probing with a sharp dental explorer remains the most common of them. Meanwhile, clinical inspection depends on the operator's subjectivity and knowledge (Sowa et al. 2011; Velusamy et al. 2019). On the other hand, external pressure promoted by the sharp dental explorer could result in damage to the outer layer enamel in initial stages of demineralization (Suzuki et al. 2019).

Dental radiography is a poor method due to its low sensitivity for an accurate diagnosis of tissue demineralization in incipient caries, since it cannot distinguish between active and arrested lesions and sometimes between noncavitated and cavitated lesions (Gomez 2015; Suzuki et al. 2019; Velusamy et al. 2019).

Due to the subjectivity of visual, tactile exams and X-ray-based methods, objective and quantitative methods for demineralization monitoring are essen-tial in modern caries management strategies. In addition, the precise diag-nosis of the demineralization can be difficult due to the hypermineralization of the outer enamel surface, which hides the subsurface lesion. In this regard, there is an increasing interest in new modalities to detect incipient caries (Sen Yavuz et al. 2021).

Optical and electronic devices have been proposed as alternative methods for incipient caries detection, such as fluorescence, quantitative light fluorescence (QLF), transillumination and electronic caries monitor (ECM) (Gomez 2015; Drancourt et al. 2019).

Optical coherence tomography emerges as an accurate and nonsubjective tool for WSLs' diagnostic that can be used in laboratory studies, but also in a clinical setting (Chong et al. 2007; Sowa et al. 2011). OCT images show high reflection and backscattering signal in areas of demineralization, if compared to sound enamel. This enables OCT devices to detect enamel demineralization as a bright lesion with increased backscattered signal (Velusamy et al. 2019). The OCT signal varies as a function of depth into enamel (A-scan intensity), which is converted in grayscale, and this data generates a histogram of the A-scan intensities. As different backscattering promotes different attenuation coefficients for the analyzed points along the A-scan, the shades of gray quantify the mineral differences of the tissues analyzed. The diagnostic is determined in a quantitative way and generates a descending slope of the A-scan analyzed (Bakhsh et al. 2017).

Different OCT systems have been used for the assessment of enamel demineralization related to orthodontic treatment, as described in Table 8.1. Four studies used SD-OCT (spectral domain optical coherence tomography) systems (Pithon et al. 2014, 2015; Şen et al., 2018, 2021). The selected studies were predominantly laboratorial (Pithon et al. 2014, 2015; Bakhsh et al. 2017; Şen et al. 2018; Velusamy et al. 2019); there were only three clinical studies (Louie et al. 2010; Nee et al. 2014; Şen et al. 2021), one of them had a clinical stage followed by a laboratorial phase, after tooth extraction for analysis (Louie et al. 2010). The authors investigated the protective effect of sealants, cements, resins, varnish or fluoride against demineralization near fixed orthodontic appliances (Louie et al. 2010; Nee et al. 2014; Pithon et al. 2014, 2015; Bakhsh et al. 2017; Şen et al. 2018; Velusamy et al. 2019).

8.6 Microimplants by OCT

A key point in orthodontics is to maintain the stability of anchorage elements, especially when the movement of other teeth are not desirable. The microimplants are considered a safe method to achieve it, by offering a simple insertion for bone anchorage. However, if not properly placed it may fail and promote cortical bone and adjacent soft tissue damages. In addition, it could disturb the patient and delay the treatment. To guarantee the success of microimplant use, it is important to provide its primary stability, which will be followed by a sustainable period of secondary stabilization. The primary stability depends solely on the mechanical interlocking of the threads of the implants with the surrounding bone (Melsen et al. 2000), but is influenced by many other factors, such as (1) the strength and type of the insertion and removal; (2) the quality and anatomy of the

TABLE 8.1

Studies Carried Out with OCT Investigating the Demineralization Related to Fixed Orthodontic Appliances

Authors	OCT system/lightsource	Type of study/samples	Investigation
Pithon et al. Pithon et al.	SD-OCT, 930 nm	Laboratory/bovine incisors	Prevention of caries lesion around brackets using varnish with CPP-ACP and fluoride sealants.
Velusamy et al.	SS-OCT, 1310 nm	Laboratory/bovine incisors	WSLs' detection around brackets bonded with different resin adhesives: nonfluoridated, fluoridated and fluoridated light cured.
Bakhsh et al.	CP-OCT, 1330 nm	Laboratory / premolars	Effect of 45S5-Bioglass on remineralization of WSLs around brackets.
Sen et al.	SD-OCT, 880 nm	Laboratory/molars and premolars	Measurement of the layer thickness of orthodontic surface sealants (Light Bond™ Sealant, Pro Seal® and Opal® Seal) using an ophthalmic OCT system.
Louie et al.	PS-OCT, with a broadband high-power superluminescent diode (SLD)	Clinical followed by laboratory study/premolars	Quantification of WSLs severity and assessment of the inhibitory effect of fluoride varnish around modified orthodontic bands.
Sen et al.	SD-OCT, 880 nm	Clinical/split mouth	Assessment of orthodontic surface sealant layer thickness and integrity (Pro Seal® and Opal® Seal) during a 12-month follow-up using an ophthalmic OCT system.
Nee et al.	CP-OCT, with a swept laser source operating with a 30 kHz a-scan sweep rate	Clinical/premolars	Monitoring the demineralization peripheral to orthodontic brackets bonded with resin or glass ionomer cement.

SD-OCT: spectral domain optical coherence tomography. SS-OCT: swept source optical coherence tomography. CP-OCT: cross-polarization optical coherence tomography. PS-OCT: polarization sensitive optical coherence tomography.

cortical bone; (3) the microdamage to the bone; (4) the design and size of the microimplants; (5) the preparation of the implantation site (drill or drill free); and (6) the operator experience (Wilmes et al. 2006; Lakshmikantha et al. 2019, 2018).

From a clinical point of view, the high torque, incorrect angulation and drilling procedure with burs may lead to large bone microcracks, decreasing the bone density (Lakshmikantha et al. 2018) and accumulating debris adjacent to the microimplant. It reduces the contact at the bone-microimplant interface and the primary stability, which increases the incidence of its dislodgement (Lee et al. 2010; Yadav et al. 2012). The classical methods to evaluate these bone alterations are the microcomputed tomography (micro-CT), the histomorphometric analysis (Wawrzinek et al. 2008), and finite element analysis (FEA) (Motoyoshi et al. 2009) – all of them considered invasive or ionizing techniques, limited to *in vitro* studies.

Two studies (Lakshmikantha et al. 2018, 2019) used a commercially available 1300 nm swept source OCT system to obtain 2D cross-sectional (250 μm depth), volumetric (3D) and *en-face* images (at 100 μm and 50 μm, respectively) of microimplants inserted at 45° and 90° in a laboratory study. 2D and *en-face* images identified the cracks, bone debris and bone elevation as a consequence of the microimplant placement with high contrast and resolution. Through the A-scan analysis it was possible to localize microcracks in depth or interface changes.

OCT captures the backscattered and reflected light from the sample. The generated image depends on the interaction between the sample (tissue characteristics and composition) and the incident light (specially the central wavelength). Microimplants' surfaces are highly reflective, since they are composed of titanium alloy, which will limit the light penetration depth. For this reason, the cortical bone in the distal area of the implant cannot be clearly seen when the microimplant is positioned (Figure 8.9). In adjacent areas, OCT provided enough depth penetration to assess debris and microcracks. According to Lakshmikantha & cols (Lakshmikantha et al. 2018), the microimplants failure rate at 45° insertion angle was higher than at 90°. The perpendicular placement of the microimplants seems to be more stable (Figures 8.9(C) and 8.9(I)). In relation to the insertion in drill or drill-free method, the bone debris occurrence was deeper in no-drilling microimplant insertion (Figure 8.9), whilst the previously drilled cavity was considered a better modality for the success of microimplants (Figure 8.9(G–L)) (Lakshmikantha et al. 2019).

Despite a good application for microimplants follow-up, it is still restricted to laboratory studies, since the central wavelength of commercially available OCT systems is not sufficient enough for deep penetration into the gingiva-bone-microimplant interface.

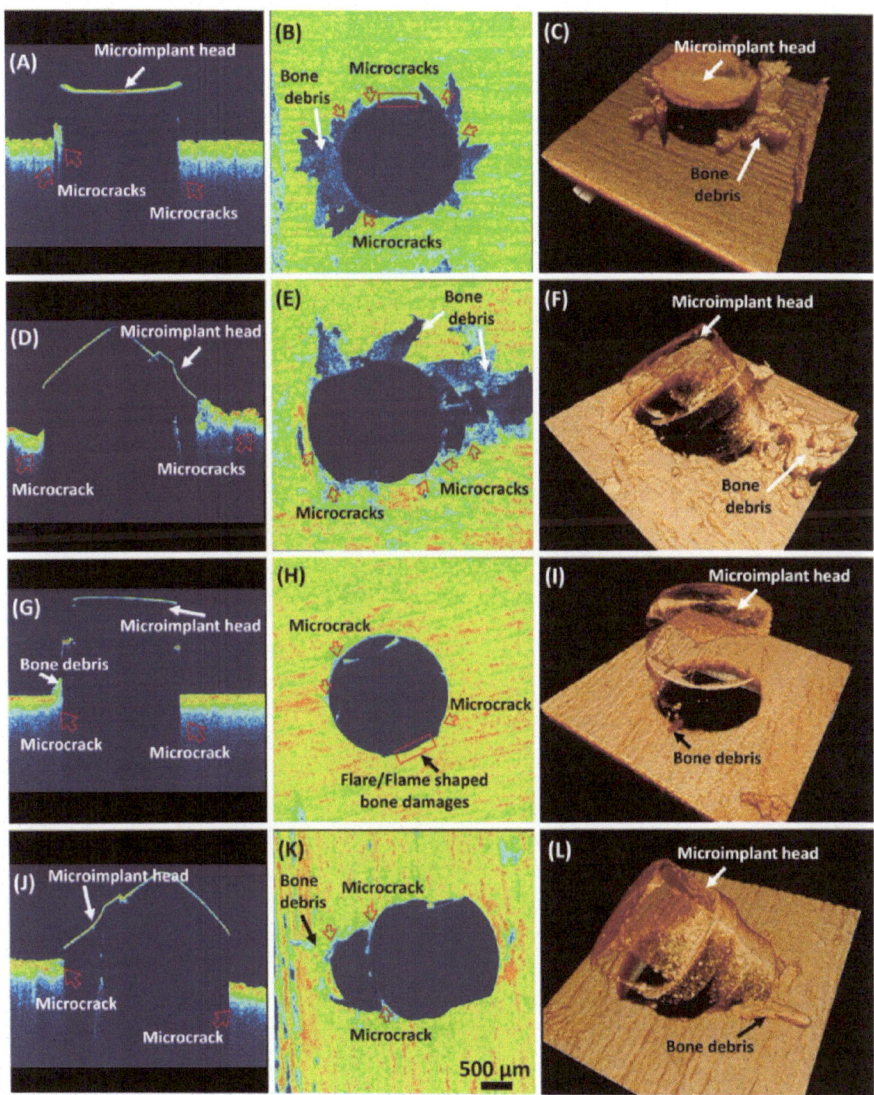

FIGURE 8.9

OCT image showing crack occurrence after microimplant insertion at 45° and 90°, with and without pre-insertion drilling. (A–C) and (D–F) are OCT images of microimplant inserted at 90° and 45°, respectively, which were not submitted to pre-insertion drilling. (G–I) and (J–L) are OCT images of microimplants inserted at 90° and 45°, respectively, after drilling. Red arrows indicate cracks, and red rectangular boxes indicate the flares/flame shaped bone damages due to the microimplant placement. Reprinted from (Lakshmikantha et al. 2019).

8.7 OCT Periodontal Analysis Related to Orthodontic Movement

Orthodontic tooth movement occurs in response to an externally applied mechanical force (Holland et al. 2019). This movement is considered a "periodontal phenomenon", as conventional orthodontic movements lead to periodontal ligament (PDL) compression, thereby activating the dynamics of crestal bone resorption and apposition (Agrawal et al. 2019).

For periodontal approach during orthodontic movements, radiographic images should show the PDL, lamina dura and periapical region, and also quantify linear measurements, such as the crestal bone levels and bone defects. These measurements are useful to identify related factors to periodontal disease and involved tissue before treatment, during and after that. In this way, radiographic images can provide critical information for diagnosis and treatment planning, which can also serve as baseline information for the assessment of treatment outcomes (Mol 2004). But although conventional radiography is a popular diagnostic aid in clinical settings, it gives us only overlapped two-dimensional images that confuse diagnosis, especially for periodontal approach (Baek et al. 2009). Also, the radiographic exam utility is limited due to its relatively low axial resolution, which could not differentiate any variation of the PDL under orthodontics forces (Na et al. 2008).

OCT has been used as an imaging tool for hard and soft tissues in dentistry for distinct purposes, providing high-resolution images that allow evaluation of the PDL changes, including responses to various orthodontic forces generated during treatment, and provide results similar to the usual histologic images of periodontal tissues (Petrescu et al. 2021). Using a homemade TD-OCT system with 10 μm of axial resolution, Baek & cols (Baek et al. 2009) carried out a study using rats and evidenced the feasibility of OCT for PDL evaluation under orthodontics forces. Tooth response could be predicted precisely by analyzing the changes of the PDL in both compressive and tensile sites tomographically. The changed periodontal ligament was imaged with OCT and digital intraoral radiography. OCT images allowed measuring the changes in the periodontal ligament from all directions; on the other hand, radiographies could not show the portions overlapped by teeth. The averages of ligament thickness in OCT were larger than those from radiography in all groups. However, several factors should be considered before real clinical application of OCT for PDL evaluation, such as the limited depth penetration of OCT, which could limit its indication to patients with thin gingival phenotype. Another study (Na et al. 2008) also observed that polarization-sensitive OCT may be helpful for PDL evaluation, since collagen, the main component of the PDL, has a well-known strong birefringence. However, the application of low intensity orthodontic forces promotes too discrete movements in PDL, which is not identified by OCT images, since it is out of its resolution.

Despite OCT has already been used in a clinical setting (Fernandes et al. 2017, 2019), to noninvasive periodontal probing and monitoring of the periodontal disease, the clinical evaluation of changes related to PDL during orthodontic treatment requires higher axial and transversal resolution of OCT systems, associated with higher central wavelengths of light source, aiming to allow deeper penetration during scanning.

The studies carried out by Baek & cols (Baek et al. 2009) and Na & cols (Na et al. 2008) obtained results not reproducible with patients, since they used an animal model (rats) whose periodontal morphologic dimensions do not correspond to those structures observed in patients.

8.8 Conclusions

Although OCT has been barely used to evaluate the after effect of materials and tissue modifications related to orthodontics in a clinical setting, it has great potential, since it is a real-time *in situ* imaging technique for monitoring patients under orthodontic treatment. The depth light penetration is sufficient to evaluate the enamel changes caused by adhesive procedures, in superficial layers, and should be explored in clinical studies. In addition, OCT can also be used along orthodontic treatment, aiming to monitor WLS development, the presence of remnant resin after bracket debonding, as well as its removal by cleanup and eventual damages promoted to enamel surface.

There are still no clinical studies with OCT to evaluate the orthodontic microimplants' behavior.

To date, the depth penetration could be an OCT limitation for clinical studies since only the superficial alterations are seen, and no information of the area under the bracket can be extracted before its removal. Also bone evaluation is nowadays limited to laboratory studies, because currently available OCT systems have no sufficient depth penetration to scan the bone under gingiva. The development of intraoral sensors with deeper light penetration and image stability become imperative to integrate OCT for clinical bone evaluation for orthodontics and other dental specialties.

References

Abbassy, M.A., Bakhsh, T.A., Bakry, A.S. 2021. A novel evaluation method for detecting defects of the bonded orthodontic bracket-tooth interface. *Biomed Res. Int.* 2021: 6634595.

Agrawal, A.A., Kolte, A.P., Kolte, R.A., Vaswani, V., Shenoy, U., Rathi, P. 2019. Comparative CBCT analysis of the changes in buccal bone morphology after corticotomy and micro-osteoperforations assisted orthodontic treatment – Case series with a split mouth design. *Saudi Dent. J.* 31: 58–65.

Baek, J.H., Na, J., Lee, B.H., Choi, E.S., Son, W.S. 2009. Optical approach to the periodontal ligament under orthodontic tooth movement: A preliminary study with optical coherence tomography. *Am. J. Orthod. Dentofac. Orthop.* 135: 252–259.

Bakhsh, T.A., Bakry, A.S., Mandurah, M.M., Abbassy, M.A. 2017. Novel evaluation and treatment techniques for white spot lesions. An in vitro study. *Orthod. Craniofacial Res.* 20: 170–176.

Chong, S.L., Darling, C.L., Fried, D. 2007. Nondestructive measurement of the inhibition of demineralization on smooth surfaces using polarization-sensitive optical coherence tomography. *Lasers Surg. Med.* 39: 422–427.

Diedrich, P. 1981. Enamel alterations from bracket bonding and debonding: A study with the scanning electron microscope. *Am. J. Orthod.* 79: 500–522.

Drancourt, N., Roger-Leroi, V., Martignon, S., Jablonski-Momeni, A., Pitts, N., Doméjean, S. 2019. Carious lesion activity assessment in clinical practice: a systematic review. *Clin. Oral Investig.* 23: 1513–1524.

Fernandes, L.O., Mota, C.C.B. d. O., Oliveira, H.O., Neves, J.K., Santiago, L.M., Gomes, A.S.L. 2019. Optical coherence tomography follow-up of patients treated from periodontal disease. *J. Biophotonics* 12: 2.

Fernandes, L.O., Mota, C.C.B.O., de Melo, L.S.A., da Costa Soares, M.U.S., da Silva Feitosa, D., Gomes, A.S.L. 2017. In vivo assessment of periodontal structures and measurement of gingival sulcus with optical coherence tomography: a pilot study. *J. Biophotonics* 10: 862–869.

Gomez, J. 2015. Detection and diagnosis of the early caries lesion. *BMC Oral Health* 15: 1–7.

Harazaki, M., Hayakawa, K., Fukui, T., Isshiki, Y., Powell, L.G. 2001. The Nd-YAG laser is useful in prevention of dental caries during orthodontic treatment. *Bull. Tokyo Dent. Coll.* 42: 79–86.

Harper, D.J., Augustin, M., Lichtenegger, A. et al. 2018. White light polarization sensitive optical coherence tomography for sub-micron axial resolution and spectroscopic contrast in the murine retina. *Biomed. Opt. Express* 9: 2115.

Holland, R., Bain, C., Utreja, A. 2019. Osteoblast differentiation during orthodontic tooth movement. *Orthod. Craniofacial Res.* 22: 177–182.

Iijima, M., Ito, S., Yuasa, T., Muguruma, T., Saito, T., Mizoguchi, I. 2008. Bond strength comparison and scanning electron microscopic evaluation of three orthodontic bonding systems. *Dent. Mater. J.* 27: 392–399.

Jumanca, D., Matichescu, A., Galuscan, A., Rusu, L.C., Muntean, C. 2018. Comparative study of acid etching on dental enamel. *Rev. Chim.* 69: 2913–2915.

Kinch, A.P., Taylor, H., Warltler, R., Oliver, R.G., Newcombe, R.G. 1989. A clinical study of amount of adhesive remaining on enamel after debonding, comparing etch times of 15 and 60 seconds. *Am. J. Orthod. Dentofac. Orthop.* 95: 415–421.

Knösel, M., Mattysek, S., Jung, K. et al. 2010. Impulse debracketing compared to conventional debonding: Extent of enamel damage, adhesive residues and the need for postprocessing. *Angle Orthod.* 80: 1036–1044.

Koprowski, R., Machoy, M., Woźniak, K., Wróbel, Z. 2014. Automatic method of analysis of OCT images in the assessment of the tooth enamel surface after orthodontic treatment with fixed braces. *Biomed. Eng. Online* 13: 48–66. https://doi.org/10.1186/1475-925X-13-48

Lakshmikantha, H.T., Ravichandran, N.K., Jeon, M., Kim, J., Park, H.S. 2018. Assessment of cortical bone microdamage following insertion of microimplants using optical coherence tomography: a preliminary study. *J. Zhejiang Univ. Sci. B* 19: 818–828.

Lakshmikantha, H.T., Ravichandran, N.K., Jeon, M., Kim, J., Park, H.S. 2019. 3-Dimensional characterization of cortical bone microdamage following placement of orthodontic microimplants using optical coherence tomography. *Sci. Rep.* 9: 1–13.

Leão Filho, J.C., Mota, C.C.B.O., Cassimiro-silva, P.F., Gomes, A.S.L. 2016. A comparative study of shear bond strength of orthodontic bracket after acid-etched and Er:YAG treatment on enamel surface. *Lasers Dent.* XXII 9692, 96920R.

Leão Filho, J.C.B., Braz, A.K.S., de Araujo, R.E., Tanaka, O.M., Pithon, M.M. 2015. Enamel quality after debonding: Evaluation by optical coherence tomography. *Braz. Dent. J.* 26: 384–389.

Leão Filho, J.C.B., Braz, A.K.S., De Souza, T.R., De Araujo, R.E., Pithon, M.M., Tanaka, O.M. 2013. Optical coherence tomography for debonding evaluation: An in-vitro qualitative study. *Am. J. Orthod. Dentofac. Orthop.* 143: 61–68.

Lee, N.K., Baek, S.H. 2010. Effects of the diameter and shape of orthodontic mini-implants on microdamage to the cortical bone. *Am. J. Orthod. Dentofac. Orthop.* 138: 8.e1–8.e8.

Leitgeb, R., Placzek, F., Rank, E. et al. 2021. Enhanced medical diagnosis for dOCTors: a perspective of optical coherence tomography. *J. Biomed. Opt.* 26: 1–47.

Lopes, D.S., Pereira, D.L., Mota, C.C. et al. 2020. Surface evaluation of enamel etched by Er, Cr:Ysgg laser for orthodontic purpose. *J. Contemp. Dent. Pract.* 21: 227–232.

Lopes, M. S. 2012. *Avaliação do Esmalte Dentário Após a Descolagem de Brackets Ortodônticos e da Remoção da Resina Remanescente.* Universidade Federal de Pernambuco.

Lopes, M.S., Mota, C.C.B.O., Pereira, D.L., Amaral, M.M., Zezell, D.M., Gomes, A.S.L. 2019. Effect of Nd:YAG laser and aluminum oxide sandblasting preconditioning on lingual enamel: Brackets shear bond strength and morphological characterization. *Opt. InfoBase Conf. Pap.* Part F142-ECBO 2019, 19–22.

Lopes, M.S., Pereira, D.L., de Oliveira Mota, C.C.B., Amaral, M.M., Zezell, D.M., Gomes, A.S.L. 2021. The lingual enamel morphology and bracket shear bond strength influenced by Nd:YAG laser and aluminum oxide sandblasting preconditioning. *Clin. Oral Investig.* 25: 1151–1158.

Louie, T., Lee, C., Hsu, D. et al. 2010. Clinical assessment of early tooth demineralization using polarization sensitive optical coherence tomography. *Lasers Surg. Med.* 42: 898–905.

Louie, T.M., Jones, R.S., Sarma, A. V., Fried, D. 2005. Selective removal of composite sealants with near-ultraviolet laser pulses of nanosecond duration. *J. Biomed. Opt.* 10: 014001.

Machoy, M., Seeliger, J., Koprowski, R., Safranow, K., Gedrange, T., Woźniak, K. 2020. Enamel Thickness before and after Orthodontic Treatment Analysed in Optical Coherence Tomography. *Biomed Res. Int.* 2020: 1–1.

Machoy, M.E., Koprowski, R., Szyszka-Sommerfeld, L., Safranow, K., Gedrange, T., Woźniak, K. 2019. Optical coherence tomography as a non-invasive method of enamel thickness diagnosis after orthodontic treatment by 3 different types of brackets. *Adv. Clin. Exp. Med.* 28: 211–218.

Melsen, B., Costa, A. 2000. Immediate loading of implants used for orthodontic anchorage. *Clin Orthod Res* 3: 23–28.

Mol, A. 2004. Imaging methods in periodontology. *Periodontol. 2000* 34: 34–48.

Motoyoshi, M., Inaba, M., Ono, A., Ueno, S., Shimizu, N. 2009. The effect of cortical bone thickness on the stability of orthodontic mini-implants and on the stress distribution in surrounding bone. *Int. J. Oral Maxillofac. Surg.* 38: 13–18.

Na, J., Lee, B.H., Baek, J.H., Choi, E.S. 2008. Optical approach for monitoring the periodontal ligament changes induced by orthodontic forces around maxillary anterior teeth of white rats. *Med. Biol. Eng. Comput.* 46: 597–603.

Nee, A., Chan, K., Kang, H., Staninec, M., Darling, C.L., Fried, D. 2014. Longitudinal monitoring of demineralization peripheral to orthodontic brackets using cross polarization optical coherence tomography. *J. Dent.* 42: 547–555.

Petrescu, S.M.S., Țuculină, M., Osiac, E. et al. 2021. Use of optical coherence tomography in orthodontics. *Exp. Ther. Med.* 22: 1–7.

Pithon, M.M., Dos Santos, M.J., Andrade, C.S.S. et al. 2014. Effectiveness of varnish with CPP-ACP in prevention of caries lesions around orthodontic brackets: An OCT evaluation. *Eur. J. Orthod.* 37: 177–182.

Pithon, M.M., Santos, M. de J., de Souza, C.A. et al. 2015. Effectiveness of fluoride sealant in the prevention of carious lesions around orthodontic brackets: An OCT evaluation. *Dental Press J. Orthod.* 20: 37–42.

Pont, H.B., Özcan, M., Bagis, B., Ren, Y. 2010. Loss of surface enamel after bracket debonding: An in-vivo and ex-vivo evaluation. *Am. J. Orthod. Dentofac. Orthop.* 138: 387.e1–387.e9.

Ravichandran, N.K., Lakshmikantha, H.T., Park, H.S., Jeon, M., Kim, J. 2021. Micron-scale human enamel layer characterization after orthodontic bracket debonding by intensity-based layer segmentation in optical coherence tomography images. *Sci. Rep.* 11: 1–15.

Rominu, R., Sinescu, C., Rominu, M. et al. 2011. The assessment of orthodontic bonding defects: optical coherence tomography followed by three-dimensional reconstruction. *Opt. Complex Syst.* OCS11 8172, 817214.

Sen Yavuz, B., Kargul, B. 2021. Comparative evaluation of the spectral-domain optical coherence tomography and microhardness for remineralization of enamel caries lesions. *Dent. Mater. J.* 40: 1115–1121.

Şen, S., Erber, R., Kunzmann, K. et al. 2018. Assessing abrasion of orthodontic surface sealants using a modified ophthalmic optical coherence tomography device. *Clin. Oral Investig.* 22: 3143–3157.

Şen, S., Erber, R., Orhan, G., Zingler, S., Lux, C.J. 2021. OCT evaluation of orthodontic surface sealants: a 12-month follow-up randomized clinical trial. *Clin. Oral Investig.* 25: 1547–1558.

Shinya, M., Shinya, A., Lassila, L.V.J. et al. 2008. Treated enamel surface patterns associated with five orthodontic adhesive systems – Surface morphology and shear bond strength. *Dent. Mater. J.* 27: 1–6.

Sinescu, C., Negrutiu, M.L., Hughes, M. et al. 2008a. Investigation of bracket bonding for orthodontic treatments using en-face optical coherence tomography. *Biophotonics Photonic Solut. Better Heal. Care* 6991, 69911M.

Sinescu, C., Negrutiu, M.L., Todea, C. et al. 2008b. Quality assessment of dental treatments using en-face optical coherence tomography. *J. Biomed. Opt.* 13: 054065.

Sowa, M.G., Popescu, D.P., Friesen, J.R., Hewko, M.D., Choo-Smith, L.P. 2011. A comparison of methods using optical coherence tomography to detect demineralized regions in teeth. *J. Biophotonics* 4: 814–823.

Sundfeld, R.H., de Oliveira, C.H., da Silva, A.M.J.D., Briso, A.L.F., Sundfeld, M.L.M.M. 2005. Resin tag length of one-step and self-etching adhesives bonded to unground enamel. *Bull. Tokyo Dent. Coll.* 46: 43–49.

Suzuki, S., Kataoka, Y., Kanehira, M., Kobayashi, M., Miyazaki, T., Manabe, A. 2019. Detection of enamel subsurface lesions by swept-source optical coherence tomography. *Dent. Mater. J.* 38: 303–310.

Üşümez, S., Orhan, M., Üşümez, A. 2002. Laser etching of enamel for direct bonding with an Er,Cr:YSGG hydrokinetic laser system. *Am. J. Orthod. Dentofac. Orthop.* 122: 649–656.

Velusamy, P., Shimada, Y., Kanno, Z., Ono, T., Tagami, J. 2019. Optical evaluation of enamel white spot lesions around orthodontic brackets using swept-source optical coherence tomography (Ss-oct): An in vitro study. *Dent. Mater. J.* 38: 22–27.

Wawrzinek, C., Sommer, T., Fischer-Brandies, H. 2008. Mikrotraumen in kortikalem Knochen nach tiefer Insertion orthodontischer Mikroschrauben. *J. Orofac. Orthop.* 69: 121–134.

Wilmes, B., Rademacher, C., Olthoff, G., Drescher, D. 2006. Einfluss der Insertionsparameter auf die Primärstabilität orthodontischer Mini-Implantate. *J. Orofac. Orthop.* 67: 162–174.

Yadav, S., Upadhyay, M., Liu, S., Roberts, E., Neace, W.P., Nanda, R. 2012. Microdamage of the cortical bone during mini-implant insertion with self-drilling and self-tapping techniques: A randomized controlled trial. *Am. J. Orthod. Dentofac. Orthop.* 141: 538–546.

Zezell, D.M., Boari, H.G.D., Ana, P.A., Eduardo, C.D.P., Powell, G.L. 2009. Nd:YAG laser in caries prevention: A clinical trial. *Lasers Surg. Med.* 41: 31–35.

9

OCT in Prosthodontics

Paulo Ney Lyra de Moraes, Marcia Cristina Dias de Moraes and Denise M. Zezell

Center for Lasers and Applications, Instituto de Pesquisas Energéticas e Nucleares, IPEN-CNEN, São Paulo, Brazil

CONTENTS

9.1 Introduction

Dental prosthesis, as a dental specialty, ranges from the partial restoration of a dental element to the total functional rehabilitation of dental arches through implant-supported prostheses (Carlsson et al. 2006).

The impact of the loss of dental elements, total or partial, is not only due to the aesthetic factor. It can lead to deformities and loss of function, which has been identified as a risk factor for dementia and cognitive (Gerritsen et al. 2010; Lin 2018; Hedberg et al. 2021).

The influence of the characteristics of dental prostheses (type of prosthesis, composition materials, shape, extension, adaptation to the remaining dental structure and oral structures (quantity of remaining dental or bone structure,

DOI: 10.1201/9781351104562-9

thickness and quality of the oral mucosa) is already widely discussed in the literature on its longevity and biocompatibility (Nassani 2017).

While the clinical evaluation of removable dental prostheses is based on clinical and visual criteria, the assessment of fixed prostheses, in addition to these criteria, is carried out by probing and periapical and/or bite-wing radiographs (Alsterstål-Englund et al. 2021).

The optical coherence tomography (OCT) technique has many medical and dental applications for diagnosis and assessment of different clinical conditions (Ali et al. 2021).

In this chapter, the use of OCT will be addressed as a conservative evaluation technique for dental prostheses, as well as for the assessment of the health of adjacent hard and soft oral tissues.

9.2 Prosthodontics

A dental prosthesis, of any type, location and size, needs to be able to recover the patient's oral functions, which include chewing, phonetics, aesthetics and support of facial tissues. It can replace a part of the dental crown; an entire crown, supported on a dental structure or on a metal or fiber core; one or more missing dental elements, through removable, fixed prostheses or through the installation of osseointegrated implants. For this, the prosthesis must be made with biocompatible material, so as not to irritate the oral tissues; be resistant to corrosion, avoiding changes in its physicochemical properties; make the accumulation of microorganisms and biofilm formation as difficult as possible; be resistant to masticatory load, maintaining its structural integrity and the patient's vertical dimension; have excellent marginal adaptation to hinder the accumulation of biofilm and consequent degradation of margins; have optical properties that mimic the oral tissues being replaced (The Glossary of Prosthodontic Terms 2017).

The evaluation of the marginal adaptation of prosthetic crowns can be carried out through probing. However, very small adaptation failures and access to the entire length around the prosthesis makes effective control difficult, leading to an increase in marginal infiltration (Kumar et al. 2020).

Intraoral and extra-oral radiographic techniques allow the assessment of marginal adaptation of single crowns and fixed prostheses. However, initial complications, even when clinical probing is included, can be very hard to detect. This is in addition to the other disadvantages in using ionizing radiation to perform the exam, and only obtaining 2D images, with limited resolution (Murat et al. 2013; Mauad et al. 2021).

It is possible to evaluate the bone support adjacent to dental elements that act as pillars of fixed partial prostheses or removable partial prostheses through radiographs. Similarly, the bone adjacent to intraosseous implants can also be monitored through radiographs, comparing the bone level at the time of implant reopening with periodic radiographs (De Bruyn et al. 2013; Coli et al. 2017; Renvert et al. 2018).

In an *in vivo* study, where 25 patients needed to undergo a surgical approach to treat periimplantitis, the authors compared the height values at the radiographic bone level with the height measured at the surgical site, obtaining significantly higher intraoperative values than those obtained through radiographs. Radiographs also do not allow an assessment of bone height on the buccal and internal surfaces (García-García et al. 2016). Casseta et al. evaluated 142 patients following the same methodology, concluding that the bone level was overestimated in the radiographic assessment compared to that observed in surgery, however, they also highlighted that the follow-up with radiographs over time was reliable in assessing the occurrence of bone loss (Cassetta et al. 2018).

In addition to intraoral and panoramic radiography, cone beam computed tomograph (CBCT) is widely used for planning the installation of implants, as it provides 3D images with a low radiation dose when compared to conventional CT scans. CBCT can also be used for monitoring implants, but in the presence of metals, artifacts occur that make post-surgical evaluation difficult. The interpretation of tomographic images is more experience than the evaluation of periapical radiographs (Bohner et al. 2017; Zhang et al. 2021).

9.3 Optical Coherence Tomography (OCT) in Prosthodontics

OCT is a non-invasive technique, which obtains real-time, contactless, high-resolution cross-sectional images based on the principle of the optical interferometer, using a non-ionizing, near infrared reflected light, to enable quantitative and qualitative *in vitro*, *ex vivo* and *in vivo* evaluation of living tissues (Huang et al. 1991).

Since the original studies of Colson et al. (Colston et al. 1998a; Colston et al. 1998b), interest in OCT in dentistry has grown, due to its potential for clinical and research use (Feldchtein et al. 1998).

Several studies have addressed changes in dental structures through OCT, even in early stages, including demineralization of enamel and dentin, occurrence of fractures and the presence of cracks, demonstrating the superiority of OCT when compared to other techniques, mainly for providing information about the depth of the observed changes (Shimada et al. 2015; Kim et al. 2017).

9.3.1 Removable Prosthesis

Edentulism is the result of a combination of factors: social, educational, cultural, as well as the influence of previous dental treatments. Oral rehabilitation, functional and aesthetic, was initially achieved through removable prostheses, either total or partial. Restoration of masticatory and phonetic functions, as well as aesthetics and facial muscle support, can be compromised by the quantity and quality of support for removable dentures, thus affecting the quality of life of patients (Carlsson 1984; Campos Sugio et al. 2021).

Despite the evolution of restorative techniques and materials, patients often still opt for rehabilitation with removable prostheses. Acrylic resin (polymethyl methacrylate – PMMA – polymer) is the most used material for the manufacture of removable dentures, despite the constant evolution of dental materials, due to its low cost, ease of handling, polishing and repair, as well as variety of colors for mimicking oral tissue (Zarb et al. 2012; Saeed et al. 2020).

The use of acrylic in dentures has already been associated with changes in the oral mucosa of patients who use removable dentures, especially for a longer period, because its physical-mechanical properties undergo changes, such as mechanical and chemical wear and influence of smoking, poor hygiene and eating habits that lead to changes in the pH of the oral environment (Moskona et al. 1992; GhiŢĂ et al. 2020).

Finished dentures, made with two types of resin, self-curing (PalaXpress, Heraeus-Kulzer, Japan) and thermopolymerizable (ACRON, GC Corporation, Tokyo, Japan) have been assessed with using Swept Source-OCT instrument (Santec Corporation, Japan: central wavelength 1260–1360 nm; 20 kHz sweep rate; axial resolution 11 μm in air and 8 μm in tissue; lateral resolution 37 μm). The image depth was up to 6 mm, depending on the optical properties of the evaluated resin, enabling the visualization of internal structural differences in the resin base of the prostheses, with greater irregularities and pores in the bases made with self-curing resin, facilitating the accumulation of biofilm, decreasing resistance and favoring pigmentation (Sumi et al. 2011).

Aquino et al. also detected and measured the biofilm development over acrylic resin samples with spectral domain-OCT (Callisto, Thorlabs Inc.: central wavelength 930 nm; 100 nm of spectral bandwidth; maximum output power of 5 mW; axial resolution of 7/5.3 μm in water/air, respectively; lateral resolution of 8 μm; depth of light penetration of 1.6 mm) (Aquino et al. 2019).

Hara et al. demonstrated the positive effect of decontaminating PMMA resin samples for the manufacture of dentures colonized by *C. albicans* and *S. mutans* by means of full-field OCT (FF-OCT, LLTech Inc., Paris, France; depth between 250 and 300 μm) with the use of unsaturated fatty acid salts (oleate, linoleate and linolenate solutions). The OCT technique allowed the verification of the detachment of the biofilm from the substrate by visualization of gaps at the interface (Hara et al. 2021).

The OCT (*en-face* OCT) technique was used to analyze dentures made by the conventional pressure-pack procedure method and dentures made with a pre-impregnated polymer glass fiber net reinforcement internally in its structure. Defects in the internal structure of the prostheses were observed that were impossible to be visualized by other methods. Such defects could result in fracture of the prostheses, or in the appearance of porosities, which could be colonized by microorganisms (Negrutiu et al. 2008).

Removable partial dentures have a metallic structure due to the mechanical stresses suffered and to provide stability. Metal alloys are normally used, and initially they had a high gold content, to avoid corrosion in the oral cavity. Currently, nickel-chrome (Ni-Cr) and cobalt-chrome (Co-Cr) alloys are the most used in removable partial dentures, for economic reasons. There is a concern about the toxicity of these elements and the possibility to cause reactions such as gingivitis and periodontitis (Council on Dental Materials, Instruments, and Equipment 1985; Reddy et al. 2011).

Changes in gingival volume can be assessed by OCT, and it is a clinical parameter to gingival health, with bleeding on probing and depth probe (Wang et al. 2020).

9.3.2 Fixed Prosthesis

A fixed prosthesis can range from the reconstruction of a dental element, presenting a loss of tooth structure greater than that recommended for the use of direct restorations, to the construction of fixed bridges in the absence of one or more dental elements. In single prosthesis like crowns, tooth preparation must consider the distribution and orientation of the masticatory load, and the need to protect the remaining tooth structure, evaluating the indication of internal filling for tooth reinforcement or the need of intraradicular cores (Potts et al. 1980; Shillingburg et al. 2007).

The thickness of dentin remaining after cavity preparation is important for the occurrence of post-operative pain and for the maintenance of the vitality of the tooth. Intraoral radiographs are usually used to determine the remaining thickness of dentin. The OCT technique (Dental SS-OCT, Prototype 2, Panasonic Healthcare, Co. Ltd, Japan: center wavelength 1330 nm $\pm$ 100 nm; lateral and axial resolutions of 20 µm and 12 µm, respectively, in air; with a hand-held probe) has been used *in vitro* to evaluate the amount of remaining dentin after preparation in the tooth structure of ten extracted human third molars, and to evaluate the optical properties of the remaining dentin. The obtained images were compared with computed microtomography (micro-CT) images (Inspexio SMX-100CT, Shimadzu Corp., Japan). With OCT it was possible to visualize the thickness of the remaining dentin <1 mm, and it was observed that the greater the thickness of the remaining dentin, the lower the intensity of the generated OCT signal (Fujita et al. 2014).

The resistance of the prostheses themselves to deformation and fractures, especially on fixed partial prostheses, depends on their composition, design and the parafunctional habits of the patients. The materials used in the manufacture of fixed prostheses have been improved, seeking for improved chemical and physical resistance, aesthetics and biocompatibility with the soft and hard tissues of the oral cavity (Eraslan et al. 2021).

Gold was one of the first metals used in the manufacture of crowns, cast metal cores and fixed partial dentures, due to its biocompatibility and excellent ability for reproducing fine detail. From the 1970s onwards, its high cost boosted the search for new alternative metal alloys. Some patients could present local reactions due to the metal present in the prosthesis, with reflection in the periodontal tissues, inducing hyperplasia and chronic inflammation (Dăguci et al. 2020; Eraslan et al. 2021). Poor quality metal alloys can be oxidized in the oral cavity, causing local irritation and loss of strength (Bacchi et al. 2013).

Marginal adaptation is critical for the success of a restoration. An acceptable clinical limit for the space between the prosthesis and the tooth was estimated at 120 μm (McLean 1971). OCT has proved to be a useful tool with clinical potential in the evaluation of the adaptation of restorations and prostheses both in the crown and in the root portion of the dental elements (Alshahni et al. 2019; Trebing et al. 2020).

The discrepancy between the marginal adaptation of direct and indirect restorations, was measured non-invasively before and after cementation through OCT. Türk et al. evaluated by means of SD-OCT (central wavelength 930 nm, bandwidth 100 nm; axial and lateral resolution of 7 μm and 8 μm respectively; image depth around 1.7 mm) the adaptation of composite restorations, made directly on prepared and isolated cavities. In order to allow its careful removal for subsequent cementation, and other restorations made indirectly, with the same material. It was possible to evaluate, in addition to the cement thickness, its structure and the interaction between the tooth and the restorations. There was a significant difference between the values obtained between the two groups, with lower values for direct restorations, both before and after cementation (Türk et al. 2016).

With the increase in aesthetic requirements, in addition to the needs for strength and biocompatibility, metal-free prostheses, especially using ceramic materials, began to gain emphasis in the dental clinic, replacing metalloplastic crowns (with PMMA as the aesthetic material). Metal-free prostheses can achieve aesethic and resistance, even in larger bridges (Lüthy et al. 2005; Pjetursson et al. 2018).

Failure in the ceramic layers of fixed prostheses can occur due to inclusion of air during the process at the laboratory. *En-face* OCT images have detected defects inside ceramic layers (Sinescu et al. 2008a).

Marginal gaps after cementation of lithium disilicate glass ceramic crowns were investigated by spectral domain (SD-OCT, with a central wavelength at

840 ± 10 nm, 26 kHz sweep rate, axial and lateral resolution of 5 and 15μm, iVue-100, Optovue), and the results were compared with the analysis made with stereomicroscope. There were no significant differences between the results, and some air was detected in some samples, at the interface of the enamel and the crown, characterizing an adhesion defect (Li et al. 2018).

In Figure 9.1 it is possible to identify changes in the OCT signal in a well-suited ceramic crown. Three peaks are displayed, which correspond to the interfaces between air and ceramic; between the ceramic and the resin-based cement; and between this cement and the tooth.

In Figure 9.2, we can also detect adhesion defects, characterized by the presence of air bubbles, with an extra peak corresponding to the interface between the cement and air, and between air and tooth.

An *in vitro* study evaluated the interface between ceramic veneers of different thicknesses in 64 extracted central incisors and prepared with different depths (unprepared – no wear; minimally invasive – no dentin exposure; semi-invasive – 50% dentin exposure; and invasive – 100% exposed dentin), after fatigue testing (thermocycle: 2000 cycles between 5 and 55°C, and mechanical load to simulate the intraoral stress situation). The samples were analyzed before and after the test with SD-OCT (Telesto II, Thorlabs GmbH, Dachau, Germany: central wavelength 1300 nm; 76 kHz; resolution of 5.5 μm in air and 4.2 μm in water; imaging depth approximately 3.5 mm), and by scanning electron microscopy (SEM, Phenom G2 pro, Phenom-World BV, Eindhoven, Netherlands). The differences between the refractive indexes and the absorption coefficients produce changes in the OCT signal. The differences in the OCT signal were higher when there was greater wear on the teeth, regardless of the ceramic thickness, which means a higher occurrence of gaps. The *in vitro* evaluation of the interface with OCT was more sensitive than the SEM analysis (Haak et al. 2021).

Failures in internal adaptation alter the main support, which in the case of failure in adaptation becomes the cement and not the underlying tooth structure. The internal and external adaptation of ceramic inlay restorations was evaluated in teeth extracted using OCT operating in the Fourier, or spectral domain (Thorlabs, NJ, USA: central wavelength 930 nm; 1.2 kHz; 512 line/frame; resolution of 7 μm in depth and 8 μm lateral resolution; imaging depth approximately 1.7 mm) and compared to the silicone replica technique. The difference in refractive index between the tooth, resin cement and inlay produces peaks in the collected signal, and the distance between these peaks corresponds to the optical path traveled by light in each material, enabling a very accurate measurement. In comparison with the silicone replica measurement technique, the measurements were smaller for the OCT, demonstrating that the OCT can be used for the accurate assessment of the internal and external adaptation of inlays (Türk et al. 2018).

The marginal adaptation, the cement interface and the gingival overlay were evaluated after the installation of ceramic laminates in a patient who had undergone periodontal plastic surgery, according to standard technique

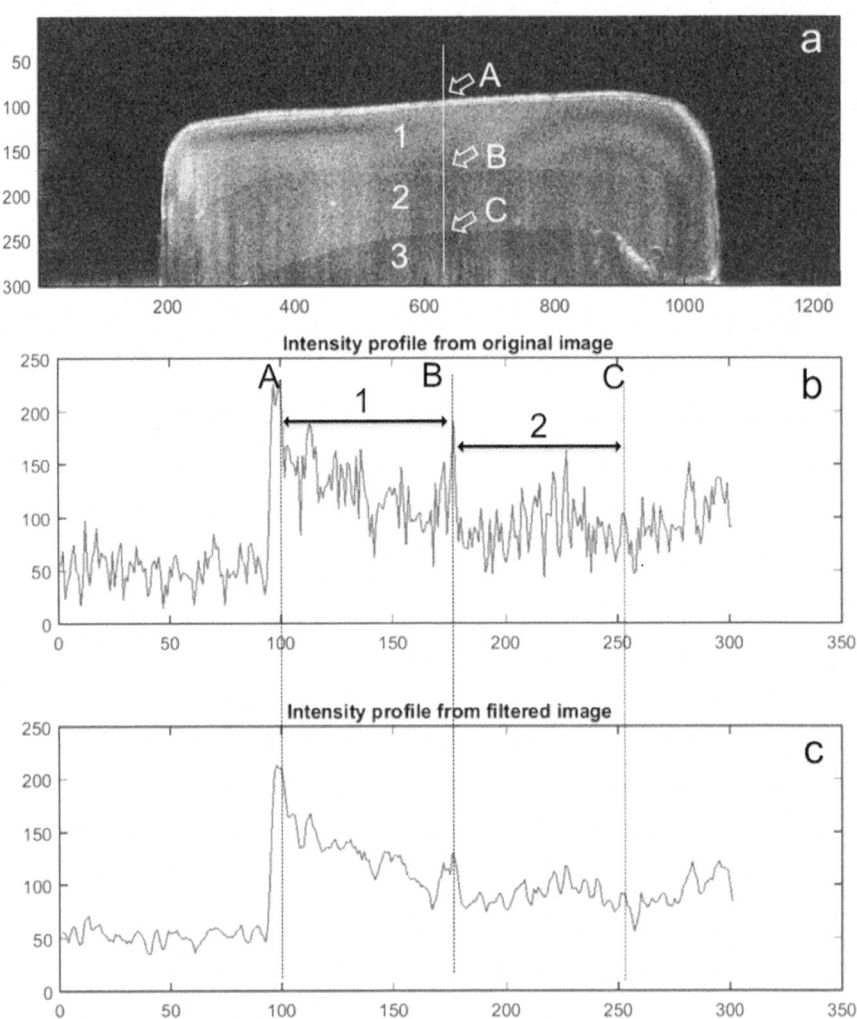

FIGURE 9.1

(a) OCT image generated from a sample. (b) A-scan obtained from the column corresponding to the dashed line in figure (a). (c) The same A-scan filtered through MATLAB. In the A-scan image it is possible to identify three peaks, corresponding to de following interfaces: A – air and ceramic veneer; B – ceramic veneer and resin-based cement; C – resin-based cement and enamel substrate. The interval distance between each peak corresponds to the distance, in pixels, between the cited structures. In this way, 1 – ceramic veneer; 2 – resin-based cement; 3 – enamel portion. Image courtesy of Tereza J. C. Dias.

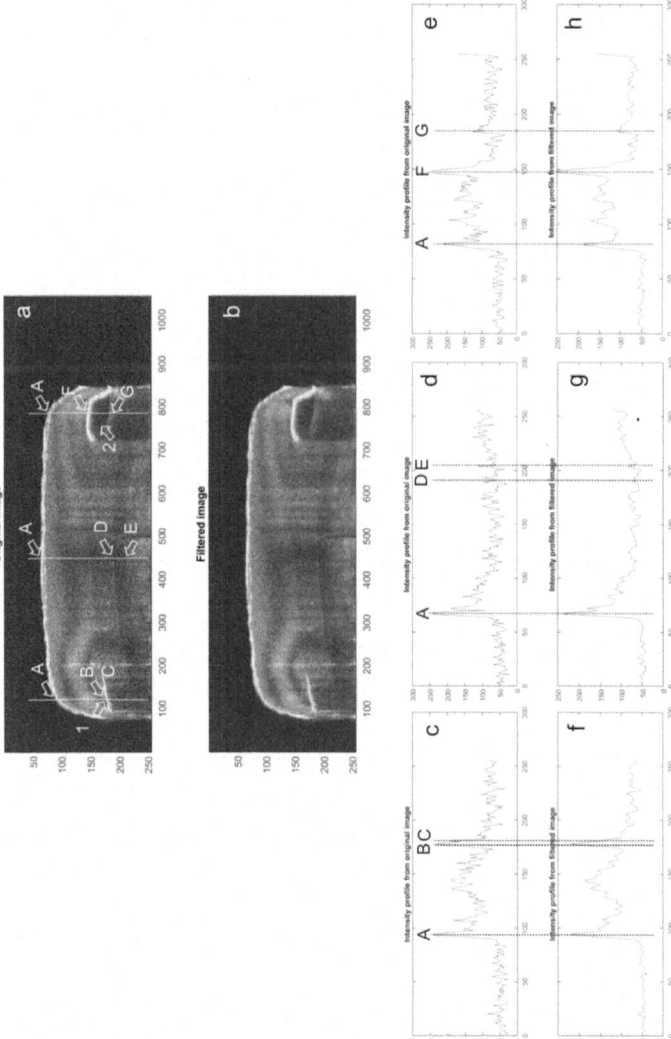

FIGURE 9.2

OCT images and A-scans obtained from three different points. (a) Original OCT image and (b), the same image filtered through MATLAB. (c), (d), (e), A-scan obtained from the columns 112, 448 and 786, respectively, in figure (a). (f), (g), (h), A-scan obtained from the columns 112, 448 and 786, respectively, in figure (b), after processing and filtering by MATLAB. 1 – a gap at the ceramic veneer–cement interface; 2 – an air bubble into the resin-based cement. Similar to that described in Figure 9.1, each peak observed in A-scan corresponds to an interface into the sample. In this way, A – air and ceramic veneer; B and C – the interfaces of the gap present in figures (c) and (f); D and E represent a well-suited interface between the ceramic veneer and RBC, and RBC and enamel substrate. F and G – ceramic veneer and air (air bubble margins). Image courtesy of Tereza J. C. Dias.

for gingival smile correction. An SS-OCT (OCS1300SS, Thorlabs, Newton, NJ, USA: central wavelength 1325 nm; 16 kHz; 512 line/frame; resolution of 25 µm in depth and 12 µm lateral resolution; imaging depth approximately 3.0 mm) recorded sagittal images in the cervical, central and incisal region of the upper right central incisor, in a standardized position at all stages, observing the enamel, dentin, enamel-dentin junction, gingiva, gingival sulcus and incisal edge. Post-operatively, images were obtained at 15 and 60 days, observing gingival regeneration and new sulcus formation around the tooth at 15 days and connective tissue maturation at 60 days. After cementation, gingival health was observed, but the presence of bubbles and gaps in the cement were visualized, demonstrating the potential of OCT as an alternative to clinical assessment and radiographs in the evaluation of indirect restorations (Graça et al. 2019).

The removal of ceramic laminate can be done with lasers operating at the correct wavelength such that the light is transmitted by the ceramic and subsequently absorbed in the cement layer under the laminate. Zanini et al. evaluated the morphological, optical and elemental analysis of enamel before cementation of the veneers, and after laser debonding. The SD-OCT analysis (Calisto, Thorlabs, Newton, NJ, USA: central wavelength 930 nm; 7 µm axial resolution in air; 8 µm transversal resolution; 1.7 mm imaging depth) showed residual cement after laser debonding, and no ablation of the surrounding enamel was observed (Zanini et al. 2021).

9.3.3 Dental Implants

9.3.3.1 Microimplants

The main indication for the use of implants is to replace lost dental elements or to perform implant-supported prostheses. However, other specialties such as orthodontics and maxillofacial prosthesis also use implants (Schierz et al. 2021).

Microimplants are devices mainly used for anchorage in orthodontics, providing an efficient support for the movement of dental elements. To achieve the objective, it is imperative that the microimplant has good primary stability, and that it remains stable during the movement period. Stability is affected by bone quality, implant design and insertion technique (Wilmes et al. 2006; Wilmes et al. 2011).

In some cases, to properly rehabilitate a patient, a multi-technique approach is necessary, and the use of microimplants can be very useful, optimizing the orthodontic movements prior to implant or prosthesis installation (Liaw et al. 2021).

Among the most common complications related to microimplants are injuries to the roots of neighboring teeth, loss of vitality and even interruption of dental vascularization due to periapex injury. Injuries to the oral mucosa at the implant placement site, tissue necrosis and perforation of the maxillary sinus wall have been reported, as well as complications after the removal of the microinserts. Among them, bleeding, microimplant fractures and exostoses (Giudice et al. 2021).

A commercial spectral OCT system (OCS1310V1; Thorlabs, Newton, NJ, USA: central wavelength at 1300 nm; spectral bandwidth of > 97 nm; axial resolution < 16 µm; lateral resolution of 25 µm; scan range of 4 mm; 3D image acquisition of 4 mm × 4 mm; depth information of 2 mm) was used to assess the effect of mechanical stress on cortical bone *in vitro* after the installation of 20 microimplants installed in bovine ribs, and compared with the analysis performed by micro-CT to validate the results. It was possible to visualize the areas of microdamage around the microimplants at different levels of damage, directions and in propagation depth up to 1 mm. Microcracks, which are the more severe form of microdamage, occurred in greater quantity around implants installed at a 45° inclination than when the installation was performed at a 90° inclination (Lakshmikantha et al. 2018).

In their previous study, Lakshmikantha et al. evaluate *in vitro* the bone microdamage during the installation of 80 microimplants (conical-shaped titanium micro implants of the AbsoAnchor System – Dentos, Daegu, Korea), in two different angulations (90° and 45°) in bovine ribs by swept source (SS) OCT (OCS1310V1; Thorlabs, Newton, NJ: 1300 nm of central wavelength; spectral bandwidth of >97 nm; axial resolution <16 µm; transverse resolution of 25 µm; scan area of 4 × 4 mm). OCT was able to detect microcracks at the cortical bone surface after the installation of the microimplants, even when with a previous perforation by a drill, as well as a bone elevation when the implant had a 45° angulation. This characterizes a stress pattern that can compromise the primary stability of the implants. The results were compared to micro-CT, the gold standard in hard tissue imaging (Lakshmikantha et al. 2019).

Dental implant-supported prostheses are considered as a safe option for oral rehabilitation. Due to its conception, of being inserted into the bone, the requirements regarding composition, design and surgical technique are even more critical than in the installation of conventional prostheses (Pal 2015). The work by Brånemark et al. was a boundary in the history of modern implantology, when they proved through optical microscopy that there was direct contact between the titanium surface of the implants and the bone of dogs (Brånemark et al. 1969).

In 1985, Brånemark et al. called "osseointegration" for this interface, as "a direct structural and functional connection between ordered, living bone and the surface of a load carrying implant, without intervening fibrous tissue" (Brånemark 1985).

Prosthetic planning must be taken into consideration during surgical planning. The anatomy of edentulous ridge, the space available for the prosthesis, the type of material to be used, the space for cleaning and the aesthetic factors, among others, need to be carefully evaluated to determine the number of implants to be installed, their inclination in the bone, as well as its distribution at the time of the surgery (Morton et al. 2018). Clearly the dimensions and characteristics of the soft tissues are crucial for the success of dental implants and the prostheses installed on them (Lee et al. 2011; Thoma et al. 2014).

Despite the histological differences between periodontal and peri-implant tissues, there is a structural similarity, such as the presence of a junctional epithelium and connective tissue. The orientation of collagen fibers in the peri-implant tissue is parallel to the implant, while in the tooth they have a horizontal orientation. Periodontal structures have already been successfully analyzed *in vitro* in different studies using OCT, enabling visual differentiation between free and attached gingiva, detection of supra and sub gingival calculus, and measurement of gingival thickness in pigs. The SS-OCT (central wavelength 1325 nm; spectral bandwidth > 100 nm; axial scan rate 16 kHz; average output power 10 mW; 25 frames per second; axial resolution in air/water of 12/9 µm and lateral resolution of 25 µm), had a better performance than the SD-OCT System (central wavelength of 930 nm; spectral bandwidth of 100 nm; maximum output power is 5 mW; axial resolution of 7 / 5.3 µm (air/water); lateral resolution of 8 µm; maximum imaging depth at 1.6 mm; axial scan rate 1.2 kHz, two frames per second). Both systems were able to visualize periodontal structures (Mota et al. 2015).

Di Stasio et al. performed measurements at six different sites in the oral cavity of 28 healthy patients, including gingiva and oral mucosa. A SS-OCT was used (VS-300, Santec™: center wavelength 1300 ± 30 nm; axial resolution in tissue ≤ 12 µm; lateral resolution 22 µm), and the authors established thickness ranges for the tissues in health mucosa, with the potential to serve as a parameter between healthy tissue and pathological changes (Prestin et al. 2012; Di Stasio et al. 2019).

The peri-implant oral mucosa consists of a differentiated stratified epithelium and underlying connective tissue, similar to the native oral mucosa. Peri-implant soft tissues, including epithelial cells and fibroblasts, constitute the first biological barrier around implants, ending approximately 1–1.5 mm from the bone level. The fibroblasts form a connective tissue rich in collagen fibers around the implants, leading to a sealing around the implant due to the quality of the newly formed tissue (Chai et al. 2013; Gómez-Florit et al. 2014).

The peri-implant tissue is less cellular and less vascularized than peri-odontal tissues. The resistance of peri-implant tissues to probing, even under healthy conditions, is lower than in periodontal tissues, increasing the risk of fiber displacement, favoring the development of peri-implant disease (Ivanovski et al. 2018).

As implantology becomes more accessible, the incidence of problems increases. One of the most common is the development of peri-implantitis, which corresponds to inflammation of the supporting tissues of the implant, clinical signs of inflammation (bleeding on probing) and/or suppuration, in combination with progressive bone loss (Heitz-Mayfield et al. 2014; Kormas et al. 2020).

Clinical follow-up after reopening the implants, or after their installation in the case of surgeries with immediate loading, is carried out through clinical probing and radiographs, which do not allow a three-dimensional evaluation of the region of interest. The evaluated aspects are radiographic bone fill (RBF), probing depth (PD), mucosal level, clinical attachment level, bleeding on probe (Khoshkam et al. 2016; Khoury et al. 2019).

Most authors consider an initial bone loss between 1.5–2 mm, in the first year after the implants come into function, as being acceptable, as it is a foreign body even after its osseointegration (Jemt et al. 2008; Papaspyridakos et al. 2012).

Peri-implantitis can be more aggressive than periodontitis, and it is necessary to intervene as soon as possible when the first clinical signs appear. Continuous monitoring of the bone crest is important to maintain the health of the peri-implant tissues (Heitz-Mayfield et al. 2010).

The contour of the implant-supported prosthesis, adaptation and polishing of the margins, as well as its correct cementation (without excess of the cement that allow the accumulation of biofilm), are important risk factors for the maintenance of peri-implant health (Korsch et al. 2015; Staubli et al. 2017; Hämmerle et al. 2018).

In an *ex vivo* study, Park et al. (2017) compared the accuracy of measurements made with OCT, microcomputed tomography (micro-CT) and histological analysis on periodontal structures in dogs. The OCT system (Prototype, LG Electronics, Seoul, Korea) was developed for the study. The swept source (AXP50124-8, Axsun Technologies, Boston, MA, USA) had a center wavelength of 1310 nm, 50 kHz repetition rate, average power of 10 mW, and sweep range of 110 nm, and image depth of 1.2–1.5 mm. It was possible to observe the contour and thickness of periodontal tissues, as well as the connective tissue. Measurement of the thickness of the gingival tissues, and the smooth perception of the distinction between epithelial and subepithelial connective tissue, were shown to be useful information both for periodontal therapy and for the success of implants, especially in aesthetic areas (Park et al. 2017).

A study determined in vitro the refractive index of water, pig gingiva and human gingiva, using a SS-OCT system (Prototype 2, Panasonic Health Care, Ehime, Japan: central wavelength 1330 nm; 100 nm bandwidth; scanning rate of 30 kHz; axial resolution 12 µm in air; lateral resolution 20 µm; light source power of the system was under 10 mW; image range 7 mm × 7 mm). The values determined were, respectively, 1.335, 1.393 and 1.397. After these values were determined, periodontal tissues were analyzed *in vivo* in 30 Asian volunteers, and it was possible to obtain cross-sectional images of gingival epithelium, connective tissue and alveolar bone, and perform gingival thickness measurement (1.06 ± 0.21 mm), epithelium (0.49 ± 0.15 mm) and depth probe (2.09 ± 0.60 mm) in the anterior region of the mandible (Kakizaki et al. 2018).

The evaluation of the gingival biotype, which influences the result of osseointegrated implants as well as periodontal and orthodontic treatments, was carried out in ten volunteers, by combining an SS-OCT system (MEMS-VCSEL laser (SL1310V1-20048, Thorlabs Inc., Newton, NJ, USA: central wavelength 1310 ± 10 nm; 7 μm of resolution in tissue; output power of 3.5 mW; LSM03 objective lens NA=0.055, 25 μm average spot size, Thorlabs Inc.) with a hand-held probe, and OCTA (OCT angiography), where for higher magnification an objective lens (LSM02 (NA=0.11, 13 μm average spot size, Thorlabs Inc.) was used to allow the visualization of gingival vasculature and the superficial capillaries, which are below the surface in the range of 50–200 μm. The OCTA imaging is obtained by the variation in the OCT signal due to the moving particles in blood. With this arrangement, it was possible to characterize the gingival microstructure and vascular arrangements during gingival inflammation, compared to health gingiva *in vivo* (Le et al. 2018).

As with the installation of microimplants, the effects of mechanical stress on sets composed of three sheets of 3 mm polyurethane each (due to the OCT's light penetration capacity) used as a bone substitute, were detected *in vitro* through OCT analysis. Testing was performed simulating the preparation of the implant bed using different tapered implant drills and drilling direction (clockwise and counterclockwise). The equipment used was a SD-OCT device (OCTG-900 – Thorlabs, Newton, NJ, USA: A-scan depth of 2.9 mm; transverse resolution of 4 μm; vertical resolution of 6 μm). Microfractures have been detected on the walls of all prepared beds. It was also possible to observe differences in the bone density of the walls, due to bone condensation promoted in the apical region by the counterclockwise direction of perforation (Delgado-Ruiz et al. 2021).

The thickness of the buccal bone seems to influence the aesthetics and health of peri-implant tissues. During the teeth extraction to immediate installation of implants, dehiscence of soft tissue and fenestration can occur (Nowzari et al. 2012; Farahamnd et al. 2017).

Sanda et al. assessed *in vitro* and *ex vivo*, implants covered by different thickness of mucosa. They installed implants in the jaws of dead pigs and evaluated the excess of cement between the implants and the abutments placed over them, with OCT (Prototype 2; Panasonic Health-care Co.; Ltd.; Ehime, Japan: central wavelength 1330 ± 10 nm; 30 kHz; resolution in 12 μm; lateral resolution 20 μm). The thickness of the pig mucosa was compared with needles, with thickness varying between 0.35 mm to 2.65 mm, and it was possible to detect the implants when the thickness ranged from 0.35 to 1.11 mm. It was also possible to visualize the excess of cement when the mucosa thickness was less than 3 mm. The implants installed in the pig's jaw are not clearly visible with OCT (Sanda et al. 2016).

Farronato et al. monitored the height of single prostheses over implants over 3 years. The implants were inserted 0.5 mm below the surface of the alveolar bone, and the thickness of the upper bone remnant was measured with a caliper. The best aesthetic result, related to the height of the crowns because of the remaining bone over time, occurred when the thickness of the bone was ≥ 1.5 mm. In addition, control radiographs of each implant were taken at the time of implant placement, at the provisional crown placement, at the time of installation of the final crown, and at 1, 2 and 3 year follow-up. However, the radiographs only provided information about the height of the proximal bone crests, without providing information about the bone height above the implant on the buccal surface (Farronato et al. 2020).

The bone/implant interface could be assessed by using an *en-face* optical coherence tomography (*en-face* OCT) to obtain 3D information of the interface between bone/implant in 26 experimental implants installed on rabbit tibia. An experimental OCT system was used, with two single-mode directional couplers, with a SLD as a light source with a central wavelength at 1300 nm. Images of the interface were successfully obtained, and the authors concluded that OCT could be suitable for the analyses of the interface between the bone and the implant (Sinescu et al. 2008b).

The risk of damage to peri-implant tissues during probing can be avoided by using OCT for monitoring of the peri-implant sulcus. In an *in vivo* study, measurements were compared in 445 sites of 23 periodontally healthy individuals using three instruments: North Carolina manual probe, Florida automated probe and SD-OCT (central wavelength at 1325 nm, 0.5 GHz; axial scan rate 16 kHz; 25 frames per second, with axial resolution in air/water of 12/9 μm and lateral resolution of 25 μm). There was an occurrence of pain during manual and automatic probing, and no pain in the measurement performed with OCT, as it is a non-invasive method. OCT has been shown to be a promising technique for the evaluation and measurement of peri-implant tissues (Fernandes et al. 2017).

The periodontal sulcus depth measurement with OCT has been compared with manual measurements, using periodontal probes. In an animal model, using pig jaws, spaces for measurement were created artificially with the aid of a probe. A SS-OCT system (Oztec Co. Ltd., Daegu, Korea), central wavelength 1,310±10 nm at a 50 kHz sweep rate, average output power was 16 mW, 500 frames per second, axial resolution in air of 8 μm/pixel and a lateral resolution of 10.03 μm/pixel was used. The authors concluded that OCT was able to assess sulcus depth and show loss of epithelial adhesion (Kim et al. 2017).

Kim et al. assessed the bone loss around implants with a SS-OCT (Oztec Co., Ltd., Daegu, Korea), central wavelength 1300 ± 10 nm, 50 kHz sweep frequency, and average output potency of 16 mW, 500 frames/s, axial resolution in the air of 7.56 μm and a lateral resolution of 10.03 μm. Although the OCT light source was not able to cross the bone table, in areas where there was bone loss it was possible to visualize the implant spires, and the extent of the vision was considered as being the depth of the peri-implant lesion. The measurements made from the OCT images and those made with direct visualization of the site after accessing the areas through a surgical flap were compared. The potential to visualize peri-implant tissues, including bone height, and to perform non-invasive measurements of the OCT was therefore confirmed (Kim et al. 2018).

The abutment composition may be responsible for microbial colonization, leading to peri-implantitis, with consequent bone loss. In a systematic review, it was found that there was less bleeding on probing (BOP) in abutments made of zirconia than when the abutments were made of titanium, which has a higher affinity for proteins and amino acids, which makes it more difficult to clean (Sanz-Martín et al. 2018).

Candida spp. are often found in larger quantities in the presence of peri-implantitis than in healthy peri-implant areas. The presence of biofilms composed of *Candida sp.*, mainly *Candida albicans*, is responsible for pain and redness in the oral cavity, and involved in periodontal disease, prosthetic stomatitis and median rhomboid glossitis.

In osseointegrated implants, the interface between the implant and the abutment is a critical area, due to the risk of excess cement residues, favoring plaque build-up, and generating stress in the cervical area of the implant. In an *in vitro* study, Kikuchi et al. evaluated the presence of gaps between implants and abutments installed in porcine mandible, with discs of variable thickness between them (50, 100, 150 and 200 μm), to serve as a control, and under different gingiva thickness (0.5, 1, 1.5 or 2 mm) with a SS-OCT with a hand-held probe (Dental SS-OCT, Prototype 2, Panasonic Healthcare, Co., Ltd., Ehime, Japan: central wavelength 1330 nm; 30 kHz sweep scan; axial resolution of 12 μm in air and lateral resolution of 20 μm). The OCT images were analyzed by ImageJ software (Ver. 1.48d) to detect increases in the intensity of the OCT signal at the interface of the implant and the abutment. Images were taken with different probe angles. OCT showed sensitivity to detect gaps at the implant-abutment interface, but the sensitivity was affected by the thickness of the gingiva placed over the samples (> 2 mm), explained by the limitation of penetration of the OCT due to the attenuation of light in tissues, due to scattering and absorption (Kikuchi et al. 2014).

Another factor to be considered for the use of OCT in monitoring the health of peri-implant tissues is the patient's tolerance for pain, as probing can cause more discomfort when performed around implants than around natural teeth (Ringeling et al. 2016; Parvini et al. 2019).

9.3.4 Digital Dentistry

In prostheses, whether in natural teeth, over osseointegrated implants, as well as in partial and total dentures, tooth or implant-supported ones, the ultimate goal is the reconstruction or replacement of teeth aiming at reestablishing function and aesthetics. Impression techniques, as well as the materials used in prostheses, are important to achieve these goals. With the technical and scientific development, these materials and techniques have also evolved, seeking faithful reproduction of the preparations, speed and lower cost, avoiding repetition due to failures in the adaptation of the prostheses at the time of installation, and damage to soft and hard tissues. The use of scanners and Computer Aided Design–Computer Aided Manufactured (CAD–CAM) technology contributes to speed up the process and to the search for better quality (Beuer et al. 2008).

Pores were found in temporary and finished fixed bridges of different materials (integral ceramics, integral polymers, metal ceramics and metal polymer bridges), through the *en-face* OCT analysis, which can also lead to fracture failures and facilitate the accumulation of biofilm (Sinescu et al. 2008a; Sinescu et al. 2008c).

The negative effects of temperature variation due to failure in the calibration of furnaces for the manufacture of metal-ceramic crowns (Duceram Kiss ceramics – DeguDent GmbH, Hanau-Wolfgang, Germany) and pressed ceramics (Ceramco iC Integrated Ceramics – Dentsply International, Inc., York, PA, USA) were evaluated using an in-house developed master-slave (MS) enhanced SS-OCT imaging system – Axsun Technologies, Billerica, MA, USA: central wavelength 1060 nm; sweeping range of 106 nm; 100 kHz sweeping speed; axial resolution in air 10 μm). The comparison of defects that occurred at different temperatures (normal operation, and 50°C difference, above and below the recommended temperature) in the two types of materials allowed the characterization of the loss of calibration of the ovens, in order to avoid defective prostheses (Sinescu et al. 2017).

Joda et al. carried out a systematic review to compare the results of prosthetic work performed by fully digital flow with conventional or mixed flow, concluding that there is little scientific evidence based on randomized clinical trials (RCTs) to recommend its use as a clinical routine, in dental prostheses and implant supported prostheses (Joda et al. 2017).

Nine intraoral scanners (IOSs) were evaluated qualitatively and quantitatively in relation to the accuracy of image acquisition of complete bimaxillary dental arches. Standard preparations on artificial epoxy resin teeth were scanned 10 times, according to the manufacturer instructions. One of the evaluated items of equipment, E4D (E4D Technologies), obtained the highest precision value (agreement among test results: average, 357.05 μm; maximum 2309.45 μm) among all, however with the highest standard deviation between its minimum and maximum values. The E4D's scanning technology uses an SS-OCT, while the other devices are based on confocal microscopy and triangulation scanning principles. Some flaws were observed in the E4D scans, such as rounding of the preparation margins, attributed to higher signal noise. Qualitatively, in *in vitro* scanning, the SS-OCT image acquisition technology did not have the same accuracy as the other systems. The equipment that requires powder coating (FastScan – IOS Technologies, Inc;

and True Definition – 3M-ESPE) had the best performance among all models (Kim et al. 2018).

A commercial SS-OCT (IVS-300, Santec Corporation, Aichi, Japan: central wavelength 1310 ± 30 nm; axial resolution of ≤ 12 μm and lateral resolution of 22 μm) was used to measure and evaluate the internal and marginal adaption of acrylic bridges, direct (TRIOS; 3Shape A/S) and indirectly (gypsum casts after conventional impressions using polyvinyl siloxane – Aquasil Ultra XLV; Dentsply Sirona; scans made with Q800, 3Shape A/S, Copenhagen, Denmark) digitized, over a prepared tooth on a phantom model. Nine impressions were made with each technique. Better internal adaptation was found in the direct digitalization, but no difference was noticed related to marginal fit between the two techniques. The authors highlighted the difficulty in measuring the area around the chamfer area of the preparation margins, probably because of the need to position the probe perpendicularly to the region to be scanned (Al-Imam et al. 2019).

A similar comparison was made in materials and techniques used for temporary crowns. Internal and external fitting of crowns made by the direct conventional technique were compared (bis-acrylic composite, fabricated manually), CAD-CAM (polymethylmethacrylate resin) and 3D impression (printed methacrylic oligomers). The methods used to compare the marginal adaptation of the provisional crows are the vinyl polysiloxane (VPS: Aquasil Ultra XLV) impression technique and SS-OCT analysis (central wavelength of 1300 nm ± 100 nm; resolution in air 7 μm; 5 frames per second). In this study, the digitally fabricated groups had better results than the manually fabricated group, and the OCT technique achieved precise measurements of the gaps. The OCT assessment and the VPS technique had low correlation for the marginal discrepancy evaluation. The internal fit was evaluated by micro-CT and VPS technique (Peng et al. 2020).

The effect of aging on restorative materials, and its impact on their failure, was analyzed using SD-OCT (Telesto II, Thorlabs, central wavelength 1310 nm; penetration depth of 2.5 mm; sensitivity ≤ 106 dB; axial/lateral resolution < 7.5 (air)/15 μm). A study sought to identify changes or irregularities in 48 thin ceramic coverings and in the cement layer over the occlusal of premolars where were installed after 1200.00 thermal-dynamics fatigue cycles (dual-axis masticatory simulator (Willytec Kausimulator, Willytec, Munich, Germany). Samples were evaluated before and after exercise testing with SD-OCT. In total, 47 survived the test, and cracks were identified in 11 of the samples through SD-OCT analysis, which varied in propagation depth. In all samples, wear due to artificial aging was observed, which did not affect the remaining tooth structure (Yazigi et al. 2018).

An *in vitro* study aimed to investigate the fatigue damage in six different CAD–CAM materials by SD-OCT with central wavelength at 880 nm, axial optical resolution of 7 μm and transverse optical resolution of 20 μm (RS-3000, NIDEK Co., Ltd., Gamagori, Aichi, Japan). The specimens were submitted to aging by mouth-motion-simulator (50–500 N, 2 Hz, 37°C), analyzed by OCT prior to aging and at every 250,000 cycles until reaching 1 million cycles. The results of the OCT measurements were compared with the results of a digital light microscope after 1 million cycles, because the destructive nature of the microscope analysis, and only the zirconia-reinforced lithium silicate and hybrid ceramic (which presented the highest damage) showed significant differences, which could have happened because of crack propagation during the sample section. The authors concluded that OCT could be suitable for monitoring fatigue damage of prosthetic materials (Schlenz et al. 2021).

9.4 Oral Probes

One of the limitations for the clinical use of OCT is the difficulty in accessing the internal areas of the oral cavity, which limits its use to the analysis of anterior oral structures, boosting research for the development of adequate probes for viewing areas of more difficult access in the oral cavity (Colston et al. 1998b; Feldchtein et al. 1998; Choi et al. 2014).

A custom cross-polarization swept source OCT (CP-OCT) system with an intraoral probe was developed, with the interferometer inside the probe (IVS-200-CPM, Santec Co. Komaki, Japan: center wavelength 1310 nm ± 104 nm; sweep rate 30 kHz; axial resolution 11 µm) to assess the enamel-composite interfaces in 22 pediatric patients, to detect the presence of secondary caries. The enamel-composite interface could be imaged and quantified with the system *in vivo* in pediatric patients, as well as the deposition of biofilm *in vitro* (Lenton et al. 2012).

In another study group, Demian et al. developed three low-cost OCT probe systems, which according to the authors could be rebuilt with minimal effort and cost. The requirements were as follows: relatively light weight; appropriate material for clinical use; heat-resistant; ease of manufacture; being durable; relative low-cost. The three models were tested in a hospital (Northwick Park Hospital in London, UK), analyzing ears, nose and throat; and in the Imaging Group of the Victor Babes University of Medicine and Pharmacy of Timisoara (Timisoara/Timis, Romania) for dental applications. After *ex vivo* analysis, the devices were tested *in vivo*, replacing the fixed scanning unit in a SD-OCT device. It was only possible to capture cross-sectional images, as they only have the scanner, but any OCT configuration (TD, SD, SS) can be used. It was also possible to use a range of wavelengths (1050–1620 nm or 650–1050 nm). In this study, in dentistry, OCT images were used to identify the different materials used in prostheses and to evaluate defects in these materials (Demian et al. 2014).

For an accurate visualization within periodontal pockets for the detection of subgingival calculus, and to make a differential diagnosis with enamel pearls on the root surface, a fiber-probe SS-OCT was developed (central wavelength 1310 nm $\pm$ 100 nm; 16 kHz rate scan; fiber diameter < 0.9 mm). The evaluation of the acquired images, associated with the analyses of the differences in the intensity of the OCT signal, allowed the authors to differentiate the dental calculus from the sound tissues, including the enamel pearls (Kao et al. 2015).

Won et al. developed a SD-OCT system (SLD-351-HP2, Superlum, Ireland: central wavelength 860 nm $\pm$ 130 nm; axial resolution 7 µm; transversal resolution 25 µm in air; imaging depth of 2.8 mm) where the probe was able to access the area of molars and premolars, including the lingual surface, and can be used in contact or without contact. The authors evaluated the effect of cleaning techniques in volunteers, comparing the gingival OCT signal intensity and dental plaque images in patients with gingivitis before and after 1 week (Won et al. 2020).

It is clear that OCT has the potential to be useful in clinical and laboratorial assessment of dental prostheses. Several applications of OCT in prosthodontics, mostly to prove its accuracy related to other techniques that are more invasive, laborious or expensive, seems to be the focus of the publications so far.

References

Ali, S., Gilani, S. B. S., Shabbir, J., Almulhim, K. S., Bugshan, A., Farooq, I. 2021. Optical coherence tomography's current clinical medical and dental applications: a review. *F1000Research*, 10: 310.

Al-Imam, H., Michou, S., Benetti, A. R., Gotfredsen, K. 2019. Evaluation of marginal and internal fit of acrylic bridges using optical coherence tomography. *Journal of Oral Rehabilitation*, 46: 274–281.

Alshahni, R. Z., Shimada, Y., Zhou, Y. et al. 2019. Cavity adaptation of composite restorations prepared at crown and root: Optical assessment using SS-OCT. *Dental Materials Journal*, 38: 779–789.

Alsterstål-Englund, H., Moberg, L.-E., Petersson, J., Smedberg, J.-I. 2021. A retrospective clinical evaluation of extensive tooth-supported fixed dental prostheses after 10 years. *The Journal of Prosthetic Dentistry*, 125: 65–72.

Aquino, M. M., Mota, C. C. B. O., Santos, J. P. C. L., Nascimento, P. L. A., Campello, S. L., Gomes, A. S. L. 2019. Optical coherence tomography as a tool to visualize biofilm formation over removable prosthesis. In *Optical Coherence Imaging Techniques and Imaging in Scattering Media III*. SPIE. 110781Y.

Bacchi, A., Consani, R. L. X., Mesquita, M. F., dos Santos, M. B. F. 2013. Stress distribution in fixed-partial prosthesis and peri-implant bone tissue with different framework materials and vertical misfit levels: a three-dimensional finite element analysis. *Journal of Oral Science*, 55: 239–244.

Beuer, F., Schweiger, J., Edelhoff, D. 2008. Digital dentistry: an overview of recent developments for CAD/CAM generated restorations. *British Dental Journal, 204:* 505–511.

Bohner, L. O. L., Mukai, E., Oderich, E. et al. 2017. Comparative analysis of imaging techniques for diagnostic accuracy of peri-implant bone defects: a meta-analysis. *Oral Surgery, Oral Medicine, Oral Pathology and Oral Radiology, 124:* 432–440.e5.

Brånemark, P. 1985. *Tissue integrated prostheses.* Quintessence Publishing. 11–76.

Brånemark, P. I., Adell, R., Breine, U., Hansson, B. O., Lindström, J., Ohlsson, A. 1969. Intra-osseous anchorage of dental prostheses. I. Experimental studies. *Scandinavian Journal of Plastic and Reconstructive Surgery, 3:* 81–100.

Campos Sugio, C. Y., Mosquim, V., Jacomine, J. C. et al. 2021. Impact of rehabilitation with removable complete or partial dentures on masticatory efficiency and quality of life: a cross-sectional mapping study. *The Journal of Prosthetic Dentistry, 16:* S0022-3913(21)00144-X.

Carlsson, G. E. 1984. Masticatory efficiency: the effect of age, the loss of teeth and prosthetic rehabilitation. *International Dental Journal, 34:* 93–97.

Carlsson, G. E., Omar, R. 2006. Trends in prosthodontics. *Medical Principles and Practice, 15:* 167–179.

Cassetta, M., Di Giorgio, R., Barbato, E. 2018. Are intraoral radiographs reliable in determining peri-implant marginal bone level changes? The correlation between open surgical measurements and peri-apical radiographs. *International Journal of Oral and Maxillofacial Surgery, 47:* 1358–1364.

Chai, W. L., Moharamzadeh, K., van Noort, R., Emanuelsson, L., Palmquist, A., Brook, I. M. 2013. Contour analysis of an implant--soft tissue interface. *Journal of Periodontal Research, 48:* 663–670.

Choi, W. J., Wang, R. K. 2014. In vivo imaging of functional microvasculature within tissue beds of oral and nasal cavities by swept-source optical coherence tomography with a forward/side-viewing probe. *Biomedical Optics Express, 5:* 2620–2634.

Coli, P., Christiaens, V., Sennerby, L., Bruyn, H. D. 2017. Reliability of periodontal diagnostic tools for monitoring peri-implant health and disease. *Periodontology 2000, 73:* 203–217.

Colston, B. W., Jr, Everett, M. J., Da Silva, L. B., Otis, L. L., Stroeve, P., Nathel, H. 1998a. Imaging of hard- and soft-tissue structure in the oral cavity by optical coherence tomography. *Applied Optics, 37:* 3582–3585.

Colston, B., Sathyam, U., Dasilva, L., Everett, M., Stroeve, P., Otis, L. 1998b. Dental OCT. *Optics Express, 3:* 230–238.

Council on Dental Materials, Instruments, and Equipment. 1985. Report on base metal alloys for crown and bridge applications: benefits and risks. *Journal of the American Dental Association, 111:* 479–483.

Dăguci, L., Dăguci, C., Dumitrescu. et al. 2020. Periodontal clinico-morphological changes in patients wearing old nickel-chromium and copper alloys bridges. *Revue Roumaine de Morphologie et Embryologie, 61:* 449–455.

De Bruyn, H., Vandeweghe, S., Ruyffelaert, C., Cosyn, J., Sennerby, L. 2013. Radiographic evaluation of modern oral implants with emphasis on crestal bone level and relevance to peri-implant health: Radiographic evaluation of oral implants. *Periodontology 2000, 62:* 256–270.

Delgado-Ruiz, R., Mahdian, M., Benezha, I., Romanos, G. 2021. Counterclockwise drilling with different tapered drills condenses the implant bed-an optical coherence tomography in vitro study. *Medicina, 57*: 940.

Demian, D., Duma, V.-F., Sinescu, C. et al. 2014. Design and testing of prototype handheld scanning probes for optical coherence tomography. *Proceedings of the Institution of Mechanical Engineers. Part H, Journal of Engineering in Medicine, 228*: 743–753.

Di Stasio, D., Lauritano, D., Iquebal, H., Romano, A., Gentile, E., Lucchese, A. 2019. Measurement of oral epithelial thickness by optical coherence tomography. *Diagnostics, 9*: 90.

Eraslan, R., Colpak, E. D., Kilic, K., Polat, Z. A. 2021. Biomechanical properties and biocompatibility of implant-supported full arch fixed prosthesis substructural materials. *Nigerian Journal of Clinical Practice, 24*: 1373–1379.

Farahamnd, A., Sarlati, F., Eslami, S., Ghassemian, M., Youssefi, N., Jafarzadeh Esfahani, B. 2017. Evaluation of impacting factors on facial bone thickness in the anterior maxillary region. *The Journal of Craniofacial Surgery, 28*: 700–705.

Farronato, D., Pasini, P. M., Orsina, A. A., Manfredini, M., Azzi, L., Farronato, M. 2020. Correlation between buccal bone thickness at implant placement in healed sites and buccal soft tissue maturation pattern: a prospective three-year study. *Materials, 13*: 511.

Feldchtein, F., Gelikonov, V., Iksanov, R. et al. 1998. In vivo OCT imaging of hard and soft tissue of the oral cavity. *Optics Express, 3*: 239–250.

Fernandes, L. O., Mota, C. C. B. O., de Melo, L. S. A., da Costa Soares, M. U. S., da Silva Feitosa, D., Gomes, A. S. L. 2017. In vivo assessment of periodontal structures and measurement of gingival sulcus with optical coherence tomography: a pilot study. *Journal of Biophotonics, 10*: 862–869.

Fujita, R., Komada, W., Nozaki, K., Miura, H. 2014. Measurement of the remaining dentin thickness using optical coherence tomography for crown preparation. *Dental Materials Journal, 33*: 355–362.

García-García, M., Mir-Mari, J., Benic, G. I., Figueiredo, R., Valmaseda-Castellón, E. 2016. Accuracy of periapical radiography in assessing bone level in implants affected by peri-implantitis: a cross-sectional study. *Journal of Clinical Periodontology, 43*: 85–91.

Gerritsen, A. E., Allen, P. F., Witter, D. J., Bronkhorst, E. M., Creugers, N. H. J. 2010. Tooth loss and oral health-related quality of life: a systematic review and meta-analysis. *Health and Quality of Life Outcomes, 8*: 126.

GhiȚĂ, R. E., Scrieciu, M., MercuȚ, V. et al. 2020. Oral mucosa changes associated with wearing removable acrylic dentures. *Current Health Sciences Journal, 46*: 344–351.

Giudice, A. L., Rustico, L., Longo, M., Oteri, G., Papadopoulos, M. A., Nucera, R. 2021. Complications reported with the use of orthodontic miniscrews: a systematic review. *Korean Journal of Orthodontics, 51*: 199–216.

Gómez-Florit, M., Xing, R., Ramis, J. M. et al. 2014. Human gingival fibroblasts function is stimulated on machined hydrided titanium zirconium dental implants. *Journal of Dentistry, 42*: 30–38.

Graça, N. D. R. L., Palmeira, A. R. de B. L. S., Fernandes, L. O. et al. 2019. In vivo optical coherence tomographic imaging to monitor gingival recovery and the adhesive interface in aesthetic oral rehabilitation: a case report. *Imaging Science in Dentistry, 49*: 171–176.

Haak, R., Siegner, J., Ziebolz, D. et al. 2021. OCT evaluation of the internal adaptation of ceramic veneers depending on preparation design and ceramic thickness. *Dental Materials, 37*: 423–431.

Hämmerle, C. H. F., Tarnow, D. 2018. The etiology of hard- and soft-tissue deficiencies at dental implants: a narrative review. *Journal of Clinical Periodontology, 45 Suppl 20*: S267–S277.

Hara, T., Sonoi, A., Handa, T. et al. 2021. Unsaturated fatty acid salts remove biofilms on dentures. *Scientific Reports, 11*: 12524.

Hedberg, L., Ekman, U., Nordin, L. E. et al. 2021. Cognitive changes and neural correlates after oral rehabilitation procedures in older adults: a protocol for an interventional study. *BMC Oral Health, 21*: 297

Heitz-Mayfield, L. J. A., Lang, N. P. 2010. Comparative biology of chronic and aggressive periodontitis vs. peri-implantitis. *Periodontology 2000, 53*: 167–181.

Heitz-Mayfield, L. J. A., Needleman, I., Salvi, G. E., Pjetursson, B. E. 2014. Consensus statements and clinical recommendations for prevention and management of biologic and technical implant complications. *The International Journal of Oral Maxillofacial Implants, 29 Suppl*: 346–350.

Huang, D., Swanson, E. A., Lin, C. P. et al. 1991. Optical coherence tomography. *Science, 254*: 1178–1181.

Ivanovski, S., Lee, R. 2018. Comparison of peri-implant and periodontal marginal soft tissues in health and disease. *Periodontology 2000, 76*: 116–130.

Jemt, T., Albrektsson, T. 2008. Do long-term followed-up Branemark implants commonly show evidence of pathological bone breakdown? A review based on recently published data. *Periodontology 2000, 47*: 133–142.

Joda, T., Zarone, F., Ferrari, M. 2017. The complete digital workflow in fixed prosthodontics: a systematic review. *BMC Oral Health, 17*:124.

Kakizaki, S., Aoki, A., Tsubokawa, M. et al. 2018. Observation and determination of periodontal tissue profile using optical coherence tomography. *Journal of Periodontal Research, 53*: 188–199.

Kao, M.-C., Lin, C.-L., Kung, C.-Y., Huang, Y.-F., Kuo, W.-C. 2015. Miniature endoscopic optical coherence tomography for calculus detection. *Applied Optics, 54*: 7419–7423.

Khoshkam, V., Suárez-López Del Amo, F., Monje, A., Lin, G.-H., Chan, H.-L., Wang, H.-L. 2016. Long-term radiographic and clinical outcomes of regenerative approach for treating peri-implantitis: a systematic review and meta-analysis. *The International Journal of Oral Maxillofacial Implants, 31*: 1303–1310.

Khoury, F., Keeve, P. L., Ramanauskaite, A. et al. 2019. Surgical treatment of peri-implantitis – consensus report of working group 4. *International Dental Journal, 69*: 18–22.

Kikuchi, K., Akiba, N., Sadr, A., Sumi, Y., Tagami, J., Minakuchi, S. 2014. Evaluation of the marginal fit at implant-abutment interface by optical coherence tomography. *Journal of Biomedical Optics, 19*: 055002.

Kim, J.-M., Kang, S.-R., Yi, W.-J. 2017. Automatic detection of tooth cracks in optical coherence tomography images. *Journal of Periodontal Implant Science, 47*: 41–50.

Kim, R. J.-Y., Park, J.-M., Shim, J.-S. 2018. Accuracy of 9 intraoral scanners for complete-arch image acquisition: a qualitative and quantitative evaluation. *The Journal of Prosthetic Dentistry, 120*: 895–903.e1.

Kim, S., Kang, S.-R., Park, H.-J., Kim, B., Kim, T.-I., Yi, W.-J. 2018. Quantitative measurement of peri-implant bone defects using optical coherence tomography. *Journal of Periodontal Implant Science, 48*: 84.

Kim, S.-H., Kang, S.-R., Park, H.-J., Kim, J.-M., Yi, W.-J., Kim, T.-I. 2017. Improved accuracy in periodontal pocket depth measurement using optical coherence tomography. *Journal of Periodontal Implant Science, 47*: 13–19.

Kormas, I., Pedercini, C., Pedercini, A., Raptopoulos, M., Alassy, H., Wolff, L. F. 2020. Peri-implant diseases: Diagnosis, clinical, histological, microbiological characteristics and treatment strategies. A narrative review. *Antibiotics, 9*: 835.

Korsch, M., Robra, B.-P., Walther, W. 2015. Predictors of excess cement and tissue response to fixed implant-supported dentures after cementation: excess cement causes Peri-implant attachment loss. *Clinical Implant Dentistry and Related Research, 17*: e45–e53.

Kumar, H. C., Kumar, T. P., Hemchand, S., Suneelkumar, C., Subha, A. 2020. Accuracy of marginal adaptation of posterior fixed dental prosthesis made from digital impression technique: a systematic review. *Journal of Indian Prosthodontic Society, 20*: 123–130.

Lakshmikantha, H. T., Ravichandran, N. K., Jeon, M., Kim, J., Park, H.-S. 2018. Assessment of cortical bone microdamage following insertion of microimplants using optical coherence tomography: a preliminary study. *Journal of Zhejiang University. Science. B, 19*: 818–828.

Lakshmikantha, H. T., Ravichandran, N. K., Jeon, M., Kim, J., Park, H.-S. 2019. 3-Dimensional characterization of cortical bone microdamage following placement of orthodontic microimplants using optical coherence tomography. *Scientific Reports, 9*: 3242.

Le, N. M., Song, S., Zhou, H. et al. 2018. A noninvasive imaging and measurement using optical coherence tomography angiography for the assessment of gingiva: an in vivo study. *Journal of Biophotonics, 11*: e201800242.

Lee, A., Fu, J.-H., Wang, H.-L. 2011. Soft tissue biotype affects implant success. *Implant Dentistry, 20*: e38–47.

Lenton, P., Rudney, J., Chen, R., Fok, A., Aparicio, C., Jones, R. S. 2012. Imaging in vivo secondary caries and ex vivo dental biofilms using cross-polarization optical coherence tomography. *Dental Materials, 28*: 792–800.

Li, W., Liu, J., Zhang, Z. 2018. Evaluation of marginal gap of lithium disilicate glass ceramic crowns with optical coherence tomography. *Journal of Biomedical Optics, 23*: 1–5.

Liaw, J. J. L., Shih, I. Y. H., Yang, S. Y. H., Tsai, F.-F., Wang, S.-H. 2021. Interdisciplinary rehabilitation for mutilated dentition with mini-implants, autotransplants, and a dental implant. *American Journal of Orthodontics and Dentofacial Orthopedics, 160*: 872–886.

Lin, C.-S. 2018. Revisiting the link between cognitive decline and masticatory dysfunction. *BMC Geriatrics, 18*: 5.

Lüthy, H., Filser, F., Loeffel, O., Schumacher, M., Gauckler, L. J., Hammerle, C. H. F. 2005. Strength and reliability of four-unit all-ceramic posterior bridges. *Dental Materials, 21*: 930–937.

Mauad, L. Q., Doriguêtto, P. V. T., de Almeida, D., Fardim, K. A. C., Machado, A. H., Devito, K. L. 2021. Quantitative assessment of artefacts and identification of gaps in prosthetic crowns: a comparative in vitro study between periapical radiography and CBCT images. *Dento Maxillo Facial Radiology, 50*: 20200134.

McLean, J. W., von Fraunhofer, J. A. 1971. The estimation of cement film thickness by an in vivo technique. *British Dental Journal, 131*: 107–111.

Morton, D., Gallucci, G., Lin, W.-S. et al. 2018. Group 2 ITI Consensus Report: Prosthodontics and implant dentistry. *Clinical Oral Implants Research, 29 Suppl 16*: 215–223.

Moskona, D., Kaplan, I. 1992. Oral lesions in elderly denture wearers. *Clinical Preventive Dentistry, 14*: 11–14.

Mota, C. C. B. O., Fernandes, L. O., Cimões, R., Gomes, A. S. L. 2015. Non-invasive periodontal probing through Fourier-domain optical coherence tomography. *Journal of Periodontology, 86*: 1087–1094.

Murat, S., Kamburoğlu, K., Isayev, A., Kurşun, S., Yüksel, S. 2013. Visibility of artificial buccal recurrent caries under restorations using different radiographic techniques. *Operative Dentistry, 38*: 197–207.

Nassani, M. Z. 2017. Aspects of malpractice in prosthodontics: malpractice in prosthodontics. *Journal of Prosthodontics, 26*: 672–681.

Negrutiu, M. L., Sinescu, C., Hughes, M. et al. 2008. Fibres reinforced dentures investigated with en-face optical coherence tomography. In J. Popp, W. Drexler, V. V. Tuchin, D. L. *Progress in Biomedical Optics and Imaging – Proceedings of SPIE*, 6991.

Nowzari, H., Molayem, S., Chiu, C. H. K., Rich, S. K. 2012. Cone beam computed tomographic measurement of maxillary central incisors to determine prevalence of facial alveolar bone width ≥2 mm: facial alveolar bone width. *Clinical Implant Dentistry and Related Research, 14*: 595–602.

Pal, T. 2015. Fundamentals and history of implant dentistry. *Journal of the International Clinical Dental Research Organization, 7*: 6.

Papaspyridakos, P., Chen, C.-J., Singh, M., Weber, H.-P., Gallucci, G. O. 2012. Success criteria in implant dentistry: a systematic review. *Journal of Dental Research, 91*: 242–248.

Park, J.-Y., Chung, J.-H., Lee, J.-S., Kim, H.-J., Choi, S.-H., Jung, U.-W. 2017. Comparisons of the diagnostic accuracies of optical coherence tomography, micro-computed tomography, and histology in periodontal disease: an ex vivo study. *Journal of Periodontal Implant Science, 47*: 30–40.

Parvini, P., Saminsky, M., Stanner, J., Klum, M., Nickles, K., Eickholz, P. 2019. Discomfort/pain due to periodontal and peri-implant probing with/without platform switching. *Clinical Oral Implants Research, 30*: 997–1004.

Peng, C.-C., Chung, K.-H., Ramos, V., Jr. 2020. Assessment of the adaptation of interim crowns using different measurement techniques. *Journal of Prosthodontics, 29*: 87–93

Pjetursson, B. E., Valente, N. A., Strasding, M., Zwahlen, M., Liu, S., Sailer, I. 2018. A systematic review of the survival and complication rates of zirconia-ceramic and metal-ceramic single crowns. *Clinical Oral Implants Research, 29 Suppl 16*: 199–214.

Potts, R. G., Shillingburg, H. T., Jr, Duncanson, M. G., Jr. 1980. Retention and resistance of preparations for cast restorations. *The Journal of Prosthetic Dentistry, 92*: 207–212.

Prestin, S., Rothschild, S. I., Betz, C. S., Kraft, M. 2012. Measurement of epithelial thickness within the oral cavity using optical coherence tomography. *Head Neck, 34*: 1777–1781.

Reddy, N. R., Abraham, A. P., Murugesan, K., Matsa, V. 2011. An invitro analysis of elemental release and cytotoxicity of recast nickel-chromium dental casting alloys. *Journal of Indian Prosthodontic Society*, 11: 106–112.

Renvert, S., Persson, G. R., Pirih, F. Q., Camargo, P. M. 2018. Peri-implant health, peri-implant mucositis, and peri-implantitis: case definitions and diagnostic considerations. *Journal of Periodontology*, 89 Suppl 1: S304–S312.

Ringeling, J., Parvini, P., Weinbach, C., Nentwig, G.-H., Nickles, K., Eickholz, P. 2016. Discomfort/pain due to pocket probing at teeth and endosseous implants: a cross-sectional study. *Clinical Oral Implants Research*, 27: 1005–1009.

Saeed, F., Muhammad, N., Khan, A. S. et al. 2020. Prosthodontics dental materials: From conventional to unconventional. *Materials Science Engineering. C, Materials for Biological Applications*, 106: 110167.

Sanda, M., Shiota, M., Imakita, C., Sakuyama, A., Kasugai, S., Sumi, Y. 2016. The effectiveness of optical coherence tomography for evaluating peri-implant tissue: a pilot study. *Imaging Science in Dentistry*, 46: 173–178.

Sanz-Martín, I., Sanz-Sánchez, I., Carrillo de Albornoz, A., Figuero, E., Sanz, M. 2018. Effects of modified abutment characteristics on peri-implant soft tissue health: a systematic review and meta-analysis. *Clinical Oral Implants Research*, 29: 118–129.

Schierz, O., Reissmann, D. R. 2021. Dental patient-reported outcomes – the promise of dental implants. *The Journal of Evidence-Based Dental Practice*, 21: 101541.

Schlenz, M. A., Skroch, M., Schmidt, A., Rehmann, P., Wöstmann, B. 2021. Monitoring fatigue damage in different CAD/CAM materials: a new approach with optical coherence tomography. *Journal of Prosthodontic Research*, 65: 31–38.

Shillingburg, H. T. 2007. *Fundamentals of fixed prosthodontics* (4th ed.). Quintessence Publishing.

Shimada, Y., Sadr, A., Sumi, Y., Tagami, J. 2015. Application of optical coherence tomography (OCT) for diagnosis of caries, cracks, and defects of restorations. *Current Oral Health Reports*, 2: 73–80.

Sinescu, C., Bradu, A., Duma, V.-F., Topala, F., Negrutiu, M., Podoleanu, A. 2017. Effects of temperature variations during sintering of metal ceramic tooth prostheses investigated non-destructively with optical coherence tomography. *Applied Sciences*, 7: 552.

Sinescu, C., Hughes, M., Bradu, A. et al. 2008b. Implant bone interface investigated with a non-invasive method: optical coherence tomography. In J. Popp, W. Drexler, V. V. Tuchin, D. L. *Proceedings of SPIE*, 6991: 69911L.

Sinescu, C., Negrutiu, M., Hughes, M. et al. 2008a. An optical coherence tomography investigation of materials defects in ceramic fixed partial dental prostheses. *Proceedings of SPIE*, 6991: 69910O.

Sinescu, C., Negrutiu, M., Todea, C., Hughes, M., Tudorache, F., Podoleanu, A. G. 2008c. Fixed partial dentures investigated by optical coherent tomography. *Coherence Domain Optical Methods and Optical Coherence Tomography in Biomedicine XII*.

Staubli, N., Walter, C., Schmidt, J. C., Weiger, R., Zitzmann, N. U. 2017. Excess cement and the risk of peri-implant disease – a systematic review. *Clinical Oral Implants Research*, 28: 1278–1290.

Sumi, Y., Ozawa, N., Nagaosa, S., Minakuchi, S., Umemura, O. 2011. Application of optical coherence tomography (OCT) to nondestructive inspection of dentures. *Archives of Gerontology and Geriatrics*, 53: 237–241.

The Glossary of Prosthodontic Terms: Ninth edition. 2017. *The Journal of Prosthetic Dentistry*, 117: e1–e105.

Thoma, D. S., Mühlemann, S., Jung, R. E. 2014. Critical soft-tissue dimensions with dental implants and treatment concepts. *Periodontology 2000, 66*: 106–118.

Trebing, C. T., Schwindling, F. S., Leisner, L., Trebing, J., Lux, C. J., Rammelsberg, P., Sen, S. 2020. Diagnostic accuracy of 870-nm spectral-domain OCT with enhanced depth imaging for the detection of caries beneath ceramics. *Journal of Dentistry, 102*: 103458.

Türk, A. G., Sabuncu, M., Ulusoy, M. 2018. Evaluation of adaptation of ceramic inlays using optical coherence tomography and replica technique. *Brazilian Oral Research, 32*: e005.

Türk, A. G., Sabuncu, M., Ünal, S., Önal, B., Ulusoy, M. 2016. Comparison of the marginal adaptation of direct and indirect composite inlay restorations with optical coherence tomography. *Journal of Applied Oral Science, 24*: 383–390.

Wang, G., Le, N. M., Hu, X. et al. 2020. Semi-automated registration and segmentation for gingival tissue volume measurement on 3D OCT images. *Biomedical Optics Express, 11*: 4536.

Wilmes, B., Drescher, D. 2011. Impact of bone quality, implant type, and implantation site preparation on insertion torques of mini-implants used for orthodontic anchorage. *International Journal of Oral and Maxillofacial Surgery, 40*: 697–703.

Wilmes, B., Rademacher, C., Olthoff, G., Drescher, D. 2006. Parameters affecting primary stability of orthodontic mini-implants. *Journal of Orofacial Orthopedics, 67*: 162–174.

Won, J., Huang, P.-C., Spillman, D. R. et al. 2020. Handheld optical coherence tomography for clinical assessment of dental plaque and gingiva. *Journal of Biomedical Optics, 25*: 116011.

Yazigi, C., Schneider, H., Chaar, M. S., Rüger, C., Haak, R., Kern, M. 2018. Effects of artificial aging and progression of cracks on thin occlusal veneers using SD-OCT. *Journal of the Mechanical Behavior of Biomedical Materials, 88*: 231–237.

Zanini, N. A., Rabelo, T. F., Zamataro, C. B., Caramel-Juvino, A., Ana, P. A., Zezell, D. M. 2021. Morphological, optical, and elemental analysis of dental enamel after debonding laminate veneer with Er,Cr:YSGG laser: a pilot study. *Microscopy Research and Technique, 84*: 489–498.

Zarb, G., Hobkirk, J., Eckert, S., Jacob, R. 2012. *Prosthodontic treatment for edentulous patients: Complete dentures and implant-supported prostheses* (13th ed.). Mosby.

Zhang, C.-N., Zhu, Y., Fan, L.-F., Zhang, X., Jiang, Y.-H., Gu, Y.-X. 2021. Intra- and inter-observer agreements in detecting peri-implant bone defects between periapical radiography and cone beam computed tomography: a clinical study. *Journal of Dental Sciences, 16*: 948–956.

10

OCT in Soft Oral Tissues I

Cláudia C. B. O. Mota,[1,2] Cecília Maria de Sá Barreto Cruz Falcão,[3]
Denise M. Zezell[4] and Anderson S. L. Gomes[3,5]

[1]Faculty of Dentistry, Centro Universitário Tabosa de Almeida, ASCES-UNITA, Brazil

[2]School of Dentistry, Universidade de Pernambuco, Campus Arcoverde, UPE, Brazil

[3]Graduate Program in Dentistry, Universidade Federal de Pernambuco, UFPE, Brazil

[4]Center for Lasers and Applications, Instituto de Pesquisas Energéticas e Nucleares, IPEN-CNEN/SP, Brazil

[5]Physics Department and Graduate Program in Dentistry, Universidade Federal de Pernambuco, UFPE, Brazil

CONTENTS

10.1 Introduction

Initially proposed by Huang & cols (Huang et al. 1991) for ophthalmology, optical coherence tomography (OCT) has been largely applied for other medical specialties, such as dermatology, pathology, cardiology, gastroenterology, rheumatology (Camus et al. 2018; Liu et al. 2018; Pires et al. 2018; Ianoși et al.

DOI: 10.1201/9781351104562-10

2019; Reddy et al. 2019). OCT is a non-invasive optical imaging technique that utilizes low-coherence interferometry to detect backscattered light from tissue to produce depth resolved images up to a few millimeters below the surface (Huang et al. 1991; Kim et al. 2018).

Due to its fast speed and high sensitivity, spectral domain OCT (SD-OCT) is currently recognized as the state-of-the-art technology for acquiring *in vivo*, cross-sectional images of ocular tissues to identify retinal morphology and abnormalities. Even the literature recognizes OCT as the gold standard for retinal imaging in ophthalmology, the high cost of clinical systems (up to $150,000) has restricted access to mostly large eye centers and laboratories (Shelton et al. 2014; Schmidt-Erfurth et al. 2017; Kim et al. 2018). Thus, the development of a low-cost, portable OCT system has been pursued to significantly increase the ease of access, particularly in low resource settings, and to expand the use of OCT to a wider range of applications, which were previously cost prohibitive.

In dentistry, the first studies using OCT were published in 1998 (Colston et al. 1998a; Feldchtein et al. 1998). Since then, several other studies have been reported, either in laboratory or clinical environment. The technique is largely applicable for early-caries diagnostic, but can also be used for evaluating tooth cracks, microleakage in the tooth-restoration interface, calculus deposition over tooth surface, and changes in the oral soft tissues, such as oral cancer and periodontal support tissues analysis (Tsai et al. 2013; Mota et al. 2015a; Han et al. 2016; Kim et al. 2017; Maslennikova et al. 2017; Quitero et al. 2019; Fernandes et al. 2019).

OCT is non-invasive, uses non-ionizing radiation and high-resolution imaging technique applicable as an alternative non-contact diagnostic method for biological tissues (Agrawal et al. 2012; Kao et al. 2015; Kim et al. 2017). Considered in the literature as an optical biopsy, OCT has 1–3 mm depth penetration in air (Shelton et al. 2014; Fernandes et al. 2017); in biological tissues it is shallower, up to 1.2 mm in depth, and depends on the optical characteristics of the samples and the optical source wavelength. OCT generates two- or three-dimensional high-resolution images, revealing in detail the microstructure of samples, based on the differences of light backscattering, without side effects for patients (Fernandes et al. 2017). Using the principle of low-coherence interferometry, it is possible to achieve a depth resolution of the order of 10–20 µm and an in-plane resolution similar to that of optical microscopes (Kao et al. 2015).

Therefore, knowing that imaging methods are widely used in diagnostic medicine, evidence points to OCT as a potential early diagnostic tool in dental health care (Mota et al. 2015a). Early diagnosis is desirable and necessary since it implies a better patient prognosis. Furthermore, non-invasive and non-ionizing diagnostic methods are of particular interest for routine use in the diagnosis and monitoring of periodontitis (Xiang et al. 2010; Fernandes et al. 2017).

10.2 Periodontics

10.2.1 Periodontal Disease: Concept and Management

Periodontitis is a prevalent multifactorial disease of the tissues surrounding the teeth, which could be associated with major oral health burden (Mota et al. 2015a; Park et al. 2017; Fernandes et al. 2019; Krause et al. 2019). In addition, it could be associated with other systemic diseases (Albandar et al. 2018), such as diabetes (Chapple et al. 2013) and cardiovascular disease (Dhadse et al. 2010).

The presence of bleeding during the probing is the primary parameter to identify the gingivitis, the initial stage of the disease (Caton et al. 2018; Lang et al. 2018; Trombelli et al. 2018) – this stage can be reverted to a health stage, but when periodontitis is already installed, the patient remains in this condition for its entire life; successful therapies should be carried out, and long-life supportive care is needed aiming to prevent the recurrence of disease (Caton et al. 2018; Chapple et al. 2018).

The staging of periodontitis is determined by considering the destruction and loss of connective tissue attachment, the amount of bone loss, the probing depth, the presence and extension of angular bony defects and furcation involvement and, in severe stages, tooth mobility and tooth loss (Mota et al. 2015a; Park et al. 2017; Caton et al. 2018; Fernandes et al. 2019; Krause et al. 2019). Figure 10.1 shows the clinical aspect of a healthy patient and those with gingivitis and periodontitis.

The main etiological factor is the biofilm deposition on the tooth surface – so it is essential to provide biofilm control for preventing periodontal diseases. The mineralized form of biofilm constitutes the calculus, a porous structure composed by inorganic content, covered by an unmineralized bacterial layer (Kao et al. 2015). In this way, periodontally healthy patients present a balanced relationship between the dental biofilm and the immunoinflammatory response (Fernandes et al. 2019).

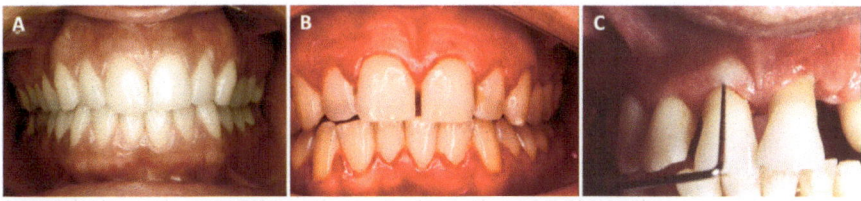

FIGURE 10.1

Intraoral photographs of patients with distinct periodontal status: (A) healthy; (B) with gingivitis and (C) with periodontitis. Image courtesy of Dr. Leógenes Santiago, ASCES-UNITA, Brazil.

Therefore, the key to success for periodontal therapy is the correct evaluation of a cleaned surface, aiming to enable thorough and substance-sparing debridement. The treatment of periodontitis involves the detection and control/removal of calculus and biofilm of the affected surfaces, being subgingival calculus the more difficult to detect due its location in periodontal pockets. Additionally, it can be confused with enamel pearls in the subgingival environment. Due to the difficulty in identifying subgingival calculus, it is relatively frequent for clinicians to lead residual calculus to deeper regions, and/or unintentionally to remove excessive amounts of root cementum during the therapy (Kao et al. 2015; Krause et al. 2019).

Another category of periodontal conditions should also be considered for patients who have undergone implant surgery. In this way, a healthy peri-implant condition is characterized by normal or reduced bone support around implants, with no visual signs of inflammation and bleeding on probing (Caton et al. 2018; Berglundh et al. 2018; Renvert et al. 2018). On the other hand, the presence of clinical signs of inflammation associated to bleeding on probing constitutes peri-implant mucositis, which is usually caused by plaque deposition, and its treatment consists of plaque removal (Caton et al. 2018; Heitz-Mayfield et al. 2018). Peri-implantitis in turn is characterized by peri-implant mucositis and subsequent progressive loss of supporting bone (Schwarz et al. 2018).

10.2.2 Current and Classical Methods for Diagnostic and Their Implications

The diagnosis of periodontal disease is mainly dependent on clinical and radiographic examination, and the periodic monitoring of the gingival sulcus will provide valuable information to determine the presence and severity of periodontal disease (Hsieh et al. 2011; Huang et al. 2012).

The most classical study to describe the dentogingival interface measurements was carried out by Gargiulo and cols (Gargiulo et al. 1961), through autopsy of patients and identified that the connective tissue attachment, junctional and sulcular epithelia measured 1.07 mm, 0.97 mm and 0.69 mm, respectively; these histologic values are still considered as reference for healthy patients.

Intraoral radiographic provides information about the root anatomy, the presence of periapical lesions, calculus deposition and remaining alveolar bone level (Kim et al. 2017; Park et al. 2017), however it may underestimate the bone loss, since it is observable on radiographs only after 30%–50% of bone resorption (Jeffcoat et al. 1995). Additionally, two-dimensional radiographs are not able to differentiate bone defects on buccal or lingual sides neither the soft tissue condition (Hsieh et al. 2011).

To support the clinician's diagnostic several technologies for calculus detection and periodontal tissue evaluation were developed in the past years, as example fiber-optic endoscopy, optical spectrometric, magnetic resonance imaging (MRI), ultrasonic imaging, light-emitting diode-based optical probe and fluorescence technology (Krause et al. 2005; Meissner et al. 2008; Park et al. 2017, Krause et al. 2019; Lee et al. 2019). Cone-beam computed tomography (CBCT) is a good way for hard and soft tissue evaluation, but its high cost and relatively low-resolution limit its application. Microcomputed tomography (micro-CT) is another non-invasive imaging technique used in dental research, able to provide submicron spatial resolution for detailing depiction of tooth morphology and accurately measure the mineral concentration in teeth samples (Kao et al. 2015; Park et al. 2017).

Periodontal probing is the most used method to quantify the periodontal condition based on the attachment loss (AL) and pocket depth (PD) values. The method is applied to diagnosis and follow-up patients under treatment, considering that one of the characteristics of periodontal disease is the presence of pockets formed by the attachment loss of connective tissues and alveolar bone surface. For healthy patients the gingival sulcus depth corresponds to an artificial space created by the introduction of the probe between the gingival tissue and the tooth surface during the examination (Polson et al. 1980; Fernandes et al. 2017; Xiang et al. 2010; Park et al. 2017).

Despite its large use, there are some limitations that should be pointed out due to its influence on the probing deep penetration, such as the inflammatory condition of the tissue, the manual pressure applied by the examiner, the probe placement and angulation, as well as the instrument caliper (Fernandes et al. 2017; Xiang et al. 2010). Still, it is important to register that periodontal probing is painful for the patient. Furthermore, periodontal probing is considered an invasive procedure due to the risk of trauma to periodontal tissues promoted by its active tip penetration (Mota et al. 2015a; Hsieh et al. 2011). Aiming to compensate the human errors, an automatic mechanical probe was developed, proposing constant force application, but it makes the patient even more uncomfortable than the manual method (Jeffcoat et al. 1995; Fernandes et al. 2017).

In this context, OCT has been investigated: it is a widely known imaging modality in biophotonics, able to provide cross-sectional images from biological tissues in real-time, with high resolution and few millimeters depth penetration (Kakizaki et al. 2018; Fernandes et al. 2019).

10.2.2.1 Important Structures to be Considered in Periodontal Diagnostic

Accurate diagnosis and follow-up of the progression of periodontitis requires not only the analysis of gingival indices, but also the combination of several methods, such as the imaging assessment, evidence of attachment loss and tooth mobility registration (Preshaw 2015; Le et al. 2018). The periodontal examination provides the clinician important information related to the type, severity and location of periodontal disease (Park et al. 2017). This exam aims to identify clinical signs of bleeding, pain and suppuration, the plaque and calculus deposition, probing depths and the extent and pattern of bone and attachment loss.

Concept of supracrestal attached tissues comprises the vertical distance between the base of the gingival sulcus and the crest of the alveolar bone. It is a critical point to be considered in esthetic plastic surgery and perio-prosthodontics, to avoid marginal gingiva inflammation (Kakizaki et al. 2018).

Changes in gingival vasculature are an important indicator in the monitoring of the severity of periodontal disease. Initial stages of the disease can present brief acute inflammation, whilst in the chronic phase the inflammatory response is characterized by vasodilatation and proliferation of the blood vessels. There are some clinical methods to score the degree of gingival inflammation using the Gingival Index, which requires probing into the already inflamed periodontal tissues and potentially induces unnecessary pain and bleeding, as for example, the papillary bleeding index, the bleeding on marginal probing, and the Eastman interdental bleeding index – but all of them are questionable due to their reliability and reproducibility (Le et al. 2018).

Periodontal phenotype influences the prognosis of periodontal therapies (for example, root coverage and implant therapy), restorative procedures, orthodontic treatment, etc (Kakizaki et al. 2018; Le et al. 2018). The appearance and anatomical structure of the gingiva might be considered a risk factor for development of changes, such as gingival recession in the presence of low gingival thickness (thin phenotype) or less likely on patients with thick gum (thick phenotype) after surgical therapy or restorative treatment. Gingival thickness variation has direct implication on the results of periodontal therapy, root coverage procedures, implant placement and surgeries for maxillary sinus elevation owing to the strong correlation between the gingival phenotype (Deepthi et al. 2012; Mota et al. 2015a; Mota et al. 2015b).

Currently, there is no consensus about the classification of periodontal phenotypes. Several methods have been used, invasive and non-invasive, to evaluate the gingival thickness, such as histologic sections, injection needles, transgingival probing, ultrasonic measurement, transparency of periodontal probing and cone-beam computed tomography. Each method has different definition for the "thick" and "thin" phenotypes (Esfahrood et al. 2013; Mota et al. 2015a; Kakizaki et al. 2018; Le et al. 2018).

10.2.3 OCT Studies

OCT has been applied in dentistry since 1998 (Colston et al. 1998a; Feldchtein et al. 1998), but since then the published studies are focused specially on early caries diagnostic (Quitero et al. 2019) and restorative materials (Han et al. 2016). After the pioneering studies of Colston and coauthors (Colston et al. 1998a; Colston et al. 1998b; Colston et al. 1998c) and Feldchtein and collaborators (Feldchtein et al. 1998) several studies have been carried out exploring the technological and commercial efforts and the applicability of OCT for periodontics. Table 10.1 briefly shows the studies reported in this chapter related to periodontal diagnostic. The laboratory studies were performed with porcine jaws (Colston et al. 1998a; Mota et al. 2015a; Mota et al. 2015b; Kim et al. 2017), canine jaw (Park et al. 2017), extracted human teeth (Feldchtein et al. 1998; Huminicki et al. 2010; Hsieh et al. 2011; Kao et al. 2015; Hsiao et al. 2021) and/or gingival samples (Hsieh et al. 2011; Hsiao et al. 2021; Surlin et al. 2021). Between the 22 selected studies, swept-source OCT constituted the largest employed systems (Hsieh et al. 2011; Mota et al. 2015a; Mota et al. 2015b; Kao et al. 2015; Kim et al. 2017; Fernandes et al. 2017; Park et al. 2017; Kakizaki et al. 2018; Le et al. 2018; Lee et al. 2019; Lai et al. 2019; Hsiao et al. 2021; Surlin et al. 2021; Townsend 2022).

Analogous to ultrasound imaging, OCT measures the intensity and time-of-flight information collected from backscattered light and uses that information to reconstruct three-dimensional reflectivity maps up to several millimeters deep in tissue. These properties, which allow OCT to perform depth-resolved imaging in human tissue while remaining non-invasive and non-ionizing, have led to a wide range of pre-clinical and clinical applications (Shelton et al. 2014).

In biological tissues, light is attenuated by optical scattering and absorption by water. Shorter wavelengths result in lower absorption by water but exhibit greater optical scattering in tissues. In dental tissues, scattering of light was considered to dominate its attenuation in the near-infrared region (Kakizaki et al. 2018).

Regarding light interaction with the periodontal tissues, Mota and coauthors (Mota et al. 2015a) affirm that in gingival tissues there is a relative homogeneity of scattering pattern, probably due to the constant water content and other constituents of the tissue. But the same behavior was not observed in hard tissues, specifically dentin and enamel, when there was calculus deposition on the tooth: the irregular and aleatory deposition of calcium phosphate promotes a strong scattering of incident light that, according to Hsieh and cols (Hsieh et al. 2011), is due to a high refractive index (2.097–0.094).

Refractive index and attenuation coefficient (product of absorption/scattering) are both important for OCT measurement. The attenuation coefficient affects the image quality of OCT, i.e., contrast of image and maximal imaging penetration depth, whereas the refractive index of tissue affects the thickness measurements by OCT (Kakizaki et al. 2018).

One of the major critical points in periodontics is the identification of subgingival calculus. Several novel methods have been developed to facilitate dental calculus detection, including fiber-optic endoscopy-based technology, spectra-optical technology, and autofluorescence-based technology (Kao et al. 2015). Particularly fluorescence-based techniques could bring a diagnostic benefit. This could be helpful in supportive therapy to avoid

TABLE 10.1

Studies Published with OCT Focusing on Periodontal Structures

Authors	Clinical or laboratorial	Subject	OCT system and central wavelength
(Colston et al. 1998a)	Laboratorial	Porcine jaw	TD-OCT at 1310 nm
(Colston et al. 1998b)	Clinical	Patients	TD-OCT at 1310 nm
(Colston et al. 1998c)	Clinical	Patients	TD-OCT at 1310 nm
(Feldchtein et al. 1998)	Laboratorial and clinical	Patients and extracted human teeth	Dual wavelength OCT at 830 nm and 1280 nm
(Huminicki et al. 2010)	Laboratorial	Extracted human teeth	Ophthalmic OCT at 850 nm
(Hsieh et al. 2011)	Laboratorial	Extracted human teeth with calculus, covered by gingiva	SS-OCT at 1310 nm
(Shelton et al. 2014)	Clinical	Patients	SD-OCT at 830 nm
(Kao et al. 2015)	Laboratorial	Extracted human teeth	SS-OCT at 1310 nm
(Mota et al. 2015a)	Laboratorial	Porcine jaw	SS-OCT at 1325 nm and SD-OCT at 930 nm
(Mota et al. 2015b)	Laboratorial and clinical	Porcine jaw and healthy patients	SS-OCT at 1325 nm
(Park et al. 2017)	Laboratorial	Canine jaw	SS-OCT at 1310 nm
(Kim et al. 2017)	Laboratorial	Porcine jaw	SS-OCT at 1325 nm
(Fernandes et al. 2017)	Clinical	Periodontally healthy patients	SS-OCT at 1325 nm
(Fernandes et al. 2019)	Clinical	Patients with periodontal disease	SS-OCT at 1330 nm
(Kakizaki et al. 2018)	Clinical	Periodontally healthy patients	SS-OCT at 1310 nm
(Le et al. 2018)	Clinical	Patients	SS-OCT at 1310 nm
(Lee et al. 2019)	Clinical	Patients	SS-OCT by combining multiple wavelengths
(Lai et al. 2019)	Clinical	Patients	SD-OCT at 860 nm
(Won et al. 2020)	Clinical	Patients	SS-OCT at 1300 nm
(Surlin et al. 2021)	Laboratorial	Gingival samples collected from patients with periodontal pockets	SS-OCT at 1310 nm
(Hsiao et al. 2021)	Laboratorial	Extracted human teeth with calculus, covered by gingiva	SS-OCT at 1305 nm
(Townsend 2022)	Clinical	Patients	

TD-OCT: time domain optical coherence tomography. SS-OCT: swept source optical coherence tomography. SD-OCT: spectral domain optical coherence tomography.

instrumentation of calculus-free root surfaces, as an intraoperative control and in the instruction and motivation of patients using the images. However, they might be unable to detect calculus unequivocally on the root surface because no subgingival illustration of the situation is possible (Krause et al. 2019).

To meet this demand, some papers proposed to investigate the application of different OCT techniques for subgingival calculus detection (Huminicki et al. 2010; Kao et al. 2015), by differentiating the calculus from enamel in OCT images, exploiting their differences in composition and consequent differences in images generated.

Regions with calculus were observed and an increase of supragingival plaque thickness was also identified in a previous study (Fernandes et al. 2019). Another study (Hsiao et al. 2021) demonstrated the feasibility of OCT for calculus examination, distinguishing dental calculus below gingiva with high detection power: dental calculus was observed in B-scan and in volumetric view, mainly in the central part of image (Figure 10.2). Calculus has an inhomogeneous constitution, with hypomineralized areas and porous – these characteristics allowed differentiation of the intensity signal of OCT images when compared to tooth enamel and enamel pearls (a rare condition of ectopic enamel, which can be clinically confused with calculus) (Kao et al. 2015).

Another study was developed (Hsieh et al. 2011) to measure the refractive indices of dental hard tissues and observed that the strong scattering properties of dental calculus is enough to distinguish it from enamel. These data were reinforced by Kao and coworkers (Kao et al. 2015), who compared OCT images from dental calculus and enamel with radiographs and micro-CT images.

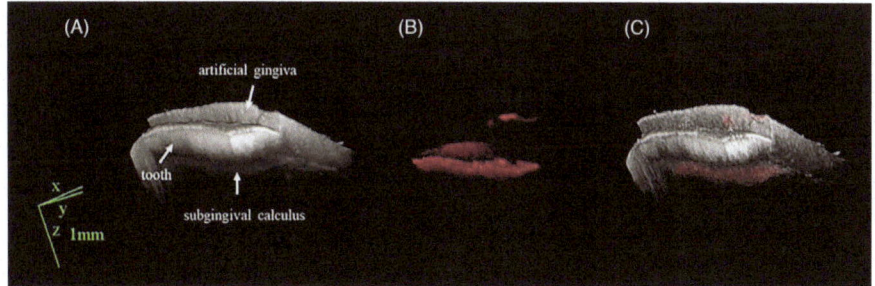

FIGURE 10.2

Representative images from a subgingival calculus in a phantom: (A) C-scan; (B) the volumetric disease activation map (DAM) and (C) the volumetric computer-aided detection (CAD). The fast-scanning direction is represented by the x-axis, the slow-scanning by the y-axis, and the axial depth direction is indicated by z-axis. Reprinted with permission from (Hsiao et al. 2021) © John Wiley & Sons.

Following the studies for calculus detection, other authors also explored the identification of periodontal structures by OCT, through laboratorial and/or clinical studies, as already shown in Table 10.1.

OCT could generate high-resolution images of hard- and soft-tissue structures of the periodontium, adding further information to the diagnostic process. The analysis of the two-dimensional OCT images allowed the identification of relevant anatomic areas of dental and periodontal regions. An *ex vivo* study (Mota et al. 2015a) examined porcine jaws with two technically different OCT systems operating in the Fourier domain, one of them operating in the spectral domain (SD-OCT) and the other one was a swept source (SS-OCT), emitting 930 nm and 1325 nm of central wavelength, respectively. Morphological differences were explored between free and attached gingiva, the supra- and subgingival calculus, gingival sulcus, and the sulcus depth and the enlargement of gingival sulcus was measured. They also measured the gingival thickness. Kim and coauthors (Kim et al. 2017) also in porcine jaws, visualized periodontal pockets and showed attachment loss and its corresponding periodontal pocket depth with manual probing. In canine jaws, OCT was able to generate high-resolution, cross-sectional images of the superficial portions of periodontal structures (Park et al. 2017). The results confirm that SS-OCT could provide more information, since a longer central wavelength allows deeper tissue penetration, besides the faster image acquisition, an essential point in the clinical setting. But the method based on spectral domain or swept source is not relevant: OCT characteristics are more important, because acquisition image rates can differ, which affect spatial resolution (Mota et al. 2015a). Hsiao and cols (Hsiao et al. 2021) suggest the choice of the wavelength at 1.31 μm is ideal for dental applications because of both the penetration depth and the resolution.

Following the study published with porcine jaws (Mota et al. 2015a), Mota and cols (Mota et al. 2015b) carried out a transitional study in two phases: *ex vivo* and clinical with periodontally healthy individuals. The aims were to identify and differentiate the free and attached gingiva, as well as determining the gingival phenotype – but now only using the SS-OCT system operating at 1325 nm of the central wavelength. OCT reveals microstructural details of the periodontal soft tissues, providing information for controlling the volume of attached keratinized gingiva, as well as enabling the observation of periodontal structures that might be associated with inflammatory processes (Gladkova et al. 2011; Mota et al. 2015a).

Through the image analysis of the animal jaws, it was possible to quantify the free gingiva and the attached gingiva, the calculus deposition over the teeth surface, as well as subgingival calculus. For the clinical studies, the gingival phenotype could be measured without the periodontal probe introduction at the gingival sulcus, confirming that OCT can be potentially useful in clinic for direct observation and quantification of gingival phenotype in a non-invasive approach. Thus, it was proposed the use of OCT as a standard technique for analysis of periodontal tissues and evaluation and determination of the gingival phenotype. OCT was efficient to identify periodontal structures: gingiva, cementum-enamel junction, and the gingival sulcus (Figure 10.3). In addition, other structures have been observed, such as the dental enamel layer, identified overlapped to dentin by dentinoenamel junction, and the free and inserted gingiva, the gingival margin, the regions of oral, sulcular and junctional epithelium, and adjacent connective tissue (Mota et al. 2015a; Mota et al. 2015b). The images allowed the qualitative and quantitative analysis of the gingiva and gingival sulcus, similar to the results obtained by Colston & cols (Colston et al. 1998a). This fact demonstrates the ability of the OCT in quantitatively assess the phenotype value and suggests the use of OCT as a standard method in evaluating the human gingival phenotype.

Kim & cols (Kim et al. 2017) examined whether the periodontal pocket could be satisfactorily visualized by OCT and suggested quantitative methods for measuring periodontal pocket depth in a porcine model (*ex vivo*). They acquired OCT images (SS-OCT 1310 nm) and determined the axial resolution for measuring the exact periodontal pocket depth using a calibration method. The OCT image acquisition is fundamentally based on the back-reflection signals of a specimen with different refractive indexes. The refractive index of tissue affects the thickness measurements by OCT (Kakizaki et al. 2018).

In the gingival sulcus, crevicular fluid is flown out from the gingival connective tissue, which has a slightly different refractive index compared to gingiva. Since a slight variation of the refractive index occurs in the depth direction, the resulting depth profile emphasizes a distinct shift of an intensity peak corresponds to the gingival sulcus (Lee et al. 2019). Since the axial resolution is affected by the medium through which the light passes, it is necessary to calculate the axial resolution in the gingiva. In addition, in order to be used in clinical practice, an optical probe should be applied not only to incisors and canines, but also to the posterior teeth and to each side of the teeth; thus, the axial resolution needs to be considered to obtain reliable values in any position. Quantitative measurements of periodontal pockets could be obtained and compared with the results from manual periodontal probing. The OCT measurements were compatible with those obtained from manual probing, allowing visualization of periodontal pockets and attachment loss. By calculating the calibration factor to determine the accurate axial resolution, quantitative standards for measuring periodontal pocket depth can be established regardless of the position of periodontal pocket in the OCT image (Kim et al. 2017).

Continuing the validation of OCT technique to periodontal probing, Fernandes and coworkers (Fernandes et al. 2017) performed a pilot study with periodontally healthy patients in a clinical setting. The study demonstrated for the first time the application of OCT imaging for clinical evaluation of gingival sulcus and adjacent tissues in periodontally healthy individuals in

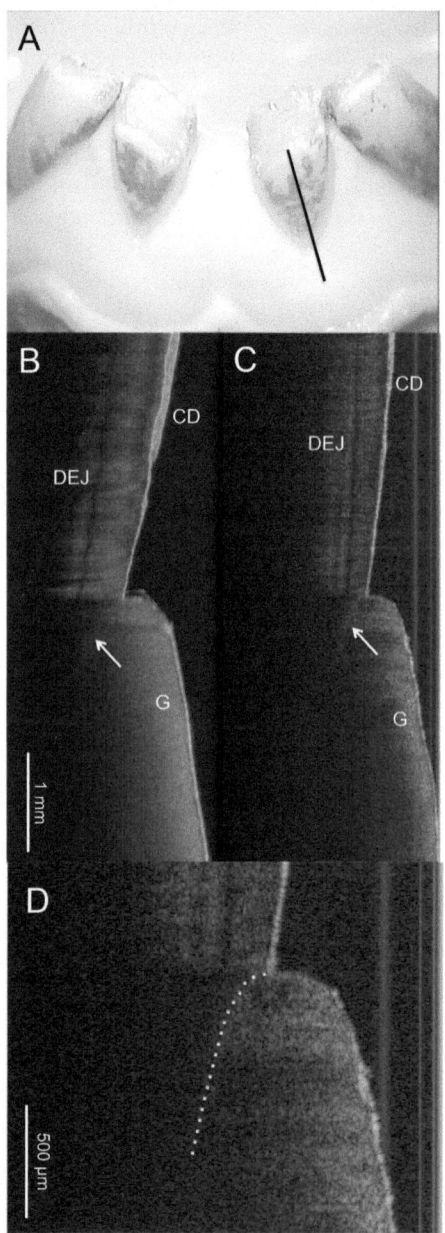

FIGURE 10.3
(A) Stereomicroscopic image (×6.5 magnification) of porcine jaw incisors after 24-hour storage in 10% formalin solution. (B) SD-OCT and (C) SS-OCT images obtained in the region corresponding to the line in (A). (D) Same as in (C), showing an expanded image highlighting the gingival sulcus, where the white dashed line was drawn as a guide. CD = calculus deposition, DEJ = dentin-enamel junction, G = gingival tissues. The arrows show the interface between free gingiva and tooth surface. Scale bars are 1 mm (B and C) and 500 mm (D). Reprinted with permission from (Mota et al. 2015a) © John Wiley & Sons – Books.

a clinical environment. Gingival sulcus depth measurements were obtained and compared to manual and conventional probes (North Carolina manual probe and Florida automated probe). A SS-OCT system (1325 nm) previously adopted to a clinical setting with a head support dispositive was used. Gingival refractive index was also determined, and discomfort/pain perception and the duration of examinations were registered for comparison among the instruments. The analysis of OCT images allowed the identification of relevant anatomic dental and periodontal regions, as shown in Figure 10.4. The average sulcus depth measured by OCT was lower than the values obtained by manual and automated probing. It was confirmed by the volunteer's perception that discomfort and pain were absent during OCT imaging, as expected for a non-invasive technique. A different pattern was observed during the probing: discomfort was referred by 34.8% of participants for manual probing and by 65.2% for automated probing. Additionally, in a range from 0 to 100, an average pain intensity of 55 was described for automated probing by four individuals who referred pain.

Preliminary research (Lee et al. 2019) demonstrated the feasible *in vivo* utilization of SS-OCT system (1310 nm) to obtain morphological visualizations and human gingival sulcus depth measurements. As seen earlier, the enlargement of the gingival sulcus is an important predictor of the presence or absence of periodontal disease: in healthy conditions, free gingiva is very close to the tooth surface. Therefore, it offers the potential for accurately identifying active periodontitis before significant alveolar bone involvement occurs. OCT technique can be well suited to a clinical environment for early and non-invasive periodontal diagnostics, also yielding quantitative information on pocket formation (depth and transverse dimension) (Xiang et al. 2010; Mota et al. 2015a).

The average values of sulcus depth measured by OCT were significantly shorter, 0.4 mm and 0.6 mm (for manual- and automated-probes, respectively), than the probing values obtained from periodontally healthy individuals (Fernandes et al. 2017). Since OCT is a non-contact and non-invasive approach, it does not compress the soft tissue and it does not disrupt the natural interface at the cementum-epithelium junction. As mentioned above, ideally these results should be compared to histology, but this second technique is not performed with patients in *in vivo* studies. However, technical limitation of this study is mitigated if we consider that the OCT results are close to that of Gargiulo and coauthors (Gargiulo et al. 1961), the only early work found with histological measurements of sulcus depth.

Apart from the cross-sectional analysis, OCT pixel intensity based numerical image classification algorithm was developed by Lee and coworkers (Lee et al. 2019) to visualize and numerically evaluate *in vivo* the depth of gingival sulcus. For this study, the volunteer used a lip retractor with its head fixed on a holder, similar to the study of Fernandes and cols (Fernandes et al. 2017). To assess the depth visualization of the

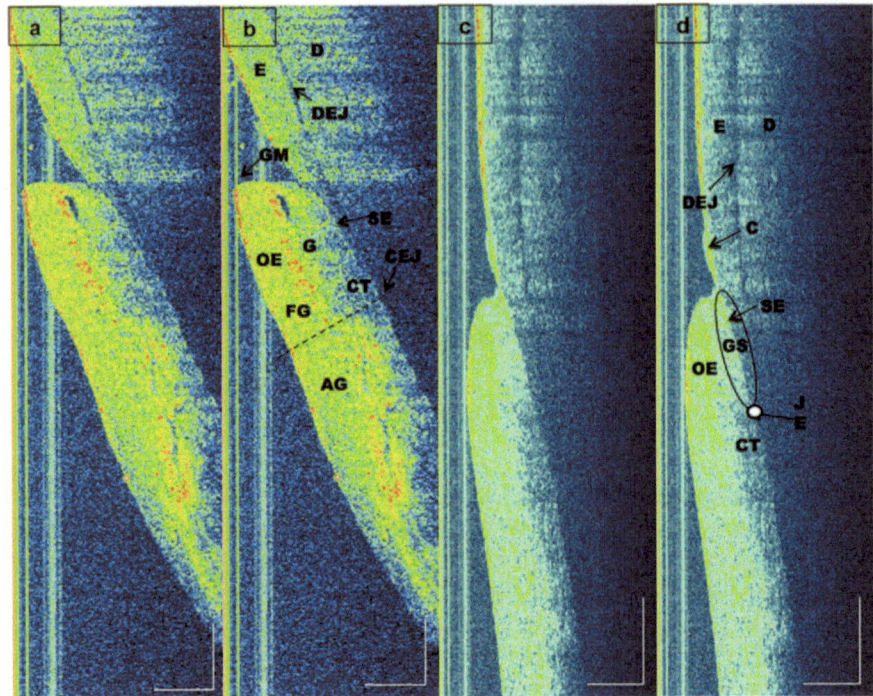

FIGURE 10.4
Images obtained by SS-OCT at 1325 nm showing the distinction between periodontal structures: the dental enamel layer (E) is shown overlapped to the dentin (D) by the dentin-enamel junction (DEJ). The cemento-enamel junction (CEJ) was clearly observed and supragingival calculus (C) was detected whenever present. The gingiva (G) could be differentiated as free gingiva (FG) and attached gingiva (AG), since AG appeared as higher scattering light areas than FG. Oral (OE) and sulcular epithelium (SE) and connective tissue (CT) could be discriminated. The gingival sulcus (GS) was delimited by identifying its contour with predictability of 100%, as well as the gingival margin (GM). Reprinted with permission from (Fernandes et al. 2017) © John Wiley & Sons – Books.

morphological structures, the A-scan profile from cross-sectional images acquired with the SS-OCT system were analyzed and revealed the inner microstructures of the crown and root. The enamel, dentin, DEJ, gum and gingival sulcus were distinguished. The developed classification algorithm could measure the gingival sulcus depth (1.15 ± 0.21 mm of the maxilla and 1.06 ± 0.27 mm of the mandible). The average total depth obtained by the system was 1.10 ± 0.26 mm. Hence, the gingival sulcus depth could be quantitatively measured by using the SS-OCT system with the developed image classification algorithm, as well as revealing a structural visualization, which ultimately confirmed the potential applicability for gingival sulcus depth real-time assessment.

The comparison of OCT to the probing method confirmed its safety and usability as an investigation tool. The gingival sulcus classification of the OCT image can be helpful as for the diagnosis of periodontal tissue conditions in the field of periodontics.

In the last stage of their study, Fernandes and coauthors (Fernandes et al. 2019) reported an important step towards the clinical use of OCT in dental practice, by following-up patients treated from periodontal disease. A total of 147 vestibular dental sites from 14 patients diagnosed with periodontal disease were evaluated prior and after treatment, using a SS-OCT and two periodontal probes (Florida probe and North Carolina) for comparison. The evaluation was performed at four stages: day 0, day 30, day 60 and day 90. It was possible to visualize in two-dimensional images the architectural components that compose the periodontal anatomy and identify the improvements in biofilm and dental calculus upon treatment. In the follow-up after the treatment, it was observed in some cases decrease of the gingival thickness associated with extinction of gingival calculus. It was also possible to visualize the improvement of the probing depth, confirmed by the OCT scanning of the same areas. The study highlighted the OCT ability to identify and monitoring of periodontal structures, constituting an important non-invasive complement or even alternative for periodontal probes for treatment follow-up.

Although previous studies have also used the technique for assessing the periodontal disease in animal models (Mota et al.2015a; Kim et al. 2017; Park et al. 2017), this was the first study that longitudinally evaluated the evolution of periodontal disease in patients (Fernandes et al. 2019).

Figure 10.5 shows an illustrative OCT image of a healthy individual (A) and a patient with periodontal disease (B). In the 2D images, it is possible to visualize the architectural components of the periodontal anatomy, both in healthy and unhealthy region. Despite the presented limitations, depth of light penetration and scan window lower than the depth of the pockets, the technique is efficient in monitoring the periodontal disease.

Kakizaki and collaborators (Kakizaki et al. 2018) aimed to observe and determine periodontal tissue profiles *in vivo*. They calculated the refractive indexes of purified water, porcine gingiva and human gingiva; then OCT scanning was carried out in mandibular anterior teeth of periodontally healthy patients, followed by intraoral photographs and manual periodontal probing. They used a prototype SS-OCT system operating at 1330 nm of central wavelength coupled to a handheld scanning probe. In the OCT images, typical dental and periodontal structures, such as enamel, dentin, root surface, epithelium, connective tissue and alveolar bone were clearly depicted, and finally, the supracrestal attached tissues were measured. The deeper light penetration was around 1.5 mm, similar to the findings of Fernandes & cols (Fernandes et al. 2019). The gingival tissue profile showed different phenotypes: thin, moderate and thick types (Figure 10.6). In the thick type, OCT images became

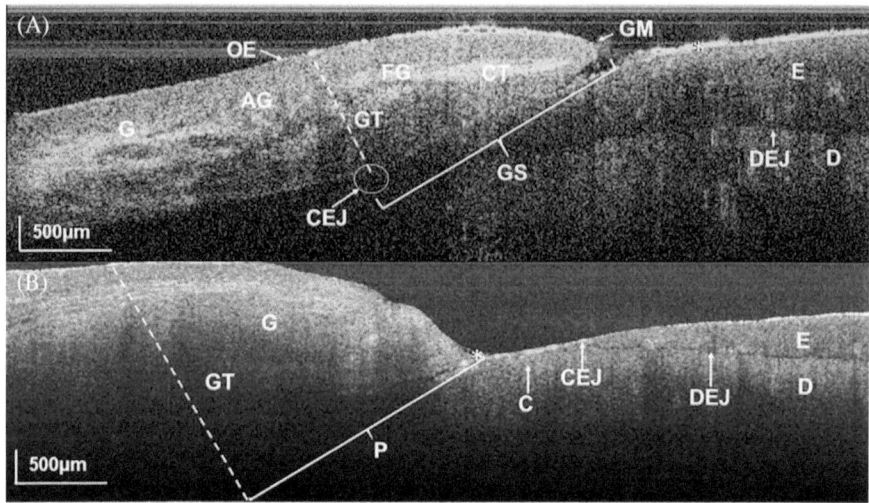

FIGURE 10.5

Images of the periodontal region of a lower incisor and its anatomical constituents obtained
from a periodontally healthy (A) and unhealthy (B) patients. In the healthy periodontium
presented in (A) it is possible to visualize the gingiva (G), enamel (E); dentin (D); gingival
thickness (GT); dentin-enamel junction (DEJ); gingival sulcus (GS), connective tissue (CT);
biofilm/dental plaque (*); cement-enamel junction (CEJ); gingival margin (GM); oral
epithelium (OE); free gingiva (FG) and attached (AG). In (B), in its turn, the same structures
present in (A) are seen, besides the cement (C) and part of the periodontal pocket (P).
The horizontal and vertical scale bars represent 500 μm. Reprinted with permission from
(Fernandes et al. 2019) © John Wiley & Sons – Books.

unclear beyond approximately 1.5 mm depth from the gingival surface. In
some cases, sulcular and junctional epithelium was also depicted. Blood
vessels within the connective tissues could be distinguished, due its lower
signal intensity if compared to the surrounding connective tissues. They
also observed in details surface characteristics of gingiva, such as stippling
and root resorption. OCT shows promise as a modality that can be used not
only for the periodontal tissue profile but also for morphometrical analysis,
including determination of supracrestal attached tissues in combination with
clinical probing. An intraoral OCT probing with a mouthpiece incorporating
a mirror enables imaging of the posterior teeth and lingual surfaces.

A non-invasive imaging technique providing depth-resolved structural
and vascular information is necessary for an improved assessment of gingival tissue and more accurate diagnosis of periodontal status. In this way,
Le and collaborators (Le et al. 2018) proposed the OCT technique to perform *in situ* imaging on human gingiva, by observing the microstructure
and vasculature in gingival tissue. Ten volunteers were recruited, and the
labial gingival tissues of upper incisors were scanned by combining SS-
OCT (1310 nm) and OCT angiography (OCTA) with up to 2 mm of depth

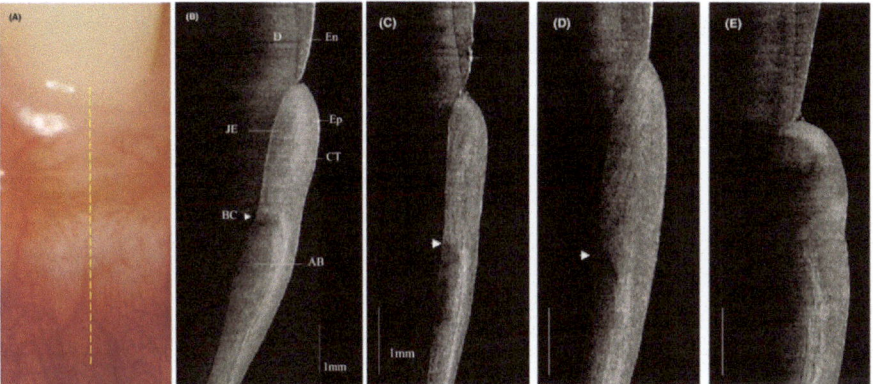

FIGURE 10.6

2D-OCT images of the typical periodontal tissue profile and distinct phenotypes of periodontal tissue. (A) Oral photograph. (B) OCT image of typical periodontal tissues scanned at the dotted line in (A). (C), (D) and (E), representative OCT images of a thin, moderate, and thick periodontal phenotypes. Enamel (En), dentin (D), gingival epithelium (Ep), junctional epithelium (JE), connective tissue (CT), alveolar bone (AB) and bone crest (BC). Alveolar bone and root surface were clearly depicted in (C) and (D), and arrowhead shows the bone crest. In (E), the alveolar bone crest and root surface were not depicted due to the limitation of imaging in depth. Reprinted with permission from (Kakizaki et al. 2018) © John Wiley & Sons – Books.

penetration, capable of resolving microcapillary loops within the gingiva. The scanning probe was a light-weight piece designed for handheld configuration. Initially employed in eye imaging, OCTA is able to separate dynamic and static signals, popularly known as vascular and non-vascular signals (Figure 10.7). Viewed with the OCT, oral epithelium appears as a highly scattering medium, producing a high OCT-intensity layer in comparison to the underlying connective tissues. Below the oral epithelium, the connective tissue is demarcated from the epithelium by the epithelial connective tissue interface, which has an alternating extension and depression pattern (which extends inward and outward from the gingival surface). This alternating pattern is well-known in periodontology as the rete pegs, or rete ridges, of the gingiva. The rete pegs can be observed under OCT B-scan as an alternating pattern of darker and brighter stripes. There are several limitations presented by OCT and especially in OCTA, namely: (1) the limited depth penetration and (2) the resolution-depth-of-field trade off. Since this technique is non-invasive, label-free, non-contact and can be implemented in real-time and with low cost, improvements in quality of oral health assessment would be significant as an adjunct tool in addition to the traditional methods. For dental clinicians, this method can be very useful in quantitative assessment of periodontal tissue (healthy or inflamed; thick or thin phenotype) before the dental procedures, such as soft tissue graft and clinical therapies.

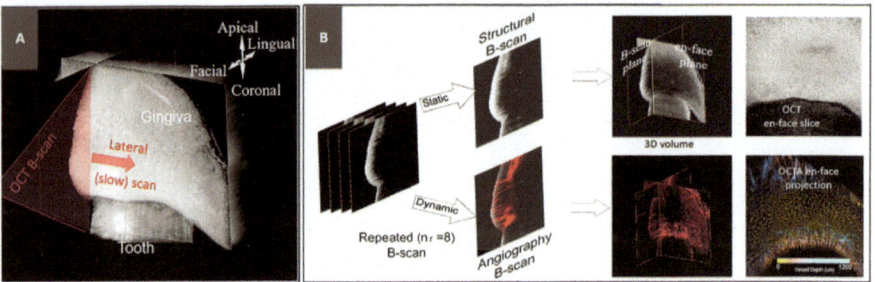

FIGURE 10.7

(A) Schematic of the scanning direction relative to the gingiva and tooth of the upper left incisor, illustrated on 3D-OCT image. (B) Scanning procedures to obtain 2D-OCT and OCTA, where the repeated B-scans at each lateral position was processed using the OMAG algorithm to separate the blood flow signal from the static tissue signal to form structural (top row) and functional vascular (bottom row) B-scans at that lateral position. Successive processing of all lateral positions forms the 3D volumetric structural and vascular information, upon which en-face slices at specific tissue depth or en-face projection can be displayed for detailed investigation. Reprinted with permission from (Le et al. 2018) © John Wiley & Sons – Books.

Townsend (Townsend 2022) conducted a clinical study by means of measuring changes in arteriolar and venular capillary flow and structure in the gingival tissues during the development of plaque-induced gingival inflammation by combining dynamic OCT, laser perfusion, and capillaroscopic video imaging. An early increase in venous capillaries is a key vascular feature of cardiovascular disease, psoriasis, Sjögren syndrome and rheumatoid arthritis – diseases significantly associated with the development of severe gingival inflammation, which leads to periodontitis. Investigations of microvascular changes in gingival inflammation might benefit from accurate capillary flow velocity measurements to assess the development of venular capillaries. OCT detected wide variation in vascular indices. The transformation of arteriolar capillaries to venular capillaries is an early feature of all diseases associated with periodontal breakdown in humans. Microvascular imaging in gingival tissues can be used to identify the transition to venular capillaries and could help our understanding of why some people develop periodontal breakdown whilst others do not. Although the image sharpness is affected by the axial resolution and signal-to-noise ratio, it is possible to vaguely discriminate between the epithelium and subepithelial connective tissue. Such information can be immensely valuable and have implications for the results of periodontal therapy, gingival augmentation procedures, root coverage, and implants in esthetic areas where the adequacy of the gingival thickness is paramount. Determining the thickness of the epithelial layer can be especially useful during the planning and execution of connective tissue grafting procedures, since this could confirm the sufficiency of undermining of the epithelium at the graft site. Furthermore, bleeding at the donor site could be reduced if palatal vessels are visualized. Several methods for evaluating gingival thickness have been proposed, such as injection needles, probe transparency and visual inspection, cannot be considered reliable due to their subjective nature. The main advantage of OCT over these techniques is that it is a quantitative high-resolution imaging method that can be used in real-time during clinical procedures (Park et al. 2017).

Brezinski and cols (Brezinski et al. 1996) showed that the contrast between different adjacent tissue is stronger when there is a greater difference in the water content within tissues. Similarly, in the study of (Park et al. 2017), the samples with subgingival calculus had higher water content than the adjacent tooth surface, resulting in an increase of signal intensity and contrast. For this reason, the authors assume that the presence of gingival crevicular fluid in an *in vivo* model contribute to better visualization of the sulcular anatomy, when compared to an *ex vivo* model.

Quantitative measurements in OCT images can be widely applied to diagnose periodontal status. Measuring the attachment level helps to assess the severity of periodontal disease and monitor improvements in treatment. Gingival thickness can be measured to determine the soft-tissue phenotype, which can affect the tissue response and treatment planning. Soft-tissue dimension is important for the successful treatment of dental implant and aesthetic restoration (Lee et al. 2011; Kim et al. 2017). They can also be used to harvest grafts during root coverage procedures and to evaluate results during wound healing period.

Primary care physicians and dentists stand at the frontline to identify the earliest indications of disease and effectively screen the general population. These professionals are required to maintain a broad knowledge of many common diseases and pathologies and typically conduct thousands of patient examinations each year. In contrast, the principal tools used for diagnosis have remained largely unchanged for decades. Technological innovation has revolutionized health care, and advances in imaging methods are leading examples for screening, detecting and monitoring disease. Due to its ability to image microstructural changes in tissue morphology, OCT is well-suited for screening in the primary care setting (Shelton et al. 2014).

10.3 Conclusions

An efficient diagnostic method able to identify early periodontal changes is fundamental for clinical success and keeping periodontal health. The identification of alterations in periodontium in the subclinical stages, and monitoring of the progression of the periodontal disease are still a great challenge in the dental clinic.

OCT is a non-invasive imaging technique that allows contact-free, non-destructive, non-ionizing, real-time imaging with high, submicron-scale resolution by analyzing the internal microstructures of samples, suitable for clinical application. OCT is able to generate 2D and 3D volumetric images, besides *en-face* reconstruction, which allows to accurately evaluate hard and soft tissues in the oral cavity, thus identifying any structural change.

A key challenge for intraoral OCT application is related to its technological advances: the development of an appropriate handheld piece, preserving the stability of the system; optimization of the chairside time for examination (software for faster image acquisition); deeper light penetration and increase of the scanning range; and reduction of the costs, without damage to the quality of images generated.

References

Agrawal, P., Sanikop, S., Patil, S. 2012. New developments in tools for periodontal diagnosis. *International Dental Journal* 62: 57–64.

Albandar, J. M., Susin, C., Hughes, F. J. 2018. Manifestations of systemic diseases and conditions that affect the periodontal attachment apparatus: case definitions and diagnostic considerations. *Journal of Periodontology* 89: S183–S203.

Berglundh, T., Armitage, G., Araujo, M. G. et al. 2018. Peri-implant diseases and conditions: Consensus report of workgroup 4 of the 2017 World Workshop on the Classification of Periodontal and Peri-Implant Diseases and Conditions. *Journal of Periodontology* 89 Suppl 1: S313–S318.

Brezinski, M. E., Tearney, G. J., Bouma, B. E. et al. 1996. Optical coherence tomography for optical biopsy: properties and demonstration of vascular pathology. *Circulation* 93: 1206–1213.

Camus, M., Beuvon, F., Barret, M. et al. 2018. Full-field optical coherence tomography: A new imaging modality for rapid on-site evaluation of resected polyps during colonoscopy. *Gastroenterology* 155: 1692–1694.

Caton, J. G., Armitage, G., Berglundh, T. et al. 2018. A new classification scheme for periodontal and peri-implant diseases and conditions – Introduction and key changes from the 1999 classification. *Journal of Clinical Periodontology* 45: S1–S8.

Chapple, I. L. C., Genco, R. 2013. Diabetes and periodontal diseases: consensus report of the Joint EFP/AAP Workshop on Periodontitis and Systemic Diseases. *Journal of Periodontology* 84: S106–S112.

Chapple, I. L. C., Mealey, B. L., Van Dyke, T. E. et al. 2018. Periodontal health and gingival diseases and conditions on an intact and a reduced periodontium: Consensus report of workgroup 1 of the 2017 World Workshop on the Classification of Periodontal and Peri-Implant Diseases and Conditions. *Journal of Periodontology* 89: S74–S84.

Colston, B. W., Everett, M. J., Da Silva, L. B., Otis, L. L. 1998c. OCT for diagnosis of periodontal disease. *Proceedings of SPIE* 3251: 52–58.

Colston, B. W., Everett, M. J., Da Silva, L. B., Otis, L. L., Stroeve, P., Nathel, H. 1998a. Imaging of hard- and soft-tissue structure in the oral cavity by optical coherence tomography. *Applied Optics* 37: 3582.

Colston, B. W., Sathyam, U., Dasilva, L., Everett, M., Stroeve, P., Otis, L. 1998b. Dental OCT. *Optics Express* 3: 230–238.

Deepthi, B. C., Shetty, S., Babu, C., Rohit, P., Mallikarjuna, D. M., Raj, R. B. 2012. Correlation between gingival phenotype, residual ridge height and the Scheneiderian Membrane. *International Journal of Oral Impantology and Clinical Research* 3:111–115.

Dhadse, P., Gattani, D., Mishra, R. 2010. The link between periodontal disease and cardiovascular disease: how far we have come in last two decades? *Journal of Indian Society of Periodontology* 14: 148–154.

Esfahrood, Z. R., Kadkhodazadeh, M., Talebi Ardakani, M. R. 2013. Gingival biotype: a review. *General Dentistry* 61:14–17.

Feldchtein, F., Gelikonov, V., Iksanov, R. et al. 1998. In vivo OCT imaging of hard and soft tissue of the oral cavity. *Optics Express* 3: 239–250.

Fernandes, L. O., Mota, C. C. B. de O., Oliveira, H. O., Neves, J. K., Santiago, L. M., Gomes, A. S. L. 2019. Optical coherence tomography follow-up of patients treated from periodontal disease. *Journal of Biophotonics* 12: e201800209.

Fernandes, L. O., Mota, C. C. B. O., de Melo, L. S. A., da Costa Soares, M. U. S., da Silva Feitosa, D., Gomes, A. S. L. 2017. In vivo assessment of periodontal structures and measurement of gingival sulcus with optical coherence tomography: a pilot study. *Journal of Biophotonics* 10: 862–869.

Gargiulo, A. W., Wentz, F. M., Orban, B. 1961. Dimensions and relations of the dentogingival junction in humans. *Journal of Periodontology* 32: 261–267.

Gladkova, N., Karabut, M., Kiseleva, E., Robakidze, N., Muraev, A., Fomina, Y. 2011. Cross polarization optical coherence tomography for diagnosis of oral soft tissues. *Proceedings of SPIE* 7884: 78840V-1.

Han, S.-H., Sadr, A., Tagami, J., Park, S.-H. 2016. Non-destructive evaluation of an internal adaptation of resin composite restoration with swept-source optical coherence tomography and micro-CT. *Dental Materials* 32: e1–7.

Heitz-Mayfield, L. J. A., Salvi, G. E. 2018. Peri-implant mucositis. *Journal of Periodontology* 89: S257–S266.

Hsiao, T.-Y., Ho, Y.-C., Chen, M.-R., Lee, S.-Y., Sun, C.-W. 2021. Disease activation maps for subgingival dental calculus identification based on intelligent dental optical coherence tomography. *Translational Biophotonics* 3: e202100001.

Hsieh, Y.-S., Ho, Y.-C., Lee, S.-Y., Lu, C.-W., Jiang, C.-P., Chuang, C.-C., … Sun, C.-W. (2011). Subgingival calculus imaging based on swept-source optical coherence tomography. *Journal of Biomedical Optics* 16: 071409.

Huang, D., Swanson, E. A., Lin, C. P. et al. 1991. Optical coherence tomography. *Science* 254: 1178–1181.

Huang, Y., Zhang, K., Yi, W., Kang, J. U. 2012. In-vivo gingival sulcus imaging using full-range, complex-conjugate-free, endoscopic spectral domain optical coherence tomography. *Proceedings of the SPIE* 8208: 820804-1.

Huminicki, A., Dong, C., Cleghorn, B., Sowa, M., Hewko, M., Choo-Smith, L.-P. 2010. Determining the effect of calculus, hypocalcification, and stain on using optical coherence tomography and polarized Raman spectroscopy for detecting white spot lesions. *International Journal of Dentistry* 2010: 879252.

Ianoşi, S. L., Forsea, A. M., Lupu, M. et al. 2019. Role of modern imaging techniques for the in vivo diagnosis of lichen planus. *Experimental and Therapeutic Medicine* 17: 1052–1060.

Jeffcoat, M. K., Wang, I. C., Reddy, M. S. 1995. Radiographic diagnosis in periodontics. *Periodontology 2000* 7: 54–68.

Kakizaki, S., Aoki, A., Tsubokawa, M. et al. 2018. Observation and determination of periodontal tissue profile using optical coherence tomography. *Journal of Periodontal Research* 53: 188–199.

Kao, M.-C., Lin, C.-L., Kung, C.-Y., Huang, Y.-F., Kuo, W.-C. 2015. Miniature endoscopic optical coherence tomography for calculus detection. *Applied Optics* 54: 7419–7423.

Kim, J.-M., Kang, S.-R., Yi, W.-J. 2017. Automatic detection of tooth cracks in optical coherence tomography images. *Journal of Periodontal & Implant Science*, 47: 41–50.

Kim, S., Crose, M., Eldridge, W. J., Cox, B., Brown, W. J., Wax, A. 2018. Design and implementation of a low-cost, portable OCT system. *Biomedical Optics Express* 9: 1232.

Kim, S.-H., Kang, S.-R., Park, H.-J., Kim, J.-M., Yi, W.-J., Kim, T.-I. 2017. Improved accuracy in periodontal pocket depth measurement using optical coherence tomography. *Journal of Periodontal & Implant Science* 47: 13–19.

Krause, F., Braun, A., Jepsen, S., Frentzen, M. 2005. Detection of subgingival calculus with a novel LED-based optical probe. *Journal of Periodontology* 76: 1202–1206.

Krause, F., Schmalz, G., Park, K. J. et al. 2019. Evaluation of calculus imaging on root surfaces by spectral-domain optical coherence tomography. *Photodiagnosis and Photodynamic Therapy* 25: 275–279.

Lai, Y.-C., Chiu, C.-H., Cai, Z.-Q. et al. 2019. OCT-based periodontal inspection framework. *Sensors* 19: 5496.

Lang, N. P., Bartold, P. M. 2018. Periodontal health. *Journal of Periodontology* 89: S9–S16.

Le, N. M., Song, S., Zhou, H. et al. 2018. A noninvasive imaging and measurement using optical coherence tomography angiography for the assessment of gingiva: an in vivo study. *Journal of Biophotonics* 11: e201800242.

Lee, A., Fu, J.-H., Wang, H.-L. 2011. Soft tissue biotype affects implant success. *Implant Dentistry* 20: e38–e47.

Lee, J., Park, J., Faizan Shirazi, M. et al. 2019. Classification of human gingival sulcus using swept-source optical coherence tomography: in vivo imaging. *Infrared Physics & Technology* 98: 155–160.

Liu, Z.-S., Peng, J., Wang, S.-L., Jiang, T., Lin, J., Meng, K. 2018. Characterization of coronary atherosclerotic plaques in a homozygous familial hypercholesterolemia visualized by optical coherence tomography. *Journal of Geriatric Cardiology* 15: 738–743.

Maslennikova, A. V., Sirotkina, M. A., Moiseev, A. A. et al. 2017. In-vivo longitudinal imaging of microvascular changes in irradiated oral mucosa of radiotherapy cancer patients using optical coherence tomography. *Scientific Reports* 7: 16505.

Meissner, G., Oehme, B., Strackeljan, J., Kocher, T. 2008. Clinical subgingival calculus detection with a smart ultrasonic device: a pilot study: clinical subgingival calculus detection. *Journal of Clinical Periodontology* 35: 126–132.

Mota, C. C. B. O., Fernandes, L. O., Cimões, R., Gomes, A. S. L. 2015a. Non-invasive periodontal probing through Fourier-domain optical coherence tomography. *Journal of Periodontology* 86: 1087–1094.

Mota, C. C. B. O., Fernandes, L. O., Melo, L. S. A., Feitosa, D. S., Cimões, R., Gomes, A. S. L. 2015b. Comparative analysis of gingival phenotype in animal and human experimental models using optical coherence tomography in a non-invasive approach. *Proceedings of SPIE* 9531: 95313S-1.

Park, J.-Y., Chung, J.-H., Lee, J.-S., Kim, H.-J., Choi, S.-H., Jung, U.-W. 2017. Comparisons of the diagnostic accuracies of optical coherence tomography, micro-computed tomography, and histology in periodontal disease: an ex vivo study. *Journal of Periodontal & Implant Science* 47: 30–40.

Pires, N. S. M., Dantas, A. T., Duarte, A. L. B. P. et al. 2018. Optical coherence tomography as a method for quantitative skin evaluation in systemic sclerosis. *Annals of the Rheumatic Diseases* 77: 465–466

Polson, A. M., Caton, J. G., Yeaple, R. N., Zander, H. A. 1980. Histological determination of probe tip penetration into gingival sulcus of humans using an electronic pressure-sensitive probe. *Journal of Clinical Periodontology* 7: 479–488.

Preshaw, P. M. 2015. Detection and diagnosis of periodontal conditions amenable to prevention. *BMC Oral Health* 15 Suppl 1: S5.

Quitero, M. F. Z., Siriani, L. K., Azevedo. et al. 2019. Optical coherence tomography and polarized light microscopy for the evaluation of artificial caries: a preliminary study. *General Dentistry* 67: e1–e6.

Reddy, N., Nguyen, B. T. 2019. The utility of optical coherence tomography for diagnosis of basal cell carcinoma: a quantitative review. *The British Journal of Dermatology* 180: 475–483.

Renvert, S., Persson, G. R., Pirih, F. Q., Camargo, P. M. 2018. Peri-implant health, peri-implant mucositis, and peri-implantitis: case definitions and diagnostic considerations: diagnostic criteria of peri-implant health and diseases. *Journal of Periodontology* 89: S304–S312.

Schmidt-Erfurth, U., Klimscha, S., Waldstein, S. M., Bogunović, H. 2017. A view of the current and future role of optical coherence tomography in the management of age-related macular degeneration. *Eye* 31: 26–44.

Schwarz, F., Derks, J., Monje, A., Wang, H.-L. 2018. Peri-implantitis. *Journal of Periodontology* 89: S267–S290.

Shelton, R. L., Jung, W., Sayegh, S. I., McCormick, D. T., Kim, J., Boppart, S. A. 2014. Optical coherence tomography for advanced screening in the primary care office: optical coherence tomography for advanced screening in the primary care office. *Journal of Biophotonics* 7: 525–533.

Surlin, P., Didilescu, A. C., Lazar, L. et al. 2021. Evaluation through the optical coherence tomography analysis of the influence of non-alcoholic fatty liver disease on the gingival inflammation in periodontal patients. *Diabetes, Metabolic Syndrome and Obesity: Targets and Therapy* 14: 2935–2942.

Townsend, D. 2022. Identification of venular capillary remodelling: a possible link to the development of periodontitis? *Journal of Periodontal & Implant Science* 52: 65–76.

Trombelli, L., Farina, R., Silva, C. O., Tatakis, D. N. 2018. Plaque-induced gingivitis: case definition and diagnostic considerations. *Journal of Periodontology* 89: S46–S73.

Tsai, M. T., Lee, J. D., Lee, Y. J et al. 2013. Differentiation of oral precancerous stages with optical coherence tomography based on the evaluation of optical scattering properties of oral mucosae. *Laser Phys* 23: 045602.

Won, J., Huang, P.-C., Spillman, D. R. et al. 2020. Handheld optical coherence tomography for clinical assessment of dental plaque and gingiva. *Journal of Biomedical Optics* 25: 116011.

Xiang, X., Sowa, M. G., Iacopino, A. M. et al. 2010. An update on novel non-invasive approaches for periodontal diagnosis. *Journal of Periodontology* 81: 186–198.

11

OCT in Soft Oral Tissues II: Oral Cancer and Other Oral Abnormalities

Luiz Alcino Gueiros and Jair Carneiro Leão

Oral Medicine Unit, Department of Clinic and Preventive Dentistry, Universidade Federal de Pernambuco, Av. Prof. Moraes Rego, Cidade Universitária, Recife, PE, Brazil

CONTENTS

11.1 Introduction

This chapter will focus on the use of OCT in the oral oncology scenario, presenting the clinical possibilities of using this method to diagnose, monitor and treat patients with oral potentially malignant disorders (OPMDs) and oral cancer. OCT is a noninvasive diagnostic method that generates real-time cross-sectional images based on the differences in tissue optical properties. OPMDs are a group of clinically suspicious conditions, of which a small percentage will undergo malignant transformation. Their presence increases the likelihood of developing oral cancer and should lead to a closer follow-up. Nevertheless, risk assessment is somewhat limited and should be based on clinical examination together with a biopsy to evaluate the presence of epithelial dysplasia (Müller 2018). Depending on the presentation, multiple-site

DOI: 10.1201/9781351104562-11

biopsy should be performed, and not rarely, repeated regularly. Even though an oral biopsy is not a major surgical intervention, repetitive interventions on the same site may promote tissue fibrosis and limit proper clinical examination. In addition, sampling bias is also a matter of concern, especially in larger lesions (Figure 11.1), and grading dysplasia still promotes a significant discussion among pathologists.

In this context, several non-invasive techniques have been suggested to evaluate the presence of epithelial dysplasia and ultimately limit the indication of oral biopsies. Among these methods, optical coherence tomography has gained attention because of its clinically relevant advantages, such as real-time radiation-free images, (relatively) easy interpretation and micron-level resolution with adequate penetration depth. Under OCT imaging, the full epithelial thickness can be evaluated on a cellular level, so that a clear comparison with histopathological analysis can be performed.

These features also make a new frontier in the evaluation of oral cancer. Oral tumors grow deep into the conjunctive tissue, so that the full tumoral thickness may be beyond OCT penetration, but still making its recognition possible (Yang et al. 2018). Besides, the surgical margin is a crucial aspect of oncological treatment, and its analysis is complex, demanding the presence of an additional physician (pathologist) in the surgical room. OCT surgical margin analysis has the potential to promote adequate surgeries by allowing the surgeon to perform margin evaluation in a real-time manner (Zaid et al. 2016).

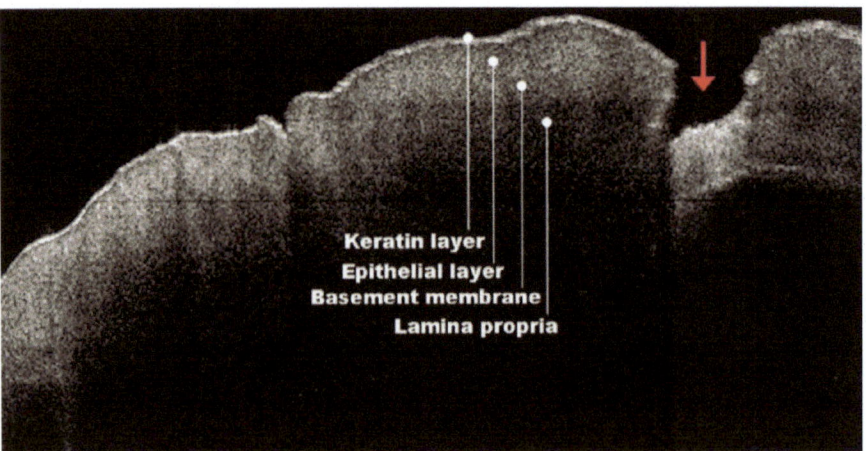

FIGURE 11.1
An OCT image of the lateral border of the tongue. There is a discontinuity in the keratin layer with epithelial layer ulceration. There is a thickening of the epithelial layer with keratosis, perhaps suggestive of epithelial dysplasia. Histologically this lesion was an area of severe epithelial dysplasia. Reprinted with permission from (Jerjes et al. 2010) © Elsevier Science & Technology Journals.

11.2 OCT in Oral Potentially Malignant Disorders

OPMDs are a heterogeneous group of conditions that share an increased likelihood of malignant transformation. Even though the malignant transformation rates present a considerable variation among these lesions, identifying high-risk lesions is still based on clinical appearance and the presence of dysplasia. Oral leukoplakia is the most common OPMD and has a 1% prevalence and reported malignant transformation rates of 2–5%, depending on the aspects mentioned above. The World Health Organization working group on oral cancer and precancer has defined that "the term leukoplakia should be used to recognize white plaques of questionable risk having excluded (other) known diseases or disorders that carry no increased risk for cancer". Clinically, they are classified as homogenous (uniformly flat, thin and exhibit shallow cracks of the surface keratin, having a low risk of malignant transformation) and non-homogenous, which show a variety of clinical presentations (speckled, nodular, and verrucous) and a significantly higher rate of malignant transformation. The size of the lesion is also a relevant aspect to be considered to evaluate the risk of malignancy.

Nevertheless, the diagnosis of leukoplakia demands a biopsy, and can only be established after excluding any other disorder. Proliferative verrucous leukoplakia (PVL) is characterized by multiple, simultaneous leukoplakias, frequently covering a wide area, and having a high risk of malignant transformation. Lastly, oral erythroplakia is characterized as "a fiery red patch that cannot be characterized clinically or pathologically as any other definable disease". These lesions have the highest risk of malignant transformation in the mouth (Müller 2018).

After long-term follow-up, multiple biopsies are often demanded since OPMDs are a dynamic process. The presence of dysplasia is a hallmark of worse prognosis but may eventually not appear at initial presentations, being observed after some time. Higher grades of epithelial dysplasia seem to indicate a higher risk of malignant transformation, but grading dysplasia is a significant matter of debate. The WHO still suggests a three-tiered grading system: mild, moderate and severe dysplasia/carcinoma *in situ*; the higher the dysplasia, the greater the epithelial involvement from the basal membrane to the upper third of the epithelium. There is also a binary system, which combines both moderate and severe dysplasia as severe cases. The main limitation of both systems is the limited inter- and intra-observer agreement, even though the binary one seems to be more precise but still demands more evidence on its use. Pathologists should evaluate both morphological and cytological alterations in order to grade dysplasia, and some of these features promote a high disagreement. Ultimately, the risk assessment of OPMLs necessarily includes an oral biopsy to exclude other lesions and determine the presence of dysplasia; evaluation may vary among pathologists. Also, early detection of malignant lesions results in less aggressive interventions and better prognosis.

In order to overcome these limitations, optical biopsies have been suggested as non-invasive methods that may have sensitivity and specificity similar conventional biopsy (Jerjes et al. 2010). Optical biopsies can be acquired through distinctive methods that provide a real-time, non-invasive, in situ optical signature. Among these methods, OCT generates microanatomical tomographic images of the epithelium, basement membrane and supporting lamina propria of the mucosa, being able to act as a diagnostic tool of OPMLs (Yang et al. 2018). When recent biopsy specimens are evaluated by OCT before 10% formalin fixation, the epithelial layers can be noted in most of the cases; epithelial thickness changes could be clearly noted, but acanthosis could not be confirmed. Also, inflammatory lesions could not be differentiated from OPMLs (Hamdoon et al. 2013).

More importantly, there seems to be an agreement among clinicians evaluating OCT images regarding the indication of biopsy – normal cases can be easily identified (Ahn et al. 2011). Besides, since disruption of the basement membrane is a defining hallmark of squamous cell carcinoma (SCC), its recognition should be sound and clear. It has been suggested that a pathologist evaluates OCT images in order to define the presence of SCC. These findings indicate that architectural changes, and not cytological atypia, are well characterized under OCT. Interestingly, *in vivo* OCT images may represent a better disease picture since there is no distortion caused by fixation.

Moreover, Doppler OCT images are able to evaluate lesional microvascular changes. When considering this information together with morphological alterations, differentiating benign from early malignant lesions becomes more accurate (Ahn et al. 2011). Although OCT has demonstrated its potential to improve the evaluation of PPOELs, additional studies are demanded to define the physical form factor and performance characteristics for clinical purposes. Also, studies with larger sample sizes and prospective evaluation are required to establish its diagnostic accuracy.

11.3 OCT in Oral Cancer Diagnosis

Oral diseases represent a significant global public health problem, having both high prevalence and major negative impacts on individuals, communities and society. Dental caries, periodontal disease and oral cancer represent the major global oral problems, and among them, the neoplastic disease has a more severe impact on the quality of life, as well as on survival. Despite significant advances in treatment modalities, the 5-year survival rate in oral and oropharyngeal squamous cell carcinoma (OSCC) is less than 60%.

Patients are still diagnosed when the disease presents an advanced staging, thus having a severe impact on prognosis and limiting survival. Even though the mouth is easily accessible to clinical examination, little has changed in the past decades. Cancer Survivorship Statistics from the US in 2019 shows that the disease is usually diagnosed in individuals older than 65 years, but people with less than 50 years tend to live longer after diagnosis (Miller et al. 2019). In this scenario, the critical point to increase patient survival is to diagnose initial cases on a regular basis.

The gold standard for diagnosing oral cancer is clinical examination followed by incisional biopsy. The oral exam is highly accurate under a trained eye (usually a specialist), but a general dentist or physician still under recognize this tumor on routine practice, especially initial lesions. On the other hand, the biopsy is an invasive procedure usually associated with patient anxiety. Sampling is a cornerstone of biopsy. Collecting a representative sample tissue at the correct site is not always a straightforward decision. And it usually takes two–three visits until the report is available. So even though a biopsy is a simple minor intervention, some inconveniences can be noted.

An ideal diagnostic method should be non-invasive and provide a cost-effective, point of care, real-time diagnosis. OCT has demonstrated its relevance to diagnosing OPMLs and its progression to oral cancer (Sunny et al. 2019). Animal carcinogenesis models have demonstrated its utility in observing disease progression, with similar results to conventional histopathological analysis (Chen et al. 2018). The technique can be used for both *in vivo* and *ex vivo* analysis, helping to perform a better selection of the biopsy site, increasing the diagnostic accuracy, as well as allowing surgical margin analysis (next topic). Since OSCC represents 90–95% of the malignant tumors of the mouth, it is of great importance to assess this tumor accurately.

A well-conducted systematic review has shown that OCT presents some correspondence with microscopy when analyzing cutaneous malignant melanomas, but an elevated sensitivity and specificity was observed when assessing basal cell carcinomas, especially when combined with the dermoscopic assessment (Ferrante di Rufano et al. 2018). Regarding OSCC evaluation, a high diagnostic accuracy was demonstrated, with a very good inter-observer agreement. On the other hand, the methods still lack adequate standardization in order to be used in routine clinical practice. There is a clear need for developing better probes to the oral cavity, and even developing better post-processing algorithms.

OCT images of initial tumors show ablation of normal microanatomy in addition to a disruption of the basal membrane (BM, Figure 11.1). The invasion of tumoral cell beyond BM characterizes an invasive tumor rather than severe dysplasia, leading to a more aggressive surgical approach. Nevertheless, differentiating it from a reactive process may not be secure under OCT, and a pathologist interpretation may be necessary. This may limit real-time diagnosis if the pathologist is not immediately available. Also, grading dysplasia achieves low agreement rates among pathologists even under an optical microscope, and it seems worthless trying to perform it under OCT. Furthermore, analysis of lesion borders can reveal the transition zone between tumoral and non-tumoral tissue. On the other hand, OCT evaluation of the 4NOQ oral carcinogenesis animal model has shown its usefulness to evaluate the pattern of microvascular change into the epithelium and its changes towards malignant transformation, especially when combined with Doppler images. This well-established cancer progression model supports OCT in evidencing initial and established lesions.

Penetration depth and lateral resolution are fundamental aspects of OCT imaging, and its clinical use may rely on them. Low-resolution images are challenging to analyze, but high-resolution images can make interpretation much more straightforward. Considering the available devices for ophthalmology, generating excellent images for clinical use is a matter of cost, not technology. Identifying altered tissue structures may be essential to differentiate normal mucosa from tumoral lesions, but subtle microscopic aspects may not be observed without excellent optical patterns.

Even though OSSC present a clear microscopic pattern, significant morphological variations may be found and eventually impair a clear OCT-microscopy correlation. Invasion pattern may significantly vary among tumors, as well as nuclear pleomorphism (Figures 11.2 and 11.3). Apart from the potential impact on prognosis, these features may turn OCT analysis even more difficult. There is a need to define the regular pattern of OSCC as well as its morphologic variations under OCT, to turn the non-invasive analysis more accurate and clearer to the clinician. To be used in routine clinical practice, OCT has to be accessible to both the clinician/surgeon and the pathologist, allowing complementary information (Davies et al. 2015).

Lastly, the clinical and trans surgical assessment of vertical and horizontal tumor extensions is somewhat limited. Incomplete tumor removal has a significant impact on prognosis, being associated with local and regional recurrence. The limited penetration of OCT limits its use in evaluating tumor depth, but the lateral extension can be clearly accessed. Nevertheless, intraoperative margin analysis by OCT has been suggested as a safe and helpful method (van Mane et al. 2018), as discussed in the next topic.

11.4 OCT in Other Head and Neck Tumors

Despite excellent diagnostic performance, OCT has overall not been adopted as a clinical tool for OPSCC diagnosis for several reasons: (1) additional training is needed to interpret the images; (2) the device is large, heavy

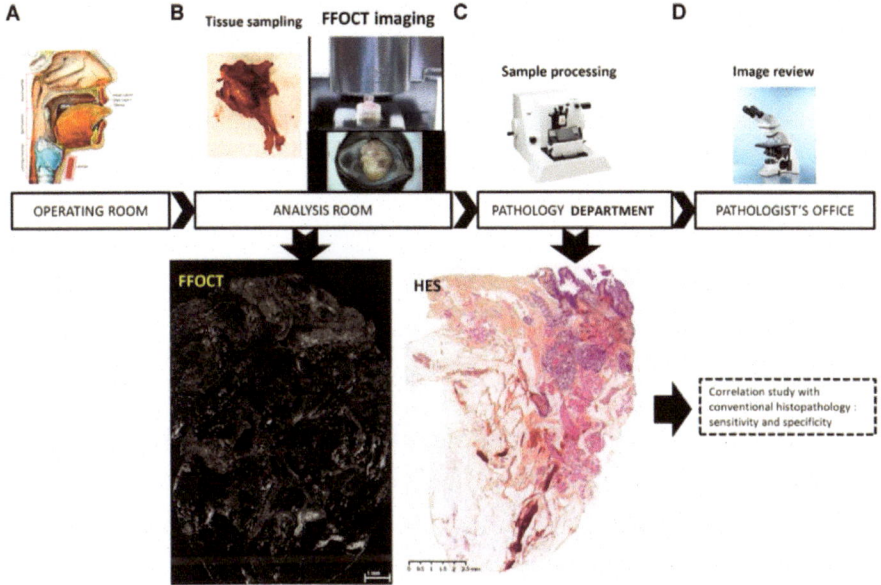

FIGURE 11.2

Synopsis of the correlation study: from sample collection to image interpretation. A total of 57 samples from 32 patients (A) were first selected by the pathologist and imaged using the full-field optical coherence tomography (FFOCT) system (B). Samples were processed afterward for further conventional histology (C). FFOCT images and histological images were blindly and randomly interpreted by two pathologists (D). Reprinted with permission from (De Leeuw et al. 2020) © John Wiley & Sons – Books.

and fragile; (3) the operating software and user interfaces are daunting; and (4) the system has an elevated cost (Heidari et al. 2020). Nevertheless, innovative approaches have been proposed by combining an OCT with some existing device. Englhard et al. (Englhard et al. 2017) have suggested the association of OCT integrated with a surgical microscope, enhancing transoperatory diagnosis and allowing detection of dysplasia and malignancies with increased accuracy (Figure 11.1). Margin analysis is also improved, and the system proved overall helpful for the intraoperative differentiation of benign and malignant tumors, but not capable of substituting the biopsies. Other combined devices, such as combined reflectance confocal microscopy (RCM)–optical coherence tomography (OCT), have been described as an excellent adjunct in the evaluation of complex head-and-neck basal cell carcinomas and guide the treatment selection and defining the extent of surgery.

Intra-opperative margin analyses of head and neck tumors are performed in frozen sections by following a multistep process. In this scenario, full-field OCT (FFOCT) is able to provide real-time images of *ex vivo* fresh samples

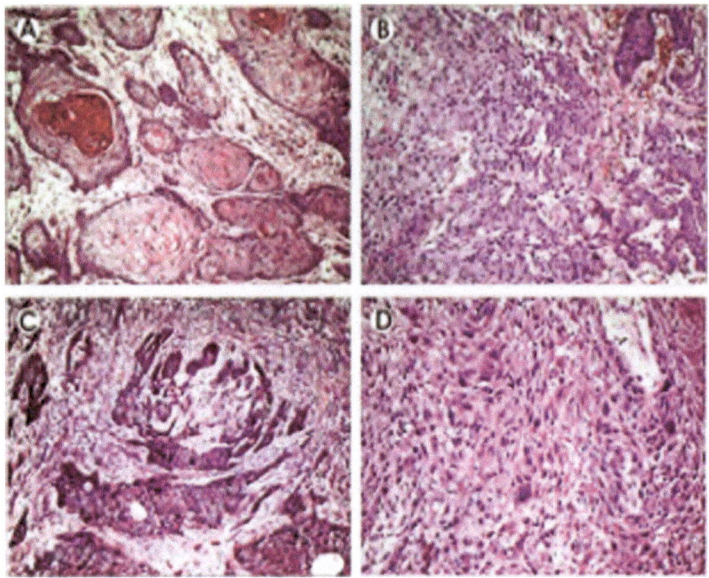

FIGURE 11.3

Differences in pleomorphic pattern in oral squamous cell carcinoma (OSCC). (A) Well-differentiated cells, resembling non-neoplastic epithelial cells. (B) Moderate nuclear pleomorphism, with less than 75% of the cells being well-differentiated. (C) Severe pleomorphism, with 25–50% of the cells being well-differentiated. (D) Extreme pleomorphism, with less than 25% of the cells being well-differentiated.

without any tissue processing (Figure 11.4). These promising results open new perspectives for studies with *in vivo* imaging of head and neck surgical margins with FFOCT associated with endoscopes, which may ultimately lead to reduced surgical time with similar oncologic outcomes (De Leeuw et al. 2020).

Thyroid cancer is the most common malignant tumor of the endocrine system. Thyroid nodules are often evaluated by fine needle aspitation cytology (FNAC), which has 15–20% of the cases termed as suspicious or inderteminate. These cases lead to thyredectomy, and only a minor portion of them are diagnosed as a malignant tumor. Real-time PCT images of the surgical site has also been demonstrated as a relevant adjuvanct to reduce surgical time. Future advances are expected to reduce the number of unnecessary total thyroidectomies because of suspicious diagnoses (Erickson-Bhatt et al. 2018). Currently, *ex vivo* analysis of fresh thyroid tissues was able to determine the presence of microscopic extrathyroidal extension, with possible impact in deterring the surgical extension if performed before thyroidectomy (Lee et al. 2016).

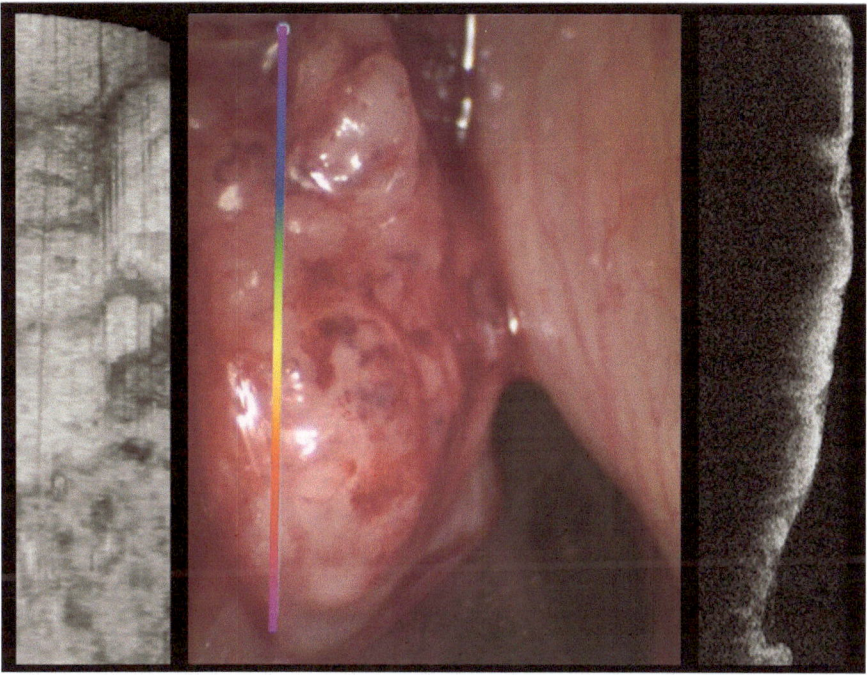

FIGURE 11.4
Examination of a patient with carcinoma of the left vocal cord. (Center) microscopic image of the larynx. (Left) OCT 3-D image of the surface of the left vocal cord. (Right) OCT image of the lesion: no basement membrane is visible. There is some hyperkeratosis. The histological examination revealed a G2 squamous cell carcinoma. Reprinted with permission from (Englhard et al. 2017) © John Wiley & Sons – Books.

11.5 OCT in Oral Cancer Margin Analysis

Incomplete tumor removal has been associated with poor prognosis and adverse outcomes as local recurrence and mortality. A clear margin is usually defined as a distance ≥ 5 mm free of tumor, but this does not consider the formalin-shrinkage effect, which reduces the specimen by 30%, representing an 8–10 mm *in situ* margin. Routinely, intraoperative inspection and palpation are used to evaluate margins, sometimes combined with margin frozen sections. This leads to a significant delay in surgical time to allow sample preparation and analysis and evaluates random areas of the surgical site. There is also a disagreement between frozen section and routine histopathological diagnosis. So even with frozen section evaluation, 5–17% of surgical resections can have positive surgical margins. So an intra-operative, point-of-procedure diagnostic tool for the assessment of tumor margin is a clinical demand, which may possibly reduce the rate of involved surgical margins and eventually improve disease outcome.

Optical margin analysis allows a fast and real-time evaluation of the whole surgical site, being an optimal alternative to routine standards of assessment. Initial studies with OCT have generated low-resolution images, but interesting results were observed even in these conditions. Using a swept-source 1310 nm OCT system with an axial and lateral optical resolution of <10 µm to evaluate *ex vivo* surgical samples showed promising results. Elevated sensitivity, specificity, and accuracy could be demonstrated, with a "very good" interobserver agreement (Davies et al. 2015). There seems to be an increased thickness of tumor-involved epithelial margins, and this finding help to overcome the limited depth of penetration of OCT. Also, evaluating *ex vivo* samples allow the direct examination of all specimen margin, but *in vivo* margin assessment may be limited in locations such as the base of the tongue and oropharynx.

Notwithstanding, *in vivo* OCT use in oral cancer have demonstrated a perfect sensitivity and specificity detection of malignant fields, with an excellent agreement with histopathology in the evaluation of tumor and dysplasia. Nevertheless, the initial studies did not evaluate the lateral or deep margins but the surgical right before surgery instead. Even in such conditions, the normal-appearing epithelium can present malignant cells that can be detected by OCT, and its almost perfect concordance with histopathology should lead to broader use of this method. OCT mapping of the surgical site should change the routine 1 cm visual tumor-free surgical margin and possibly increase surgical results. However, its 2 mm depth evaluation impairs its application to tumor sites extending beyond this limit (van Mane et al. 2018).

A multipurpose OCT system has been used to evaluate the mouth and oropharynx during surgical endoscopy, so it can also be adapted to evaluate the *on-site* surgical margins. Also, OCT can be used to perform an accurate demarcation of these margins, especially when combined with an algorithm-based prediction. The malignant tumor under clinically normal mucosa would be included in the surgical specimen, improving patient outcomes. Nevertheless, there is still a place for advancing the probes and improve its feasibility, so that the full mouth can be clearly evaluated. Moreover, there is no data comparing OCT with intraoperative frozen biopsy, which represents the current way of accessing tumor margins.

11.6 Conclusions

OCT has been demonstrated as a promising non-invasive method for monitoring and even diagnosis PMOL, oral cancer and its surgical margins.

Mapping biopsy site, follow up of PMOL, and defining surgical margins can be significantly improved under OCT analysis. However, the image analysis should be performed by a trained professional, and some innovations on image algorithm analysis should improve its feasibility, as already done in ophthalmology. To be used in clinical practice, OCT probes need to easily access every site of the mouth, and some advances should be made in this sense.

References

Ahn, Y. C., Chung, J., Wilder-Smith, P., Chenb, Z. Multimodality approach to optical early detection and mapping of oral neoplasia. 2011. *Journal of Biomedical Optics* 16: 076007.

Chen, P. H., Wu, C. H., Chen, Y. F. et al. 2018. Combination of structural and vascular optical coherence tomography for differentiating oral lesions of mice in different carcinogenesis stages. *Biomedical Optics Express* 9: 1461–1476.

Davies, K., Connolly, J. M., Dockery, P., Wheatley, A.M., Olivo, M., Keogh, I. 2015. Point of care optical diagnostic technologies for the detection of oral and oro-pharyngeal squamous cell carcinoma (SCC). *Surgeon* 6: 321–329.

De Leeuw, F., Abbaci, M., Casiraghi, O. et al. 2020. Value of full-field optical coherence tomography imaging for the histological assessment of head and neck cancer. *Lasers in Surgery and Medicine* 52: 768–778.

Englhard, A. S., Betz, T., Volgger, V. et al. 2017. Intraoperative assessment of laryngeal pathologies with optical coherence tomography integrated into a surgical microscope. *Lasers in Surgery and Medicine* 49: 490–497.

Erickson-Bhatt, S. J., Mesa, K. J., Marjanovic, M. et al. 2018. Intraoperative optical coherence tomography of the human thyroid: feasibility for surgical assessment. *Translational Research* 195: 13–24.

Ferrante di Ruffano, L., Dinnes, J., Deeks, J. J. et al. 2018. Optical coherence tomography for diagnosing skin cancer in adults. *Cochrane Database of Systematic Reviews* 12: CD013189.

Hamdoon, Z., Jerjes, W., Upile, T. et al. 2013. Optical coherence tomography in the assessment of suspicious oral lesions: an immediate ex-vivo study. *Photodiagnosis and Photodynamic Therapy* 10:17e27.

Heidari, A. E., Pham, T. T., Ifegwu, I. et al. 2020. The use of optical coherence tomography and convolutional neural networks to distinguish normal and abnormal oral mucosa. *Journal of Biophotonics* 13: e201900221.

Jerjes, W., Upile, T., Conne, B. et al. 2010. In vitro examination of suspicious oral lesions using optical coherence tomography. *British Journal of Oral and Maxillofacial Surgery* 48: 18–25.

Lee, H. S., Shin, S. W., Bae, J. K. et al. 2016. Preliminary study of optical coherence tomography imaging to identify microscopic extrathyroidal extension in patients with papillary thyroid carcinoma: OCT for extrathyroidal extension. *Lasers in Surgery and Medicine* 48: 371–376.

Miller, K. D., Nogueira L., Mariotto, A.B. et al. 2019. Cancer treatment and survivor-
    ship statistics. *CA: A Cancer Journal for Clinicians* 69: 363–385.
Müller, S. 2018. Oral epithelial dysplasia, atypical verrucous lesions and oral poten-
    tially malignant disorders: focus on histopathology. *Oral Surgery, Oral Medicine,
    Oral Pathology and Oral Radiology* 125: 591–602.
Sunny, S. P., Agarwala, S., Jamesb, B. L. et al. 2019. Intra-operative point-of-procedure
    delineation of oral cancer margins using optical coherence tomography. *Oral
    Oncology* 92: 12–19.
van Mane, L., Dijkstra, J., Boccara, C. et al. 2018. The clinical usefulness of optical
    coherence tomography during cancer interventions. *Journal of Cancer Research
    and Clinical Oncology* 144: 1967–1990.
Yang, E. C., Tan, M. T., Schwarz, R. A., Richards-Kortum, R. R., Gillenwater, A.M.,
    Vigneswaran, N. 2018. Noninvasive diagnostic adjuncts for the evaluation of
    potentially premalignant oral epithelial lesions: current limitations and future
    directions. *Oral Surg Oral Med Oral Pathol Oral Radiol.* 125: 670–681.
Zaid, H., Waseem, J., Gordon, M., Amrita, J., Colin, H. 2016. Optical coherence tom-
    ography in the assessment of oral squamous cell carcinoma resection margins.
    Photodiagnosis and Photodynamic Therapy 13: 211–217.

12

OCT in Nanodentistry

Mariana Torres[1] and Anderson S. L. Gomes[2]

[1]*Carvalho – INL – International Iberian Nanotechnology Laboratory, Braga, Portugal*

[2]*Physics Department and Graduate Program in Dentistry, Universidade Federal de Pernambuco, Recife, PE, Brazil*

CONTENTS

12.1 Introduction

Nanotechnology is a fascinating field of science where all the disciplines of natural sciences converge at the nanoscale, such as physics combined with life sciences, engineering, chemistry, materials science and computational approaches (Melo et al. 2013; Padovani et al. 2015; Foong et al. 2020), working with materials with at least one dimension less than 100 nm (particles with size above 100 nm are classified as sub-micron). This area developed in such a way that it is already being used in several knowledge fields, with social and economic applications, including health benefits (Salamanca-Buentello et al. 2021), therefore, making a big impact.

Dentistry is a medical field, which is also constantly evolving. Multidisciplinary approaches have led to the advancement of oral medicine in prevention, diagnostics and therapeutics. Nanotechnology has also influenced this area in many different ways (Rathee et al. 2014; Sasalawad et al. 2014; Bhardwaj et al. 2014; Aeran et al. 2015; Ellis 2017; Sinha et al. 2017).

DOI: 10.1201/9781351104562-12

From dental materials (Yadav et al. 2013; Miraz et al. 2015; Khurshid et al. 2015), e.g., nanoscale hydroxyapatite, restorative dentistry and orthodontic adhesives (Yamagata et al. 2012), to silver nanoparticles due to their anti-bactericidal properties (Corrêa et al. 2015; Noronha et al. 2017; Teixeira et al. 2018; Yin et al. 2020), all of them have been receiving increasingly attention. For example, man-made biomaterials synthesized at the nanoscale, for instance hydroxyapatite (HAp) and fluor-hydroxyapatite (FHAp or FAp), have been studied in several occasions (Wan et al. 2007; Grigorjeva et al. 2015) and is already widely used commercially.

Many studies have emphasized the developments of nanomaterials in dentistry regarding their therapeutic applications, including chemistry, synthesis, properties and therapeutic benefits over conventional materials (Hannig et al. 2010; Sinha et al. 2017; Desai et al. 2020). Nanomaterials can be prepared, synthesized or grown in many different ways and their final format can determine the best application for it. From the point of view of imaging techniques, nanomaterials, particularly nanoparticles of different materials and shapes, have already played an important role in dentistry. Within the scope of this chapter, we will treat how nanomaterials have been exploited with optical coherence tomography (OCT) and how OCT can perform imaging with 10's to 100's nm resolution.

In section 2, we will give a broad insight into nanodentistry in general. In section 3 we will describe and review recent work with OCT applied to nanomaterials in dentistry and in section 4 we will review how OCT can be managed to provide 10's to 100's nm resolution, concluding in section 5.

12.2 Nanodentistry

Many areas of science, throughout history, have taken advantage of tools and techniques that allowed the design of material properties at a finer scale. The interest in nanomaterial research for regenerative medicine is growing and spreading for different fields (Khang et al. 2010). Many areas of science have taken advantage of tools and techniques that allowed the design of material properties at a finer scale. The interest in nanomaterial research for regenerative medicine is growing and spreading for different fields.

Nanotechnology is the exploitation of matter at molecular and atomic levels, which has revolutionized the field of dentistry. Nanodentistry is based on four approaches (as depicted in Figure 12.1) and can be defined as a promising discipline that provides nanotechnology based on next generation devices and tools for use in oral healthcare. This has shown a great potential for clinical translation (Hannig et al. 2010; Ellis 2017; Sinha et al. 2017; Seth

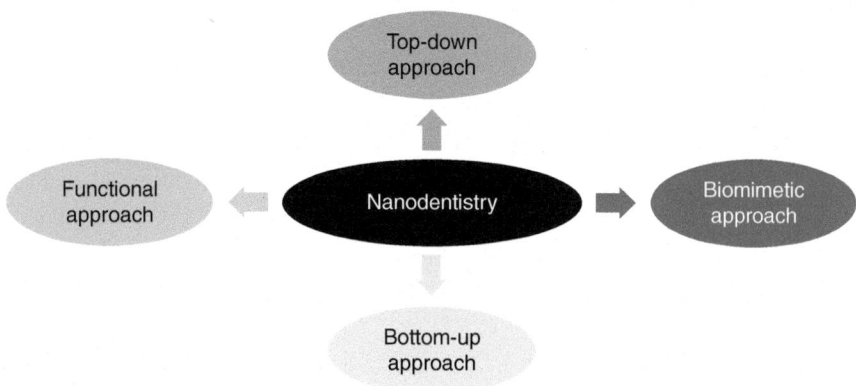

FIGURE 12.1
Different methodologies of nanodentistry.

et al. 2017; Foong et al. 2020; Desai et al. 2020; Adeola et al. 2020; Raura et al. 2020; Brun et al. 2020). In this section we will focus on the nanobiomaterials for dental applications and its different usages.

Regarding the different approaches or methods of nanodentistry, they deal not only with the fabrication methodology, but also with the final application of the nanomaterial. The top-down method synthesizes particles in the conventional manner, making them smaller using mechanical, chemical or other forms of energy, starting from bulk materials and then break them into smaller pieces. The biomimetic method focuses on preserving the structure and function of the natural teeth (or biological tissue), focusing mainly in preserving a healthy structure, applying materials that closely duplicates the natural structure. Bottom-up method synthesize the material from atomic or molecular species via chemical reactions, allowing for the precursor particles to grow in size. On the other hand, the functional method does not give importance to the method of production of a nanomaterial, it emphasizes on its specific use. The so-called dental nanobiomaterials are fabricated by well-developed nanofabrication processes (Sinha et al. 2017), and from the economic point-of-view, the bottom-up approach is cheaper than the top-down, also producing much less waste or sub-products.

As a result of the growth and development of the nanofabrication processes, nowadays it is possible to have access to organic or inorganic nanostructures. Currently it is possible to obtain dielectric, semiconductive or metallic nanoparticles of different structures and shapes (Figure 12.2). One can produce nanoparticles, nanoshells, nanorods, even intricate structures of nanodimensions, etc. These make the physical properties of these nanomaterials' morphology-dependent. Therefore, nanomaterials with such excellent properties have been extensively investigated in a wide range of biomedical applications, in particular for all the areas of oral medicine, as dentistry.

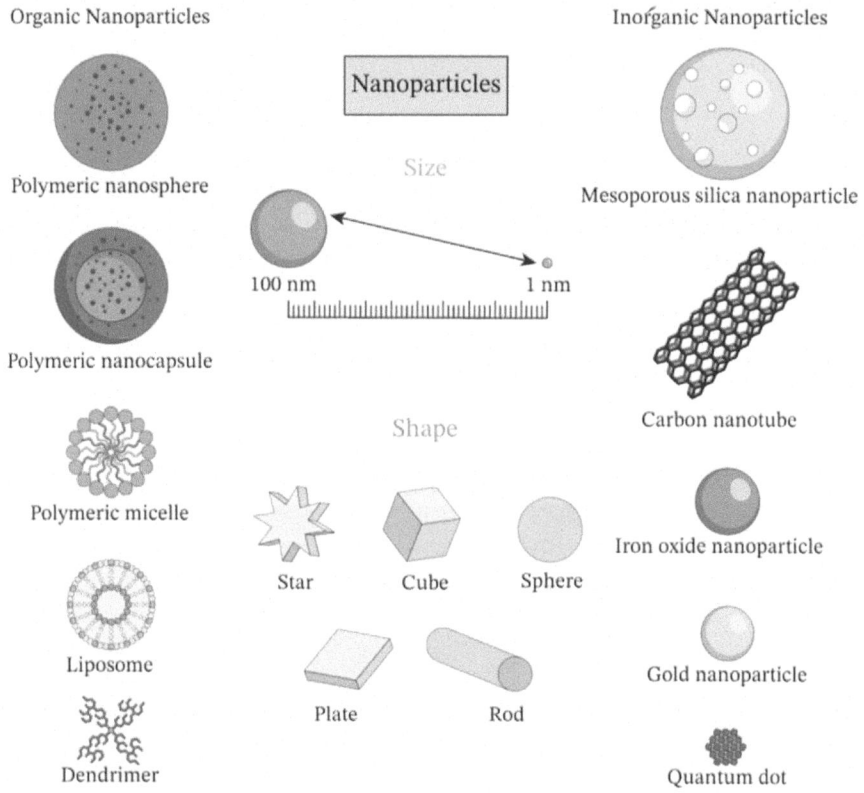

FIGURE 12.2
Different types and shapes of nanoparticles. Reprinted with permission from Lesson Explainer: Nanoparticles © Nagwa Limited.

It is not too early to consider, evaluate or attempt to shape the potential outcomes of nanodentistry. It will certainly lead to highly efficient and effective personalized dental treatments. Nanotechnology seems to be where the world is directed if technology remains advancing. This will open a huge range of possibilities and advantages for both dentists and patients (Mirsasaani et al. 2019).

12.3 OCT Applied to Nanodentistry

OCT is one of the most prominent biomedical techniques for diagnosing pathologies due to some of their unique advantages (Drexler and Fujimoto 2015; Fujimoto et al. 2016): non-invasive, the amplitude of penetration depth and spatial resolution, real-time assessment. Nowadays, artificial intelligence methods (Aggarwal et al. 2021) has even increased its application branches. This section focuses on OCT applied to nanodentistry. The literature about OCT and its nuances, methodologies and detection differences is vast and keeps growing rapidly. In this book, you can find more about the technique in Chapter 2 and references therein, with very accurate sources of information.

The applications of OCT in dentistry have also been reviewed on a number of occasions, from applications in the areas of tooth decay (caries, attrition and abrasion), periodontal diseases, oral cancer and other dental-related diseases (Hsieh et al. 2013). For tissue imaging, OCT has been applied from the evaluation of dental restorations on enamel (de Melo et al. 2005) to gingival recovery and adhesive interface in aesthetic oral rehabilitation involving periodontal plastic surgery and ceramic laminate veneers (Graça et al. 2019). It can also be employed to assess the changes made by nanostructures in dental tissue or dental materials.

Dental OCT provides the benefits of low cost, non-invasive, non-radiative and high resolution. With conventional OCT, clinicians can obtain structural images besides blood flow and structure orientation using functional-OCT methods. OCT can not only diagnose periodontal disease and precancerous lesions (see Chapters 10 and 11), as well as aid in the early diagnosis of caries (see Chapter 3), since it can distinguish mineral changes at early demineralization stages. Subgingival calculus can also be detected, allowing minimum invasive therapy to be performed. Nonetheless, through early detection of oral cancer, OCT benefits treatment outcomes and survival rates of the patients. This imaging technique has proven to provide countless benefits.

OCT in nanodentistry can also be seen from two perspectives: to study nanostructured material changes in oral medicine; or having the OCT operating in such way to visualize nanostructures. This section will focus on the first perspective, OCT operating to improve the sensitivity or detect structures in the nanometer regime. Meanwhile, observing and evaluating nanomodification in the dental tissue or materials used in dentistry will be discussed in the next section.

Commercially available OCT system can be easily employed to assess nanostructures within samples. As an example, a pioneer application reported gold nanoparticles (AuNP) formed *in situ* and used immediately as a contrast agent for dental OCT (Braz et al. 2012). To achieve that, gold ions were dispersed in the primer of a commercially available dental bonding system and the modified adhesive applied in the dentin. An innovative *in situ* photothermal reduction procedure and a photopolymerized dental bonding material were applied simultaneously, inducing the production of spherical AuNP inside the dentinal layers and tubules. The diameter of the AuNP was determined to be in the range of 40 to 120 nm, while it is known that the dentin tubule's diameters ranged from 500–4000 nm. Due to the presence of AuNP highly scattering regions were observed in the OCT images. As a result, the tubules become detectable and more visible by the presence of the AuNP, which act as contrast agents to enhance the OCT image, results are shown in Figure 12.3. The gold NPs formed in the dentinal tubules was verified by conventional image techniques such as SEM or TEM (Figure 12.3 – Top), and the cross-sectional OCT image of the dental bonding structure showed the presence of AuNP within the imaged volume (Figure 12.3 – Bottom). The OCT images show highly scattering portions and high levels of direct light backscatter, due to the presence of the AuNP, without them the OCT image is not resolved, nor can reach such depth (Braz et al. 2012).

Another example of OCT in nanodentistry exploits RED NP, a novel core-shell nanoparticle design developed and exploited for different optical imaging techniques as contrast agent for dental adhesion evaluation (Braz et al. 2018). These particles can be used for both OCT and photoluminescence for dental adhesive evaluation. The synthesized nanomaterial was based on a rare-earth-doped nanoparticle as the core and a highly refractive TiO_2

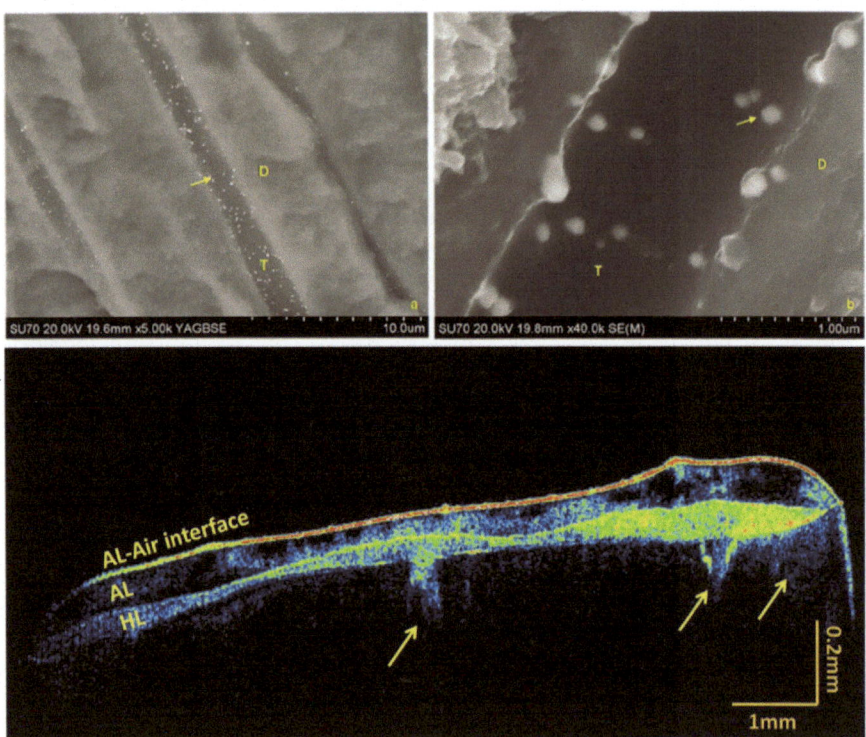

FIGURE 12.3
(Top) SEM images of dentinal tubules, showing the gold NP and (Bottom) OCT image of the dentinal tubules, only possible due to the presence of gold NPs. Reprinted with permission from Braz et al. (2012).

nanolayer as the shell. Figure 12.4 summarizes the procedure, where the role of these NPs is emphasized, showing also pictorial and TEM pictures of the nanostructure. This reference shows that the TiO_2 shell nanolayer provided enhanced contrast for OCT, whereas the RED core up-converts excitation light from 975 nm to an emission peaked at 800 nm for photoluminescence imaging. These core-shell nanoparticles when dispersed in the primer of a commercially available dental bonding system, allow the identification of the dental adhesive layers with OCT.

Figure 12.4 C shows the OCT images in gray and yellowish scale, indicating high concentration of nanoparticles inside the dentinal tubules. The presence of the RED NP was estimated to induce an enhancement of 67% in the scattering coefficient, which significantly increased the OCT contrast. Also, Figure 12.4 D shows how the up-conversion photoluminescence in the NIR spectrum region is suitable for image of deep dental tissue, highlighting carious regions in the tooth enamel. The potential of this specialty NP added to dental materials show promising *in vivo* diagnostics with the use of different imaging techniques.

Silver nanoparticles are well-known as biocompatible and already employed in nanodentistry, mostly as anti-bactericidal agents (Corrêa et al. 2015; Noronha et al. 2017; Carneiro et al. 2018; Teixeira et al. 2018). Nonetheless, the role of optical clearing agents in biotissue imaging is a very active subject (Tuchin et al. 1997; Costantini et al. 2019; Tuchin et al. 2022). The physical process of optical clearing consists of the immersion/permeabilization of biocompatible chemical substances in biological tissues (Tuchin et al. 1997; Corrêa et al. 2015; Noronha et al. 2017; Carneiro et al. 2018; Teixeira et al. 2018; Costantini et al. 2019; Das et al. 2022) to provide deeper penetration depth for imaging and other healthcare purposes. The clearing effect is obtained via a series of properties of these substances on the biosample, such as the compatibility of refractive indices, cell dehydration and the increase of collagen solubility arising from osmotic properties of the material. Optical clearing effect was studied in another nanodentistry application of OCT, where silver and TiO_2 nanostructures were exploited to improve caries diagnostic and imaging contrast of tooth hard tissues (Carneiro et al. 2017; Carneiro et al. 2018). Nano-silver-fluoride nanoparticles also have remineralizing potential for tooth enamel and OCT was used to prove that they showed the best effect against caries compared to conventional fluoride treatments (Silva et al. 2019).

When analyzing a tooth surface with an OCT device, the presence of caries lesions typically promotes a large increase in light scattering due to demineralization, therefore limiting the light penetration and reducing the signal before it even reaches the dentin-enamel junction (Maia et al. 2016). For that application, nanostructured optical clearing agents may provide deeper penetration and improve OCT image quality, while an agent that modifies the diffusion properties of a sample may improve the image contrast (Braz et al. 2012). More recently, silver nanoparticles (AgNP) in aqueous solution

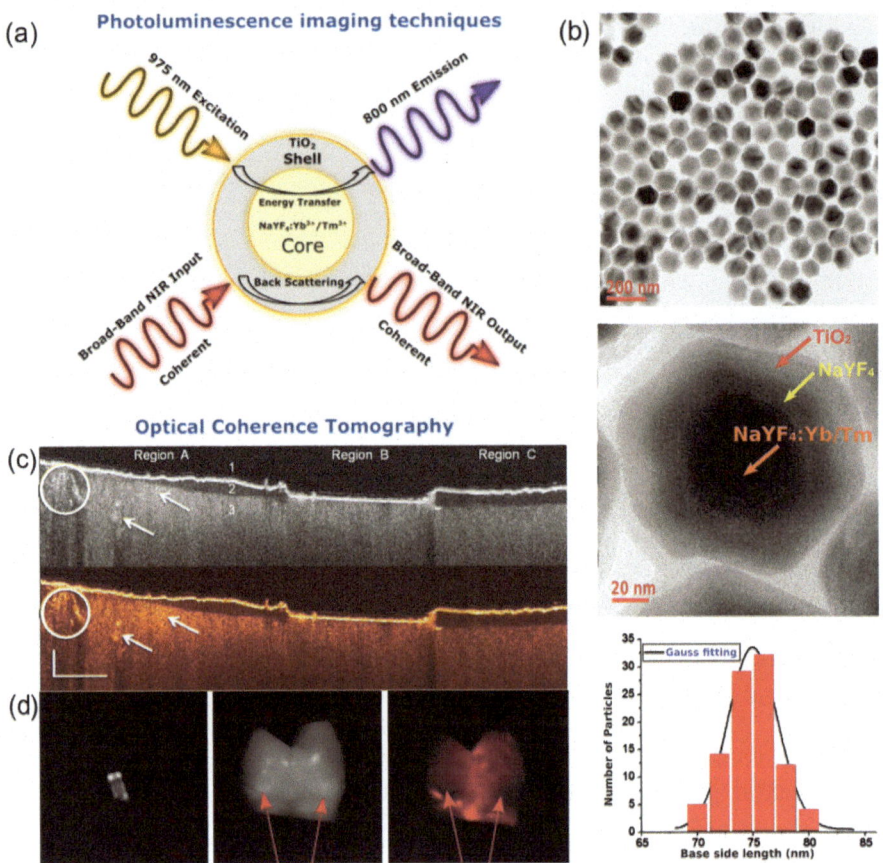

FIGURE 12.4

(A) Illustration of TiO_2-coated core–shell nanoparticle developed. (B) TEM image of the synthesized hexagonal-prism-shaped core–shell TiO_2-coated ($NaYF_4$: Yb 60%, Tm 0.5%)/ $NaYF_4$ core–shell nanoparticle. Scale bar presents 200 nm in the left image and 20 nm in the middle image. Histogram image in (B) shows the side-length distribution of the hexagonal particles. (C) OCT images displayed in grayscale (upper) and yellow scale (below). The arrows and circles indicate the high concentration of nanoparticles inside the dentinal tubules. Three different regions were prepared for the sample: region A, adhesive with nanoparticles; region B, no adhesive (control); region C, adhesive without nanoparticles. 1, air; 2, adhesive layer; 3, hybrid layer. Scale bar, 100 µm (vertical) and 1 mm (horizontal). (D) From left to right: image of core–shell nanoparticles (CSNp) solutions deposit on a glass slide; tooth placed on the glass slide covering the CSNp sample; right, photoluminescence imaging of the tooth. Adapted with permission from (Braz et al. 2018) © John Wiley & Sons – Books.

and diluted in glycerol have been exploited as clearing agents for a diagnostic of occlusal incipient caries lesions. The presence of the AgNP highlights the enamel birefringence and defines initial demineralization areas, presenting OCT images with higher contrast between healthy and demineralized regions (Carneiro et al. 2018).

Besides AgNP, gold nanoparticles and nanorods (AuNP and AuNR, respectively) have also been exploited as contrast agent for OCT image enhancement, as reported in reference (Das et al. 2022) whose results were obtained with a commercial OCT system. In the article, they divided the samples into six groups: control group (G1), glycerol only (G2), AuNP (G3), AuNP diluted on glycerol (G4), AuNR (G5) and AuNR diluted on glycerol (G6). The spherical gold nanoparticles were produced by the authors, treating hydrogen tetrachloroaurate ($HAuCl_4$) with polyvinylpyrrolidone (PVP) in boiling water. The resulting colloidal gold nanoparticles are spherical and have 2.0±1.0 nm dispersed in the aqueous solution, the spectrally measured peak plasmon resonance at 550 nm confirmed the gold nanosphere characteristic. The nanorods were purchased and had 50 nm diameters and 160 nm length, also dispersed in aqueous solution, with two plasmon resonance peaks (520 nm and 825 nm) corresponding to the transverse and longitudinal plasmon resonances, respectively.

The acquired OCT images were analyzed using a software developed by the authors to measure the optical attenuation coefficient, μ. The software used the average A-scan of each region of interest (ROI) window to fit an exponential decay, based on the Beer–Lambert law, $I_{(z)} = I_0 \exp(-\mu z)$, where $I_{(z)}$ is the intensity as a function of depth, z, and μ. As already discussed (see Chapter 2), the μ coefficient quantitatively characterizes the decay of OCT signals when light propagates through the tissue. Thus, it is possible to use attenuation coefficient to discriminate between different types of tissues and their state of health (see ref. (Das et al. 2022) and refs therein). The results shown in Figure 12.5 represent 2D OCT images, or B-scans (left column), and the A-scan graphics (right column) of the ROI corresponding to the pit area in G1 (control), G3 (AuNP) and G6 (AuNR + glycerol). The central line shows where the A-scan was measured. Both G3 and G6 evidenced great difference in the attenuation coefficient compared with the control group.

The quantitative average values of μ, obtained from this reference data shows an increase in the light attenuation in all carious tested groups when compared with the control group G1 ($\mu=0.184$). It was observed that groups G3 and G6 had a higher μ (0.224) on the carious surface. On the other hand, at the sound areas, gold nanorods diluted in glycerol (G6), presented values of $\mu = 0.168$, similar to that obtained from the isolated samples in the presence of glycerol isolated G2 ($\mu = 0.169$). The message of all those results is that OCT is indeed able to provide quantitative measurements for carious and health teeth, and nanomaterials are well suited as contrast agents.

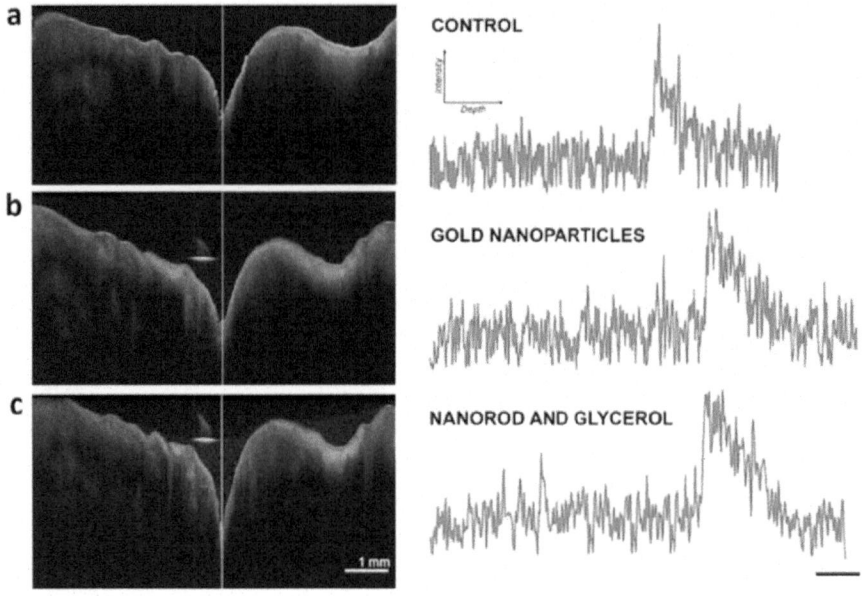

FIGURE 12.5

OCT B-scan images across occlusal surface of a molar, followed on the right-side by the corresponding light intensity decay obtained from an A-scan of the region of interest (ROI) in the central pit area, according to the optical clearing agent used on the surface: (a) G1-Control; (b) G3-AuNPs; and (c) G6-AuNRs in glycerol. From (Das et al. 2022).

Bioceramics such as hydroxyapatite (HAp) are extensively used in medical applications, mainly as an interface between implants and living tissues in orthopaedic and dentistry. In an application example (Strąkowska et al. 2015; Głowacki et al. 2017), two samples were analyzed with OCT: a reference HAp solution and a similar HAp solution with silver nanoparticles. The authors compared the different samples of sol-gel derived hydroxyapatite placed in Petri dishes using a polarization-sensitive OCT. The obtained cross-sectional visualizations of every sample were examined and compared to the pure HAp sample. Every other sample was compared with it to evaluate the distribution of the silver nanoparticles inside the hydroxyapatite matrix. The resulting OCT images showed well-detailed scattering characteristics at any depth. Their aim was to analyze the concentration and dispersion of this nanodopants in the bioceramic matrix. Also, they monitored the quality of the HAp coating and deposition process repetition with the same PS system and obtained good results. One of the main applications of HAp is on the reduction of tooth sensitivity, filling the dentinal tubules to block the hydro-dynamic mechanism and pain stimulation (Low et al. 2015) and, as exposed before, OCT is a trustworthy tool to study tooth remineralization (Taha et al. 2018). In terms of restorative and preventive dentistry, nanohydroxyapatite has significant demineralizing effects on initial enamel lesions, certainly superior to conventional fluoride and good results on reducing the sensitivity of the teeth (Pepla et al. 2014).

Both endogenous and exogenous contrast agents have been widely used to increase the contrast of OCT techniques to label and visualize specific molecules in biological tissues (Wang et al. 2022). There are far more kinds of extrinsic (exogenous) contrast agents than intrinsic (endogenous) ones, as can be seen from the examples given earlier in this section. Examples of endogenous contrast agents include melanin and hemoglobin, while exogenous molecules include dyes, as methylene blue and indocyanine green, gas vesicles and nanomaterials, our focus in this chapter. An exogenous contrast agent is targeted if it only strengthens the molecular contrast of specific regions. Meanwhile, an untargeted contrast agent will enhance the image contrast of a sample in general. This means that the molecular contrast from imaging agents within the biological tissues could be mistaken by the background scattering or speckle pattern from a sample.

Most of the reported contrast agents of molecular contrast OCT are still untargeted, but some types of contrast agents like gold nanoshells and nanoparticles with protein or poly shells can be functionalized to target specific cell sites, e.g., by the use of biomarkers. Among them, AuNP are of particular interest as they have good biocompatibility and can vary in size, shape and optical properties quite easily. Nanoparticles, especially gold nanoparticles, have a strong depolarization effect and therefore can easily be used as exogenous contrast agents. Photothermal OCT (PT-OCT) also benefits from a wide range of contrast agents, although gold nanostructures are the most popular ones due to their resonance in the NIR optical window and can easily be used for photothermal therapy (Wang et al. 2022). Nevertheless, every OCT technique has its own choices of molecular contrast agents (Yang 2005).

Despite these promising features, the potential use for molecular contrast OCT imaging has not been fully explored yet. Essentially because for any prospective molecular contrast agent, its characteristics such as synthesis, stability, toxicity, biocompatibility and biodegradability should be methodically researched, as this would make up the first step towards clinical applications and it takes time and extensive research, as well as long-term-effect studies (Yang 2005; Wang et al. 2022). In the next section, we will discuss how it is possible to use the OCT to get molecular information.

12.4 Nanosensitive OCT

The growing need to understand the molecular mechanisms of diseases has prompted the revolution in molecular imaging techniques along with nanomedicine development. Conventional OCT provides unique anatomic images but little molecular or nanosensitive information. However, given the widespread adoption of OCT in research and clinical practice, it is strongly desired to combine it with molecular and nanosensitive changes. A range of relevant approaches has been reported already. In this section, we review these recent advances, mentioning nanoparticle-based contrast agents and the modifications on OCT to obtain sub-diffraction limit information with nanosensitivity capability and their applications. Given the extensive background around the subject, we will focus to the main concepts.

OCT is a biomedical imaging and diagnosis technique rapidly developing that provides real-time 2D/3D scans depicting morphological structures of living tissue with unique micron-scale resolution and 2~3 mm depth penetration (Walther et al. 2011). It just fills a place between confocal reflectance microscopy and diffuse optical tomography. Compared to other optical imaging methods, OCT can generate sharp, reliable and cost-effective images using light intensities far below the recommendation of the American National Standard (ANSI). However, OCT is usually considered more of a structural than a functional imaging method. One of the main shortcomings of commercial OCT machines is their low resolution and sensitivity to structural changes (typically occurring below 10 microns). The best ultra-high-resolution OCT has sensitivity to structural changes and depth resolution up to 1 micron. Since numerous applications of interest rely upon primary changes at the nanoscale level, OCT would definitively benefit from improved structural resolution and sensitivity. But then again, since the early 1990s, reports on nanomedical research using OCT have been gradually increasing.

The spectral OCT (S-OCT) technique has proven to have the potential for microstructure and molecular evaluation at the nanoscale level (Morgner et al. 2000; Robles et al. 2011; Spicer et al. 2019; Kamińska et al. 2020). Many researchers have worked in the Fourier-domain OCT techniques to achieve nanoscale sensitivity, taking advantage of the phase-detection capability of the technique (Wang et al. 2010; Yi et al. 2013), including a technique called inverse spectroscopic OCT (ISOCT), which quantify the mass-density correlation function to detect structural changes ranging from ~30 to ~450 nm. An application example is shown in Figure 12.6, where the authors determine the attenuation coefficient map and distribution of different molecules in corals using ISOCT (Spicer et al. 2019). They achieve it upon quantification of the wavelength-dependent backscattering coefficient $\mu_b(\lambda)$ and the scattering coefficient μ_s.

But it was Martin Leahy's research group in Ireland that presented a reliable spectroscopic contrast method to achieve nanoscale measurements (Alexandrov et al. 2014a; Alexandrov et al. 2014b; Alexandrov et al. 2014c), a method they called nanosensitive OCT (nsOCT).

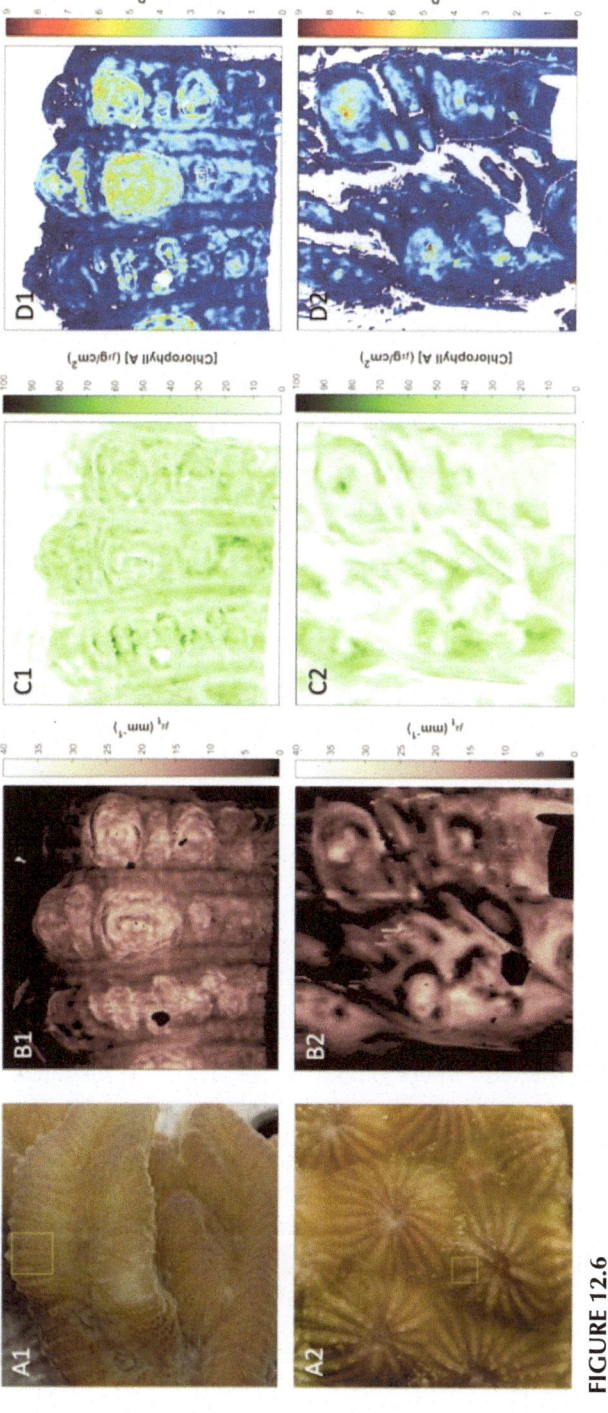

FIGURE 12.6

Top-down projection maps of optical and structural properties of corals takes with ISOCT. Photographs of (A1) Merulina ampliata and (A2) Diploastrea heliopora with box demarcating region scanned with ISOCT. (B1,B2) En face ISOCT projection maps of total attenuation coefficient μ_t, (C1,C2) chlorophyll a concentration and (D1,D2) D value for Merulina and Diploastrea, respectively. Maps (B1,C1,D1) are 2.56 × 2.56 mm; maps (B2,C2,D2) are 1.85 × 1.85 mm. From (Spicer et al. 2019).

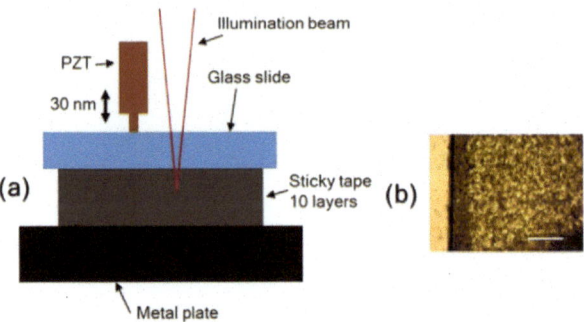

FIGURE 12.7.1

(a) Schematic of nanoscale structural changes within the sample (multilayer sticky tape);
(b) image of one layer of the tape, scale bar is 200 μm. Reprinted with permission from
(Alexandrov et al. 2014c) © Royal Society of Chemistry.

The nsOCT was developed and demonstrated taking advantage of the reasonable control of the micrometer resolution data from the Fourier-domain OCT to resolve images in the nanoscale (100's of nm). Their method uses the spectral encoding of spatial frequency (SESF) approach (Alexandrov et al. 2012) to reconstruct the structural information about the axial profile of the three-dimensional spatial frequency for each image point, transforming spectral amplitudes to axial spatial frequency amplitudes for sub-bands' decomposition. The development SESF approach has opened the opportunity to map the axial structural information into each pixel of a 2D image, quantitatively, with nanoscale sensitivity. The spatial period profile of a given point in the sample is calculated based on the sub-bands' energy distribution. It enables a conventional OCT with a resolution of 30 μm × 30 μm × 12 μm to detect the difference between two layers of nanospheres as small as 30 nm. In the set of Figures 12.7.1 to 12.7.3, an example of structural changes of a multilayer sticky tape sample demonstrates the capability of the nsOCT to detect nanometric displacements (30 nm). The nsOCT directly translate information about a particular structure from the Fourier domain to the image domain and map this information into the corresponding location within the 3D OCT image. As a result, sub-micron axial structure can be visualized at the nanoscale, making it possible to detect structural changes within a scattering sample as small as 30 nm. Its sensitivity is more than 300 times higher than any previous OCT generation. Therefore, it may monitor the movements or changes of nanostructures, e.g., wound healing within the cornea (Lal et al. 2020). The nsOCT sensitivity is limited by the spectral resolution, the collected range of spatial frequencies is limited by spectral range and both can go far beyond what they have demonstrated. The ability of nsOCT to probe human skin *in vivo* has also been shown (Das et al. 2020) and we expect that the technique could be applicable in the early detection and treatment of many diseases.

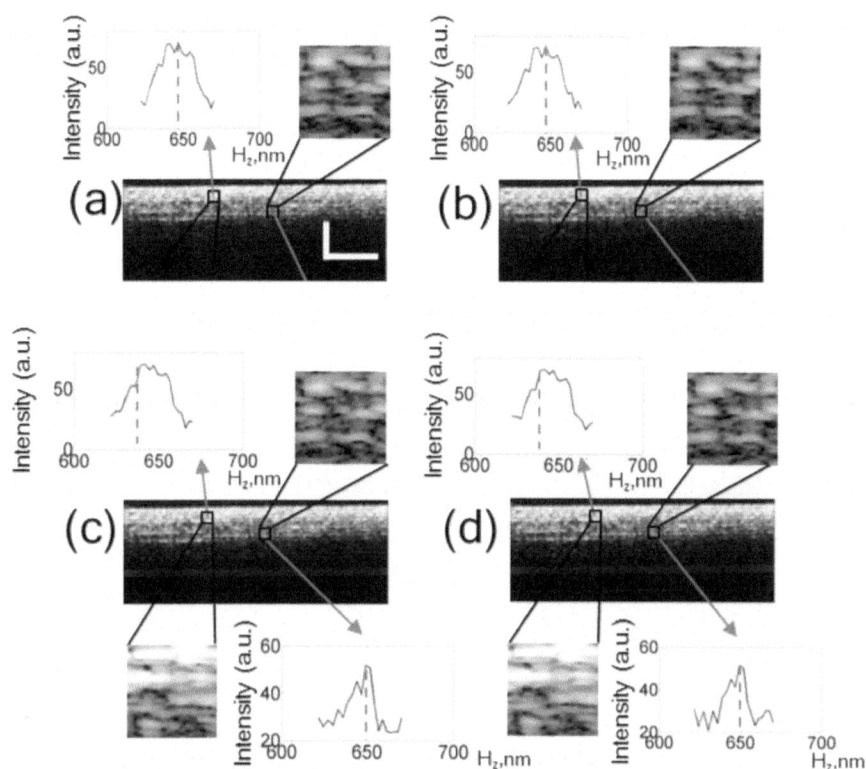

FIGURE 12.7.2

OCT images of multilayer scattering tape with axial spatial period profiles and magnified portions for two selected locations. (a,b) before and (c,d) after top surface displacement of 30 nm. Images (a,c) are second frames and images (b,d) are fiftieth frames. Lateral and depth scale bars are 500 μm. Reprinted with permission from (Alexandrov et al. 2014c) © Royal Society of Chemistry.

Conventional OCT has a fairly restricted capacity to track biochemical distribution and changes within living organisms. It is because OCT cannot distinguish the signals from different molecules and the background nor detect incoherent processes like Raman scattering or fluorescence emission. To address this issue, significant effort has been taken to develop sophisticated strategies that can provide additional *ex vivo, in vitro* and *in vivo* molecular information to OCT devices (Yang 2005). For many different techniques, to make images of living samples with molecular or nanoselectivity, it usually requires the use of labels, or contrast agents. In the case of OCT, its combination with contrast agents can enhance its diagnostic capabilities, and nanoparticles are peculiarly suitable as contrast agents for reflection-based or scattering-based imaging methods.

Currently, S-OCT also benefits from the fast development of nanotechnology. Many nanoparticles, such as gold nanorods, nanoshells and nanocages, have

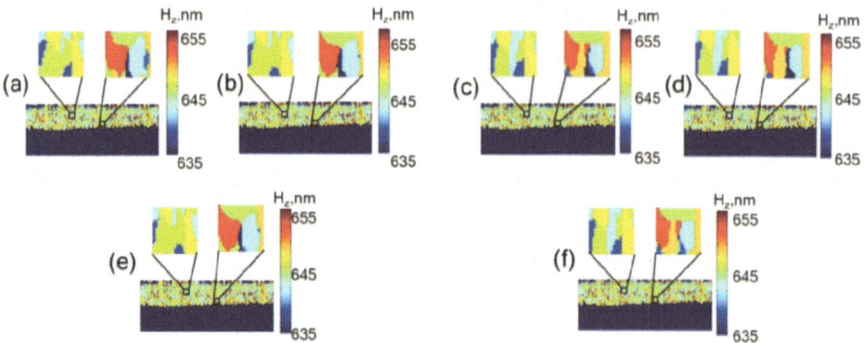

FIGURE 12.7.3

nsOCT images of multilayer scattering tape with magnified portions for two selected locations. (a, b, e) before and (c, d, f) after top surface displacement of 30 nm. Images (a, c) are second frames, images (b, d) are fiftieth frames and images (e, f) are averaged images for 49 frames. Reprinted with permission from (Alexandrov et al. 2014c) © Royal Society of Chemistry.

been validated as optically and chemically stable S-OCT contrast agents for a widespread application in the biomedical field. At the same time, variations of S-OCT, such as spectroscopic optical coherence refraction tomography (SOCRT), have been developed. The SOCRT technique reconstructs spectroscopic images from S-OCT scans at different angles for higher spatial resolution, showing excellent potential to measure nanostructures (Zhou et al. 2020). As the S-OCT signal is computed by taking the light bandwidth spectra and dividing it using the number of pixels for every A-scan, broader bandwidth light sources can improve the resolution of S-OCT. Thus, using visible light instead of NIR light in S-OCT is potentially a better way to identify molecules in biological tissues. Although, the contrast agents with strong absorption peaks in the NIR region are still the most promising ones, particularly for deeper imaging purposes. Besides, plasmon-resonant nanoparticles with high extinction coefficients have been introduced to provide molecular information with this technique. Given the facility of making different sizes and geometry, the absorption peak of gold nanostructures can be tuned to match the OCT light source. Upconversion nanoparticles were also demonstrated as good molecular probes (Mohan et al. 2021).

Polarization sensitive-OCT (PS-OCT) is a valuable tool to measure both the size and shape of nanoscale structures, such as nanoparticles. A reported example used a PS-OCT to measure nanoparticles and assessed its performance with disk-like and spherical particles, simulating the particle size and shape from their scattering parameters (Schneider et al. 2013). Their results suggested that spherical particles tend to maintain the polarization state of the scanning light, while non-spherical particles are likely to reflect light with changed polarization states. In others reported examples using PS-OCT, it was demonstrated the diffusion and concentration of gold nanorods from their depolarization signatures (Lippok et al. 2017) and presented a non-destructive way to assess the characterization of thin hydroxyapatite layers outside metal particles (Strąkowska et al. 2015). There are also a series of exciting applications of PS-OCT with contrast agents, especially AuNP, which present strong depolarization effect. PS-OCT is capable of measuring their dynamic scattering signals and polarization properties, while analyzing the relation between the degree of depolarization and the nanoparticle concentration. Nanoscale viscoelastic properties' studies using PS-OCT have also profited from the plasmon-resonant and highly anisotropic properties of AuNP (Wang et al. 2022).

12.5 Conclusions

Nanodentistry has achieved tremendous progress in the past years. It is expected that nanotechnology will change dentistry, healthcare and human life more profoundly than many developments of the past. To date, there has been an exponential increase in studies using nanotechnology for dental applications and it is not too early to consider, evaluate and attempt to shape potential effects of nanodentistry. Nanotechnology has been used for dental applications in several forms and optical coherence tomography has proven to take enormous advantages of these applications. From the development of nanomaterials for treatment and diagnosis (OCT contrast agents), to the detection of structural modifications in the nanoscale and molecular detection, OCT has been exploited in the nanoworld. Nanodentistry will lead to efficient and highly effective personalized dental treatments, as it seems to be where the world is headed if technology keeps advancing. This will open a huge range of opportunities of benefit for both the dentist and the patient.

References

Adeola, H.A., Sabiu, S., Adekiya, T.A., Aruleba, R.T., et al. 2020. Prospects of nanodentistry for the diagnosis and treatment of maxillofacial pathologies and cancers. *Heliyon* 6: e04890.

Aeran, H., Kumar, V., Uniyal, S. and Tanwer, P. 2015. Nanodentistry: is just a fiction or future. *Journal of Oral Biology and Craniofacial Research* 5: 207–211.

Aggarwal, R., Sounderajah, V., Martin, G. et al. 2021. Diagnostic accuracy of deep learning in medical imaging: a systematic review and meta-analysis. *npj Digital Medicine* 4: 1–23.

Alexandrov, S., Subhash, H. and Leahy, M. 2014a. Nanosensitive optical coherence tomography for the study of changes in static and dynamic structures. *Quantum Electronics* 44: 657–663.

Alexandrov, S., Subhash, H., Zam, A. and Leahy, M. 2014b. Nano-sensitive optical coherence tomography (nsOCT) for depth resolved characterization of 3D submicron structure. *Proceeding of SPIE* 8934: 89340Z.

Alexandrov, S.A., Subhash, H.M., Zam, A. and Leahy, M. 2014c. Nano-sensitive optical coherence tomography. *Nanoscale* 6: 3545–3549.

Alexandrov, S.A., Uttam, S., Bista, R.K., Staton, K., et al. 2012. Spectral encoding of spatial frequency approach for characterization of nanoscale structures. *Applied Physics Letters* 101: 033702.

Bhardwaj, A., Bhardwaj, A., Misuriya, A. et al. 2014. Nanotechnology in dentistry: present and future. *Journal of International Oral Health* 6: 121–126.

Braz, A.K.S., de Araujo, R.E., Ohulchanskyy, T.Y. et al. 2012. In situ gold nanoparticles formation: contrast agent for dental optical coherence tomography. *Journal of Biomedical Optics* 17: 066003.

Braz, A.K.S., Moura, D.S., Gomes, A.S.L., Ohulchanskyy, T.Y., et al. 2018. TiO2 - coated fluoride nanoparticles for dental multimodal optical imaging. *Journal of Biophotonics* 11: e201700029.

Brun, A., Moignot, N., Colombier, M.L. and Dursun, E. 2020. Emerging nanotechnology in non-surgical periodontal therapy in animal models: a systematic review. *Nanomaterials* 10: 1–22.

Carneiro, V.S.M., Mota, C.C.B.O., Gomes, A.S.L. et al. 2017. Optical clearing agents associated with nanoparticles for scanning dental structures with optical coherence tomography. In: *Conference on Lasers and Electro-Optics* JW2A.52.

Carneiro, V.S.M., Mota, C.C.B.O., Souza, A.F. et al. 2018. Silver nanoparticles as optical clearing agent enhancers to improve caries diagnostic by optical coherence tomography. *Proceedings of SPIE, Colloidal Nanoparticles for Biomedical Applications XIII* 10507: 1050719.

Corrêa, J.M., Mori, M., Sanches, H.L. et al. 2015. Silver nanoparticles in dental biomaterials. *International Journal of Biomaterials* 2015: 485275.

Costantini, I., Costantini, I., Cicchi, R. et al. 2019. In-vivo and ex-vivo optical clearing methods for biological tissues: review. *Biomedical Optics Express* 10: 5251–5267.

Das, A., Raposo, G.C.C., Lopes, D.S. et al. 2022. Exploiting nanomaterials for optical coherence tomography and photoacoustic imaging in nanodentistry. *Nanomaterials* 12: 506.

Das, N., Sergey, A., Zhou, Y. et al. 2020. Nanoscale structure detection and monitoring of tumour growth with optical coherence tomography. *Nanoscale Advances* 2: 2853–2858.

de Melo, L.S.A., de Araujo, R.E., Freitas, A.Z. et al. 2005. Evaluation of enamel dental restoration interface by optical coherence tomography. *Journal of Biomedical Optics* 10: 064027.

Desai, K., Somasundaram, J., S, L.R. 2020. Nanodentistry – an overview. *European Journal of Molecular & Clinical Medicine* 7: 2879–2887.

Drexler, W., Fujimoto, J.G. 2015. *Optical Coherence Tomography*. Springer Cham International Publishing, 2nd edition.

Ellis, P.J. 2017. Nanodentistry: the benefits of nanotechnology in dentistry and its impact on oral health. *Journal of Student Science and Technology* 10: 45–50.

Foong, L.K., Foroughi, M.M., Forutan Mirhosseini, A. et al. 2020. Applications of nano-materials in diverse dentistry regimes. *RSC Advances* 10: 15430–15460.

Fujimoto, J., Swanson, E. 2016. The development, commercialization, and impact of optical coherence tomography. *Investigative Ophthalmology and Visual Science.* 57: OCT1–OCT13.

Głowacki, M.J., Gnyba, M., Strąkowska, P. et al. 2017. Metrology and measurement systems examination of sol-gel derived hydroxyapatite enhanced with silver nanoparticles using OCT and Raman spectroscopy. *Metrology and Measurement Systems* 24: 153–160.

Graça, N.D.R.L., Palmeira, A.R. de B.L.S., Fernandes, L.O. et al. 2019. In vivo optical coherence tomographic imaging to monitor gingival recovery and the adhesive interface in aesthetic oral rehabilitation: a case report. *Imaging Science in Dentistry* 49: 171.

Grigorjeva, L., Smits, K., Millers, D., Jankovia, D. 2015. Luminescence of Er/Yb and Tm/Yb doped FAp nanoparticles and ceramics. *IOP Conference Series: Materials Science and Engineering.* 77: 1–6.

Hannig, M., Hannig, C. 2010. Nanomaterials in preventive dentistry. *Nature Nanotechnology.* 5: 565–569.

Hsieh, Y.-S., Ho, Y.-C., Lee, S.-Y. et al. 2013. Dental optical coherence tomography. *Sensors* 13: 8928–8949.

Kamińska, A.M., Strąkowski, M.R., Pluciński, J. 2020. Spectroscopic optical coherence tomography for thin layer and foil measurements. *Sensors* 20: 5653.

Khang, D., Carpenter, J., Chun, Y.W. et al. 2010. Nanotechnology for regenerative medicine. *Biomedical Microdevices* 12: 575–587.

Khurshid, Z., Zafar, M., Qasim, S. et al. 2015. Advances in nanotechnology for restorative dentistry. *Materials* 8: 717–731.

Lal, C., Alexandrov, S., Rani, S. et al. 2020. Nanosensitive optical coherence tomography to assess wound healing within the cornea. *Biomedical Optics Express,* 11: 3407–3422.

Lippok, N., Villiger, M., Albanese, A. et al. 2017. Depolarization signatures map gold nanorods within biological tissue. *Nature Photonics* 11: 583–588.

Low, S. B., Allen, E.P., Kontogiorgos, E.D. 2015. Reduction in dental hypersensitivity with nano-hydroxyapatite, potassium nitrate, sodium monoflurophosphate and antioxidants. *The Open Dentistry Journal* 9: 92–97.

Maia, A.M.A., de Freitas, A.Z., de L. Campello, S. et al. 2016. Evaluation of dental enamel caries assessment using quantitative light induced fluorescence and optical coherence tomography. *Journal of Biophotonics* 9: 596–602.

Melo, M.A.S., Guedes, S.F.F., Xu, H.H.K., Rodrigues, L.K.A. 2013. Nanotechnology-based restorative materials for dental caries management. *Trends in Biotechnology.* 31: 459–467.

Miraz, M.H., Ali, M., Excell, P.S., Picking, R. 2015. A review on Internet of Things (IoT), Internet of Everything (IoE) and Internet of Nano Things (IoNT). In: *2015 Internet Technologies and Applications (ITA)* 219–224.

Mirsasaani, S.S., Hemati, M., Dehkord, E.S. et al. 2019. Nanotechnology and nanobiomaterials in dentistry. In: *Nanobiomaterials in Clinical Dentistry.* Elsevier. 19–37.

Mohan, M., Poddar, R. 2021. Ex-vivo molecular imaging with upconversion nanoparticles (UCNPs) using photo thermal optical coherence tomography (PTOCT). *Photodiagnosis and Photodynamic Therapy* 33: 102027.

Morgner, U., Drexler, W., Kärtner, F.X. et al. 2000. Spectroscopic optical coherence tomography. *Optics Letters*. 25: 111.

Noronha, V.T., Paula, A.J., Durán, G. et al. 2017. Silver nanoparticles in dentistry. *Dental Materials* 33: 1110–1126.

Padovani, G.C., Feitosa, V.P., Sauro, S. et al. 2015. Advances in dental materials through nanotechnology: facts, perspectives and toxicological aspects. *Trends in Biotechnology* 33: 621–636.

Pepla, E., Besharat, L.K., Palaia, G. et al. 2014. Nano-hydroxyapatite and its applications in preventive, restorative and regenerative dentistry: a review of literature. *Annali di Stomatologia* 5: 108.

Rathee, M., Bhoria, M. 2014. Nanodentistry: the emerging tiny tools – a review. *International Journal of Biosciences and Nanosciences* 1: 63–67.

Raura, N., Garg, A., Arora, A., Roma, M. 2020. Nanoparticle technology and its implications in endodontics: a review. *Biomaterials Research* 24: 1–8.

Robles, F.E., Wilson, C., Grant, G., Wax, A. 2011. Molecular imaging true-colour spectroscopic optical coherence tomography. *Nature photonics* 5: 744–747.

Salamanca-Buentello, F., Daar, A.S. 2021. Nanotechnology, equity and global health. *Nature Nanotechnology* 16: 358–361.

Sasalawad, S.S., Naik, S.N., Shashibhushan, K.K., Poornima, P. 2014. Nanodentistry: the next big thing is small. *International Journal of Contemporary Dental and Medical Reviews* 1–6.

Schneider, S., Krämer, A., Eppler, F. et al. 2013. Polarization-sensitive optical coherence tomography for characterization of size and shape of nano-particles. In: *CLEO: 2013*. AF1J.4.

Seth, N., Khan, K. 2017. Dentistry at the nano level: the advent of nanodentistry. *International Healthcare Research Journal*. 1: 3–9.

Silva, A.V.C., Teixeira, J. de A., Melo Júnior, P.C. de. 2019. Remineralizing potential of nano-silver-fluoride for tooth enamel: an optical coherence tomography analysis. *Pesquisa Brasileira em Odontopediatria e Clínica Integrada*. 19: 1–13.

Sinha, N., Kulshreshtha, N.M., Dixit, M. et al. 2017. Nanodentistry: novel approaches. In: *Nanostructures for Oral Medicine*. Elsevier. 751–776.

Spicer, G.L.C., Eid, A., Wangpraseurt, D. et al. 2019. Measuring light scattering and absorption in corals with inverse spectroscopic optical coherence tomography (ISOCT): a new tool for non-invasive monitoring. *Scientific Reports* 9: 1–12.

Strąkowska, P., Trojanowski, M., Gardas, M. et al. 2015. Nano-particle doped hydroxyapatite material evaluation using spectroscopic polarization sensitive optical coherence tomography. *Proceedings of SPIE 9312, Optical Coherence Tomography and Coherence Domain Optical Methods in Biomedicine XIX*, 9312: 93122X.

Taha, A.A., Fleming, P.S., Hill, R.G., Patel, M.P. 2018. Enamel remineralization with novel bioactive glass air abrasion. *Journal of Dental Research*. 97: 1438–1444.

Teixeira, J.A., Costa E Silva, A.V., dos Santos, V.E. et al. 2018. Effects of a new nano-silver fluoride-containing dentifrice on demineralization of enamel and streptococcus mutans adhesion and acidogenicity. *International Journal of Dentistry* 2018: 1351925.

Tuchin, V. v., Maksimova, I.L., Zimnyakov, D.A. et al. 1997. Light propagation in tissues with controlled optical properties. *Journal of Biomedical Optics* 2: 401–417.

Tuchin, V. v., Zhu, D., Genina, E.A. 2022. *Handbook of Tissue Optical Clearing: New Prospects in Optical Imaging.* 1st edition. Boca Raton, CRC Press.

Walther, J., Gaertner, M., Cimalla, P. et al. 2011. Optical coherence tomography in biomedical research. *Analytical and Bioanalytical Chemistry.* 400: 2721–2743.

Wan, Y.Z., Huang, Y., Yuan, C.D. et al. 2007. Biomimetic synthesis of hydroxyapatite/ bacterial cellulose nanocomposites for biomedical applications. *Materials Science and Engineering: C.* 27: 855–864.

Wang, A., Qi, W., Gao, T., Tang, X. 2022. Molecular contrast optical coherence tomography and its applications in medicine. *International Journal of Molecular Sciences* 23: 3038.

Wang, R.K., Nuttall, A.L. 2010. Phase-sensitive optical coherence tomography imaging of the tissue motion within the organ of Corti at a subnanometer scale: a preliminary study. *Journal of Biomedical Optics*, 15: 056005.

Yadav, S.K., Khan, Z.A., Mishra, B. 2013. Impact of nanotechnology on socio-economic aspects: an overview. *Reviews in Nanoscience and Nanotechnology.* 2: 127–142.

Yamagata, S., Hamba, Y., Nakanishi, K. 2012. Introduction of rare-earth-element-containing ZnO nanoparticles into orthodontic adhesives. *Nano Biomedicine* 4: 11–17.

Yang, C. 2005. Molecular contrast optical coherence tomography: a review. *Photochemistry and Photobiology* 81: 215–237.

Yi, J., Radosevich, A.J., Rogers, J.D. et al. 2013. Can OCT be sensitive to nanoscale structural alterations in biological tissue? *Optics Express* 21: 9043–9059.

Yin, I.X., Zhang, J., Zhao, I.S. et al. 2020. The antibacterial mechanism of silver nanoparticles and its application in dentistry. *International Journal of Nanomedicine* 15:2555–2562.

Zhou, K.C., Qian, R., Farsiu, S., Izatt, J.A. 2020. Spectroscopic optical coherence refraction tomography. *Optics Letters* 45: 2091.

13

Summary and Perspectives for OCT in Dentistry

Anderson S. L. Gomes,[1,*] **Denise M. Zezell,**[2,†] **Cláudia C. B. O. Mota**[3,‡] **and John M. Girkin**[4,§]

[1]*Universidade Federal of Pernambuco, Physics Department and Graduate Program in Dentistry, Av Prof. Luis Freire s/n, Recife, Pernambuco, Brazil*

[2]*Center for Lasers and Applications, Nuclear and Energy, Research Institute, IPEN-CNEN/ SP, Av Lineu Prestes, São Paulo, Brazil*

[3]*Centro Universitário Tabosa de Almeida, Faculty of Dentistry, Avenida Portugal, Caruaru, Pernambuco, Brazil*

[4]*Durham University, Physics Department, South Road, Durham, United Kingdom*

[*]*anderson@df.ufpe.br*

[†]*zezell@usp.br*

[‡]*claudiabmota@gmail.com*

[§]*j.m.girkin@durham.ac.uk*

CONTENTS

The twenty-first century is being recognized as the century of photonics and it is also known as the century of multidisciplinary work, particularly in sciences. Photonics is a ubiquitous, enabling technology and the basis for many multidisciplinary tasks, from environmental sensing to optical communications. On the other hand, noninvasive imaging methods are required for diagnostics in health care, from primary to bedside, with real-time processing and at distance evaluation.

This book was written considering this new reality, and exploits photonics as an enabling technology and optical coherence tomography (OCT) as a tool to implement several new multidisciplinary insights developed

DOI: 10.1201/9781351104562-13

by researchers worldwide. The book focuses on OCT applied to dentistry, which was first employed in 1998 (Colston et al. 1998) a few years after the introduction of OCT in ophthalmology (Huang et al. 1991) as the pioneer work that opened a fantastic avenue in imaging for medical and nonmedical applications (de Boer et al. 2017)

OCT as a technique has developed and expanded in such a way that, nowadays, is a commercially available technique (Fujimoto et al. 2016) and simultaneously is under scientific development, particularly with implementation of artificial intelligence and other modern techniques (Nguyen et al. 2021)

13.1 The Chapters

As mentioned above, this book deals with OCT in dentistry. In Chapter 1, a brief review on basics in optics is given, and an overview of a diversity of optical imaging methods was written such that the reader can have a broader view of the possibilities in optical imaging. Further insights in optical bioimaging can be found in (Qian et al. 2022). In Chapter 2, a review on the basics and general applications in OCT is brought to the reader in a nutshell, heavily based on the 2015 book by Drexler and Fujimoto (Drexler et al. 2015).

Chapters 3 through 12 cover the applications of OCT in dentistry, hopefully including all aspects of dental OCT published so far, although certainly not exhaustive in the referenced work. Every chapter starts with an insight into the dental aspect and then how OCT is applied to it. Chapter 3 described the use of OCT in cariology, one of the most employed uses of OCT in dentistry. Early diagnosis of carious and noncarious lesions, as well as in monitoring the progression or reversal of these lesions, is reviewed in that chapter.

Chapter 4 reviewed how OCT is employed to evaluate how restorative dental materials based on composite resin, which are often used in operative dentistry, prosthodontics, pediatric, and endodontic fields of dentistry, perform once placed in the hard tissue under study or treatment. More recent publications in this aspect can be found in (Bakhsh et al. 2020a, 2020b; Shi et al. 2020; Santana et al. 2020; El-Basha 2020; Turkistani et al. 2020; Zeng et al. 2021; Kantovitz et al. 2021; Zhou et al. 2021).

In Chapter 5, further insight of OCT use in dental materials evaluation is presented, from a laboratory perspective. The chapter focuses on the investigated structure and the OCT method used. Recent work on this subject can be found in (Iijima et al. 2021; Merle et al. 2022; Schlenz et al. 2021; Zang et al. 2022)

Chapter 6 deals with OCT in endodontics, which is the part of dentistry that deals with the morphology, physiology and pathology of the human dental pulp and periapical tissues. After a brief background on clinical aspects of endodontics, the chapter brings the state-of-the-art in OCT applied to endodontics.

In Chapter 7, the use of OCT in pediatric dentistry is described. As pediatrics is the part of dentistry that cares about all alterations on the hard and soft tissue of children, the reviewed work covers different aspects of OCT uses in different dentistry fields, with particular emphasis on caries assessment and periodontics.

Chapter 8 deals with OCT in orthodontics, since monitoring changes in dental and support tissues that receive and dissipate forces imprinted on them, due to orthodontics tools, depends on instruments that access these tissues accurately and continuously without causing damage. OCT is particularly appropriate for this application, as reviewed in that chapter.

Chapter 9 reports on OCT in prosthodontics, which deals with dental prosthesis, a dental specialty whose applications range from the partial restoration of a dental element to the total functional rehabilitation of dental arches through implant-supported prostheses. In this chapter, the use of OCT will be addressed as a conservative evaluation technique for dental prostheses, as well as for the assessment of the health of adjacent hard and soft oral tissues.

Chapters 10 and 11 described what is perhaps one of the most widespread applications of OCT in dentistry – its application in soft oral tissues. Chapter 10 deals with periodontal diseases and their assessment through OCT, while Chapter 11 expands the OCT uses for the oral cavity including cancer and other types of abnormalities.

Finally, in Chapter 12 we bring the use of OCT in a novel specialty in dentistry, known as nanodentistry. Still, in the laboratory environment, this area is yet an important application that evolved from nanoscience and nanotechnology as a whole and is no longer just a future bearing area, but in many other fields is already a daily reality. Therefore, the translation of OCT applications from the lab environment is closer than we suspect. This chapter brings the state-of-the-art of OCT in nanodentistry, which opens several new avenues, as will be pointed out in the perspectives.

13.2 Perspectives for OCT in Dentistry – The Author's View

From a *perspective* point of view, it is the author's opinion that the main expectation for OCT in dentistry is its wide clinical use. Several of the specialties in dentistry described in this book, which employ OCT as a diagnostic tool, have found niches of clinical applications. Figure 13.1 shows a commercial OCT system, not designed for dental applications and without a dental probe, being used with limitation to the anterior teeth in noninvasive periodontal assessment. Most certainly we anticipate that using appropriate

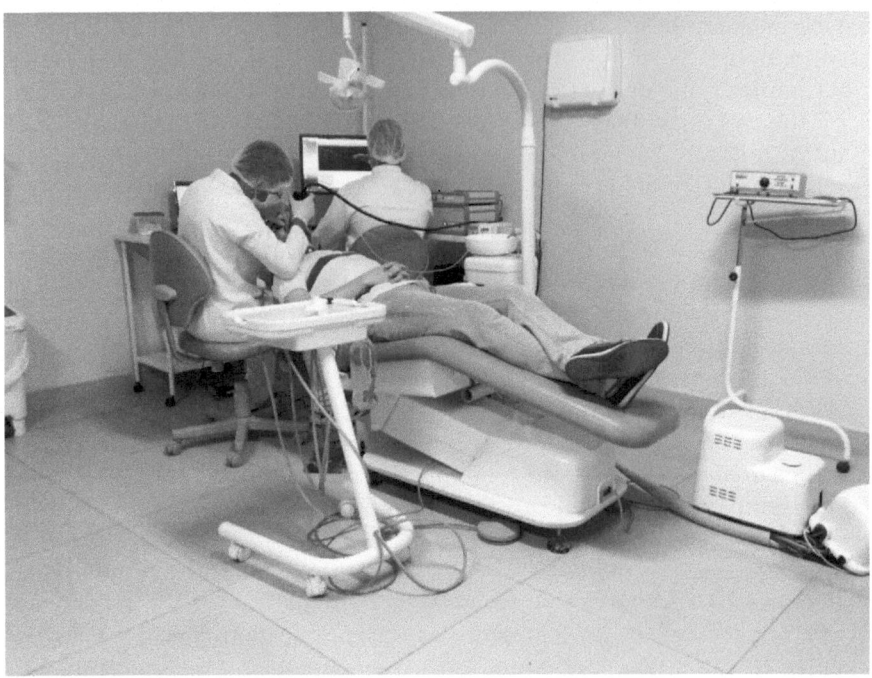

FIGURE 13.1
Commercial OCT system being used for periodontal diagnostic in dentistry. Courtesy C Mota,
ASCES/UNITA, Brazil.

probes (Haak et al. 2019; Song et al. 2021; Walther et al. 2022) such a picture can become a reality. Naturally, to be widespread and have scalability,
the cost-benefit (pricewise) needs to come down, but one thing leads to the
other. General OCT systems for lab work have already become much more
affordable (down to ~ US$10k price) and with more companies selling OCT
systems.

Another important point is resolution, and in that area nanoOCT, even
relying on available systems, which provide micrometer axial resolution, can
be one way to further investigate and apply. That can also lead to molecular
imaging with OCT.

Penetration depth, another important point, may be more difficult to
improve due to the basic limitations such as tissue absorption and scattering.
Even mitigation procedures, such as optical clearing agents, cannot improve
a factor of 10 or more in penetration depth. Miniaturization is another technological desire and is certainly in perspective for the short term.

Finally, multimodality systems based on OCT, such as OCT+Raman (Wang
et al. 2016) or OCT+photoacoustics, keeping the optical basis and expanding,
for instance, penetration depth, while keeping an axial resolution is a most

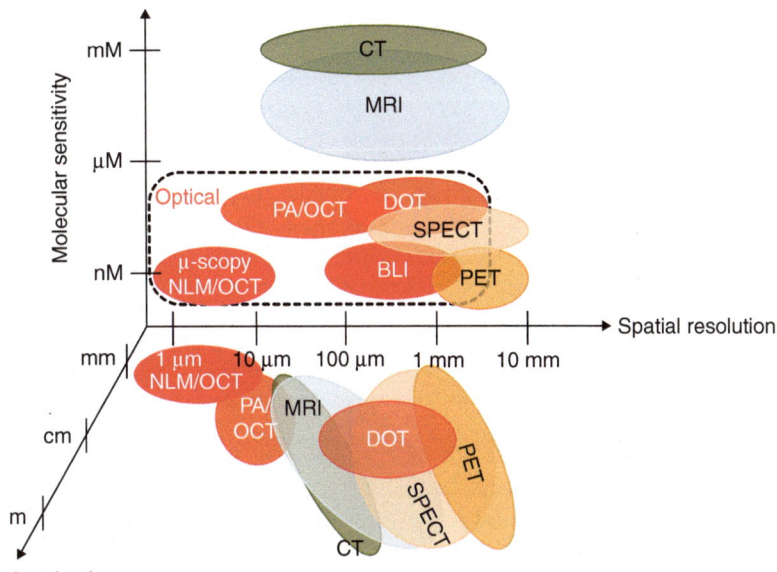

FIGURE 13.2

Medical imaging technologies as a function of penetration depth, molecular sensitivity and spatial resolution; MRI, magnetic resonance imaging; CT, computed tomography: SPECT, spectroscopic CT; PET, positron emission tomography; PA/OCT, multimodal photoacoustics-OCT; NLM/OCT, multimodal nonlinear microscopy-OCT; BLI, bioluminescence imaging; DOT, diffuse optical tomography.

Source: From (Leitgeb et al. 2018).

expected future step, and Figure 13.2 shows how these possibilities may be exploited. Other multimodality possibilities do exist, but those mentioned above can be used clinically.

References

Bakhsh, T.A., Sadr, A., Shimada, Y., Turkistani, A., Abuljadayel, R., Tagami, J. 2020a. Does lining class-II cavities with flowable composite improve the interfacial adaptation? *J. Adhes. Sci. Technol.* 34: 400–416.

Bakhsh, T.A., Tagami, J., Sadr, A. et al. 2020b. Effect of light irradiation condition on gap formation under polymeric dental restoration; OCT study. *Z. Med. Phys.* 30: 194–200.

Colston, B.W., Everett, M.J., Da Silva, L.B., Otis, L.L., Stroeve, P., Nathel, H. 1998. Imaging of hard- and soft-tissue structure in the oral cavity by optical coherence tomography. *Appl. Opt.* 37: 3582.

de Boer, J.F., Leitgeb, R., Wojtkowski, M. 2017. Twenty-five years of optical coherence tomography: the paradigm shift in sensitivity and speed provided by Fourier domain OCT [Invited]. Biomed. *Opt. Express* 8: 3248.

Drexler, W., Fujimoto, J.G. 2015. *Optical Coherence Tomography: Technology and Applications*, 2nd Edition. ed. Springer.

El-Basha, E. 2020. Assessment of composite leakage using optical coherence tomography: a systematic view. *J. Adv. Clin. Exp. Dent.* 57(1): 20–32.

Fujimoto, J., Swanson, E. 2016. The development, commercialization, and impact of optical coherence tomography. *Investig. Ophthalmol. Vis. Sci.* 57: OCT1–OCT13.

Haak, R., Ahrens, M., Schneider, H. et al. 2019. A handheld OCT probe for intraoral diagnosis on teeth. *Opt. InfoBase Conf. Pap.* Part F142-ECBO 2019, 7–9.

Huang, D., Swanson, E.A., Lin, C.P. et al. 1991. Optical coherence tomography.. *Sci. Reports* 254: 1–4.

Iijima, T., Kurokawa, H., Takamizawa, T. et al. 2021. Prevention of acidic attack on tooth enamel surfaces using polishing paste containing ion-releasing filler. *Dent. Mater. J.* 40: 1352–1358.

Kantovitz, K., Cabral, L., Carlos, N. et al. 2021. Impact of resin composite viscosity and fill-technique on internal gap in class I restorations: an OCT evaluation. *Oper. Dent.* 46: 537–546.

Leitgeb, R.A., Baumann, B. 2018. Multimodal optical medical imaging concepts based on optical coherence tomography. *Front. Phys.* 6: 114–130.

Merle, C.L., Fortenbacher, M., Schneider, H., et al. 2022. Clinical and OCT assessment of application modes of a universal adhesive in a 12-month RCT. *J. Dent.* 119: 104068.

Nguyen, T.T., Larrivée, N., Lee, A., Bilaniuk, O., Durand, R. 2021. Use of artificial intelligence in dentistry: current clinical trends and research advances. *J. Can. Dent. Assoc.* 87: 17.

Qian, J., Feng, Z., Fan, X., Kuzmin, A., Gomes, A.S.L., Prasad, P.N. 2022. High contrast 3-D optical bioimaging using molecular and nanoprobes optically responsive to IR light. *Phys. Rep.* 962: 1–107.

Santana, M.L.C., Paiva, L.F.S., Carneiro, V.S.M., Gomes, A.S.L., Cenci, M.S., Faria-E-Silva, A.L. 2020. Fracture resistance of extensive bulk-fill composite restorations after selective caries removal. *Braz. Oral Res.* 34: 1–8.

Schlenz, M.A., Skroch, M., Schmidt, A., Rehmann, P., Wöstmann, B. 2021. Monitoring fatigue damage in different CAD/CAM materials: a new approach with optical coherence tomography. *J. Prosthodont. Res.* 65: 31–38.

Shi, G., Zhang, Y., Zhu, Y. et al. 2020. Use of spectral domain optical coherence tomography to detect internal defects of resin composites in carious teeth after restorations. *J. Mod. Opt.* 67: 1509–1515.

Song, G., Jelly, E.T., Chu, K.K., Kendall, W.Y., Wax, A. 2021. A review of low-cost and portable optical coherence tomography. *Prog. Biomed. Eng.* 3 .

Turkistani, A., Nasir, A., Merdad, Y. et al. 2020. Evaluation of microleakage in class-II bulk-fill composite restorations. *J. Dent. Sci.* 15: 486–492.

Walther, J., Golde, J., Albrecht, M. et al. 2022. A handheld fiber-optic probe to enable optical coherence tomography of oral soft tissue. *IEEE Trans. Biomed. Eng.* 69. PP, 1.

Wang, J., Zheng, W., Lin, K., Huang, Z. 2016. Development of a hybrid Raman spectroscopy and optical coherence tomography technique for real-time in vivo tissue measurements. *Opt. Lett*. 41: 3045.

Zang, H.L., Ai, S.N., Liang, Y.H. 2022. Microtensile bond strength to sealer-contaminated dentin after using different cleaning protocols. *J. Dent. Sci.* 17: 122–127.

Zeng, S., Huang, Y., Huang, W. et al. 2021. Real-time monitoring and quantitative evaluation of resin in-filtrant repairing enamel white spot lesions based on optical coherence tomography. *Diagnostics 11*. 11: 2046–2059.

Zhou, Y., Matin, K., Shimada, Y., Wang, G., Sadr, A., Tagami, J. 2021. Detection and analysis of early degradation at resin-dentin interface by optical coherence tomography (OCT) and confocal laser scanning microscope (CLSM). *J. Dent.* 106: 103583.

Index